PEDIATRIC RADIOLOGY CASE BASE

PEDIATRIC RADIOLOGY CASE BASE

The Baby Minnie of Pediatric Radiology

Joanna J. Seibert, M.D.

Charles A. James, M.D.

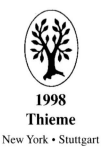

1998
Thieme
New York • Stuttgart

Thieme New York, Inc.
333 Seventh Avenue
New York, NY 10001

Pediatric Radiology Casebase
Joanna J. Seibert, M.D.
Charles A. James, M.D.

Library of Congress Cataloging-in-Publication Data

Pediatric Radiology Casebase : "the Baby Minnie of pediatric
    Radiology" / [edited by] Joanna J. Seibert, Charles A. James.
        p.   cm.
    Includes bibliographical references and index.
    ISBN 0-86577-697-0 (TNY). — ISBN 3-13-107891-X (GTV)
    1. Pediatric radiology—Case studies.   I. Seibert, Joanna J.
II. James, Charles A.
    [DNLM: 1. Diagnostic Imaging—in infancy & childhood—case
studies.   2. Technology, Radiologic—case studies.   WN 240 C337
1997]
    RJ51.R3C37   1997
618.92'00757—dc21
    DNLM/DLC
    for Library of Congress   97-25643
                                                          CIP

For information about the interactive CD-ROM, *Pediatric Radiology*, J. J. Seibert, M.D., and C. A. James, M.D., please call Customer Service at 1-800-782-3488.

Important note: Medical knowledge is ever-changing. As new research and clinical experience broaden our knowledge, changes in treatment and drug therapy may be required. The authors and editors of the material herein have consulted sources believed to be reliable in their efforts to provide information that is complete and in accord with the standards accepted at the time of publication. However, in view of the possibility of human error by the authors, editors, or publisher of the work herein, or changes in medical knowledge, neither the authors, editors, publisher, nor any other party who has been involved in the preparation of this work, warrants that the information contained herein is in every respect accurate or complete, and they are not responsible for any errors or omissions or for the results obtained from use of such information. Readers are encouraged to confirm the information contained herein with other sources. For example, readers are advised to check the product information sheet included in the package of each drug they plan to administer to be certain that the information contained in this publication is accurate and that changes have not been made in the recommended dose or in the contraindications for administration. This recommendation is of particular importance in connection with new or infrequently used drugs.

Some of the product names, patents, and registered designs referred to in this book are in fact registered trademarks or proprietary names even though specific reference to this fact is not always made in the text. Therefore, the appearance of a name without designation as proprietary is not to be construed as a representation by the publisher that it is in the public domain.

Printed in the United States of America

5 4 3 2 1

TNY ISBN 0-86577-697-0
GTV ISBN 3-13-107891-X

Dedication

To our children, who reminded us to treat each patient as our own child.

To our patients and their parents, who continually challenge us to learn more in order to heal.

To our residents and fellows, who challenge us to be current in our specialty in order to learn from and teach them.

To pediatricians and pediatric specialty physicians, who make pediatric radiology such a pleasant and fulfilling profession.

To the radiology department and staff of Arkansas Children's Hospital, people who have supported us and taught us how to work together as part of a team in order to deliver excellent healthcare.

Contents

HEAD AND NECK
Janice W. Allison

GASTROINTESTINAL
Sally G. Klein

GENITOURINARY
Richard E. Leithiser, Jr.

BONE
Charles A. James

CHEST
Theodora Vanderzalm

Editors

Joanna J. Seibert, MD
Professor of Radiology and Pediatrics, University of Arkansas for Medical Sciences (UAMS)
Radiologist, Arkansas Children's Hospital
Director of Radiology at Arkansas Children's Hospital
Little Rock, Arkansas

Charles A. James, MD
Associate Professor of Radiology, UAMS
Radiologist, Arkansas Children's Hospital
Little Rock, Arkansas

Co-Editors

Janice W. Allison, MD
Assistant Professor of Radiology, UAMS
Radiologist, Arkansas Children's Hospital
Little Rock, Arkansas

Debbie A. Desilet-Dobbs, MD
Instructor, UAMS
Radiologist, Arkansas Children's Hospital
Little Rock, Arkansas

Charles M. Glasier, MD
Professor of Radiology, UAMS
Radiologist, Arkansas Children's Hospital
Little Rock, Arkansas

Sally G. Klein, MD
Associate Professor of Radiology, UAMS
Radiologist, Arkansas Children's Hospital
Little Rock, Arkansas

Richard E. Leithiser, Jr., MD
Associate Professor of Radiology, UAMS
Radiologist, Arkansas Children's Hospital
Little Rock, Arkansas

Theodora Vanderzalm, MD
Associate Professor of Radiology, UAMS
Radiologist, Arkansas Children's Hospital
Little Rock, Arkansas

Foreword

This is a fun book that Ben Felson would have thoroughly enjoyed reading. Dr. Felson, the former head of Radiology at the University of Cincinnati, was the finest radiologist with whom I've been associated and one of the nicest men I've ever met. This book uses the Aunt Minnie approach (namely, that the reader will recognize the diagnosis as he recognizes his Aunt Minnie), which is often attributed to Dr. Felson. Dr. Felson in turn indicated that Dr. Ed Neuhauser, former Chief of Boston Children's, used this method first. This approach remains an important component of imaging diagnosis. In addition to Felson's incredible diagnostic abilities, he had an infectious enthusiasm for learning that permeated all of his staff, including the residents. Teachers live on through their pupils. Ben, through his Aunt Minnie approach, lives on in this fine book by the outstanding pediatric radiologists at Arkansas Children's Hospital.

The authors have collected many pediatric roentgen classics. To maximize the benefit of the book, the reader might consider attempting to make a diagnosis by viewing just the first image. If unsuccessful on that image, go on to the next, again trying to establish the answer. If you haven't gotten the diagnosis after looking at all the images, then go back, read the history, and look at the images again. Resist the temptation to look ahead at the answer. If you are not sure of what the condition is after reviewing the illustrations and history, read the descriptions of the images. After deciding on your diagnosis, look at the answer. There are excellent discussions in which the authors summarize current literature and provide helpful information on each condition.

I have connections with the two editors and Dr. Felson. Joanna Seibert is a dear friend whom I've known many years; Charles James was a very fine resident with us in St. Louis; and I trained under Dr. Ben Felson.

William A. McAlister, M.D.
Mallinkrodt Institute of Radiology
St. Louis, MO

Preface

The radiologist faces many challenges when dealing with pediatric patients. As with all areas of radiology, tricks of the trade evolve from experience. By presenting clinical cases, we hope to impart a variety of important teaching points that will hopefully guide all those involved in pediatric imaging.

This book is one of several in the CASEBASE series. The clinical cases in these books directly reflect what radiologists will see in practice and offer practical guidelines to make accurate diagnoses. By using a logical sequence to present the workup of patients, the reader will understand the decision-making behind each diagnosis. The cases vary in complexity and should appeal to radiologists at different levels of experience.

We have divided the cases into nine anatomical sections: neuroradiology, head and neck, gastrointestinal, genitourinary, bone, chest, cardiac, interventional, and syndromes. Each section discusses pathology and also includes normal variants and artifacts. Cases within each section represent congenital or developmental abnormalities, infection, trauma, tumors, or metabolic disorders. Each case is organized by clinical presentation, radiographic findings, diagnosis, discussion, and further reading.

We believe that this approach is ideal for all radiology and pediatric residents in training and preparing for examinations. We have deliberately omitted the diagnosis from the first page of each case so that the reader can review the clinical presentation and images for self assessment before reading the correct diagnosis and explanatory discussion covering pathophysiology of the disease and the differential diagnosis.

Many years ago, Dr. Ben Felson from Cincinnati described certain radiographic cases as "Aunt Minnies"; if you have met Aunt Minnie once, you will recognize her again. Many of the cases in this book can be described as "Baby Minnies." In addition to more challenging cases, you will see Baby Minnies in this casebook and hopefully recognize them again.

For more experienced radiologists and pediatricians, this book can be used as a quick reference using the table of contents or index to identify specific cases. Indeed, we hope that general radiologists and pediatricians will find this format useful in daily practice to quickly review practical guidelines presented as 'Pearls' and 'Pittfalls'. For those radiologists preparing for examinations, this comprehensive compilation of cases should also serve as an excellent resource to review a variety of cases that are seen in daily pediatric radiology practice.

Acknowledgments

We would like to thank Dr. Ina Tonkin of Le Bonheur Hospital in Memphis for reviewing the cardiac section and Dr. William McAlister of Mallinckrodt Institute in St. Louis for reviewing the syndrome section. We are indebted to the media services at Arkansas Children's Hospital and University of Arkansas for Medical Sciences for the photographic work. We also thank Jane Pennington at Thieme for her trust in us and constant guidance. We thank the department of Radiology at UAMS and our chair, Dr. Ernest Ferris, as well as the radiology staff of Arkansas Children's Hospital for supporting us in this project. Finally, we could not have completed this book without the expertise of our editorial secretary, Ms. Marcia Phillips.

PEDIATRIC RADIOLOGY CASE BASE

NEURORADIOLOGY

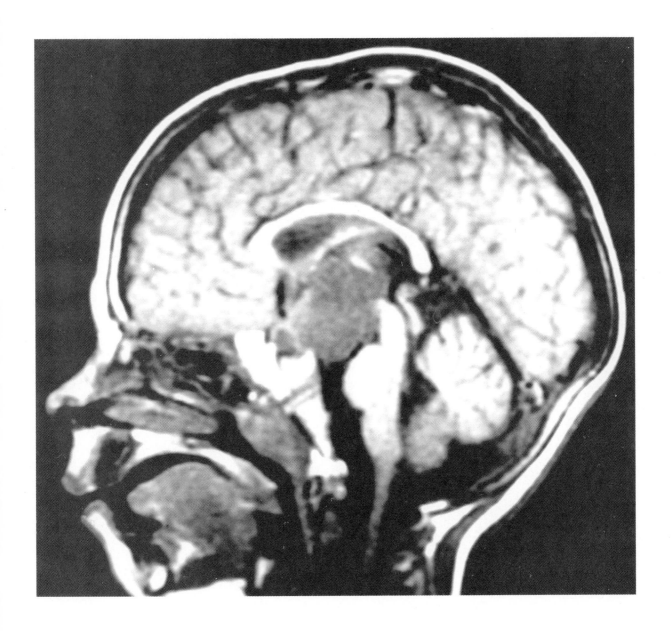

Case 1

Clinical Presentation

Developmentally normal 3-month-old infant with elongated calvarium.

Radiographic Studies

Lateral skull radiograph (Fig. 1A) shows elongation of the anteroposterior (AP) measurement of the calvarium. This deformity of the skull is known as scaphocephaly or dolichocephaly. On plain radiography, the Towne projection (Fig. 1B) most commonly shows the bony sutural bar with associated osseous bridge (white arrows, Fig. 1B), palpable clinically as a midsagittal ridge on the calvarium. Most superior "bone window" computed tomography (CT) slice shows abnormal, straight, knife-edge–like suture posteriorly (black arrows, Fig. 1C) with linear bony sclerosis anteriorly (black arrowheads, Fig. 1C).

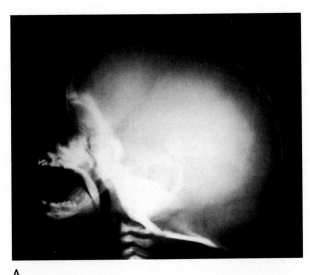

A

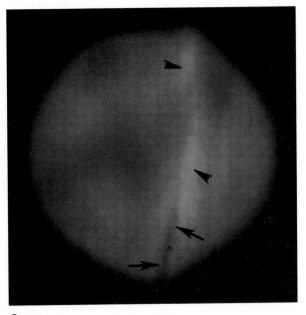

C

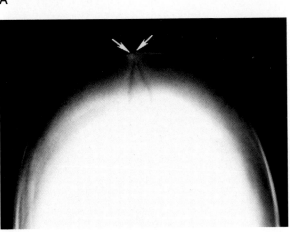

B

Diagnosis Sagittal Craniosynostosis

Discussion and Differential Diagnosis

Skull radiography in infants with suspected sagittal synostosis is performed to document the clinical diagnosis. Computed tomography or magnetic resonance imaging (MRI) is performed to exclude intracranial anomalies that are occasionally found in infants with primary craniosynostosis. A common cause of dolichocephaly not related to sagittal synostosis is positional molding producing mild dolichocephaly in premature infants. This is probably related to their spending long periods in the supine position with the head turned to the side on respiratory support in the neonatal nursery. Positional molding is not associated with actual bony bridging of the sagittal suture. Premature sutural closure is frequently secondary to severe, diffuse encephalomalacia related to hypoxic-ischemic encephalopathy or other perinatal insults. In these patients, sutural hyperostosis is usually absent, severe microcephaly is present, and neuroimaging studies show extensive destructive changes in the cerebral hemispheres.

Further Reading

1. Silverman FN, Kuhn JP. *Essentials of Caffey's Pediatric X-ray Diagnosis.* Chicago: Yearbook Medical Publishers; 1990:14–21.

Case 2

Clinical Presentation

An 800-gram, 32-week-gestation infant who required ventilatory support for hyaline membrane disease.

Radiographic Studies

Semicoronal image from cranial ultrasound examination at 1 week of age shows increased clumpy echogenicity in the periventricular white matter bilaterally (black arrows, Fig. 2A). Subsequent ultrasound examination 3 weeks later shows discrete cyst formation (white arrows, Fig. 2B) in the periventricular white matter corresponding to the echogenic areas seen in the previous examination. Axial image from long TE, long TR pulse sequence demonstrates mild ventricular dilatation with cyst formation in the periatrial white matter (black arrows, Fig. 2C). Axial long TE, long TR MR image in another patient shows irregularly enlarged outline of the lateral ventricles secondary to excavation of the white matter with high signal in the remaining periventricular white matter probably representing gliosis (Fig. 2D).

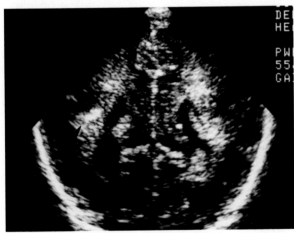

A

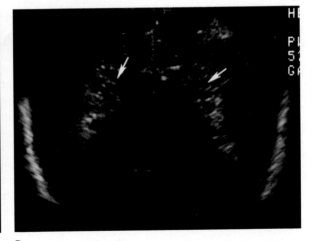

B

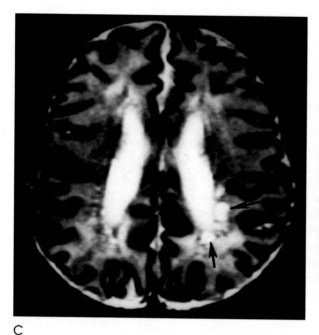

C

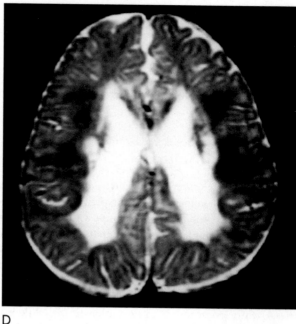

D

Diagnosis Periventricular Leukomalacia (PVL)

Dicussion and Differential Diagnosis

Diagnostic considerations in infants with periventricular white matter echodensities on cranial sonography include diffuse cerebral edema and TORCH (*t*oxoplasmosis, *o*ther agents, *r*ubella, *c*ytomegalovirus, *h*erpes simplex) infections. Periventricular leukomalacia is typically found in preterm infants, particularly in those requiring ventilatory support and with cardiopulmonary instability. Damage to the periventricular white matter in PVL is probably related to the vascular border zones in the frontal and peritrigonal white matter and to episodes of hypoxia and hypotension that invariably occur in sick preterm infants. Diffuse cerebral edema is most frequently seen in asphyxiated full-term newborns and usually lacks the "clumpy" appearance of echodensities seen with typical PVL. TORCH infections are less commonly seen in the preterm infant and may show striations in the basal ganglia and thalamus, subependymal cysts, and focal periventricular echodensities with posterior shadowing representing calcification.

Further Reading

1. Carson SC, Hertzberg BS, Bowie JD, Burger PC. Value of sonography in the diagnosis of intracranial hemorrhage and periventricular leukomalacia: a postmortem study of 35 cases. *AJNR Am J Neuroradiol* 11:677–683, 1990.

PEARLS

- Focal, dense increased echogenicity in the periventricular white matter may be the earliest sonographic sign of PVL.

- Cystic PVL at birth denotes intrauterine injury.

- MRI is the most sensitive imaging examination.

PITFALLS

- Serial ultrasound scans may be necessary for diagnosis. Small subependymal cysts should not be confused with PVL, which by definition involves the periventricular white matter.

Case 3

Clinical Presentation

A 13-year-old girl with low back pain relieved by aspirin.

Radiographic Studies

Frontal radiograph of the lumbar spine shows sclerosis in the right side of the fifth lumbar vertebra (black arrows, Fig. 3A). Posterior view from a bone scan demonstrates increased activity on the right side of L5 (black arrow, Fig. 3B). Axial high-resolution CT image (Fig. 3C) shows an oval, lytic lesion in the right lamina of L5 with a central soft tissue nidus and surrounding bony sclerosis. Axial short TE, short TR MR image at L5 demonstrates expansion of the right L5 lamina with extremely low signal corresponding to the area of sclerosis seen on plain films and CT (Fig. 3D).

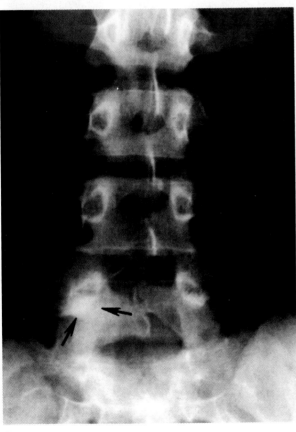

A

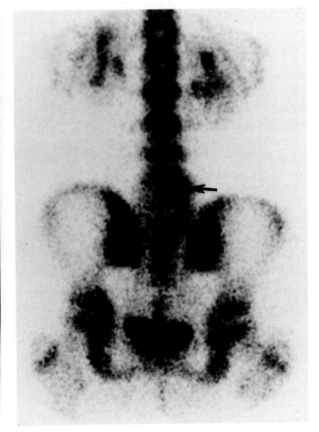

B

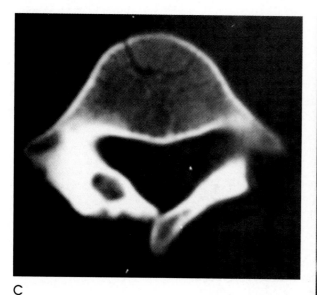

C

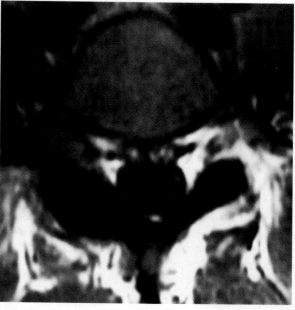

D

Diagnosis   Osteoid Osteoma

Discussion and Differential Diagnosis

Osteoid osteoma most commonly occurs in the femur and spinal column, particularly the posterior elements. Radiographic findings include a small lytic lesion that may contain a bony or soft tissue density vascular nidus, frequently with associated bony sclerosis. There may be associated soft tissue edema. Increased joint fluid may be found in periarticular lesions. Differential diagnostic considerations include primarily chronic infection such as Brodie abscess, stress fracture, or Langerhans' cell histiocytosis. Osteoblastoma is distinguished from osteoid osteoma by size (the lucent center of an osteoblastoma is classically larger than 1.5 cm) and by the fact that there is usually less reactive adjacent sclerosis in osteoblastoma. High-resolution CT and bone scan show the most characteristic findings in osteoid osteoma. Focal intense increased activity in the central vascular nidus is a classic bone scan finding. CT typically shows a less than 1.5 cm lytic lesion that may contain a contrast-enhancing central nidus and surrounding bony thickening.

Further Reading

1. Bloem JL, Kroon HM. Osseous lesions in imaging of bone and soft tissue tumors. *Radiol Clin North Am* 31(2):261–278, 1993.

Case 4

Clinical Presentation

A 7-year-old girl with bilateral decreased visual acuity.

Radiographic Studies

Axial high-resolution short TE, short TR MR image through the globes and optic chiasm shows severely hypoplastic intracranial optic nerves bilaterally (black arrows, Fig. 4A) as well as a thin optic chiasm. Coronal short TE, short TR MR image at the level of the suprasellar cistern (Fig. 4B) demonstrates absence of the septum pellucidum and again shows the thinned optic chiasm.

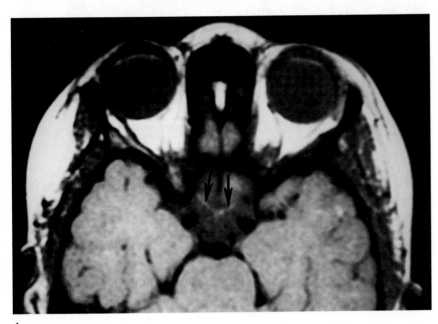

A

PEARLS

• High-resolution imaging in the coronal plane is necessary to reliably diagnose optic nerve hypoplasia.

PITFALLS

• Absent septum pellucidum may be seen without optic hypoplasia or other anomalies. The septum pellucidum is often absent in patients with severe hydrocephalus, especially those who have undergone multiple cerebrospinal fluid diversion procedures with damage to septal tissue from shunt catheter placement.

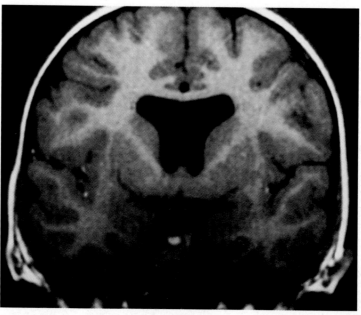

B

Diagnosis Septo-optic Dysplasia

Discussion and Differential Diagnosis

Optic nerve hypoplasia may occur as an isolated abnormality but frequently occurs in the presence of other cerebral abnormalities, especially absent septum pellucidum, posterior pituitary ectopia, neuronal migration anomalies such as schizencephaly and perinatal cerebral hemispheric injury. Thinning of the corpus callosum is present in some patients. Patients with posterior pituitary ectopia, and to a lesser extent, absence of the septum pellucidum, have an increased incidence of neuroendocrine abnormalities. Optic nerve hypoplasia is usually diagnosed clinically. High-resolution cranial MR imaging is used to confirm the presence of intracranial optic nerve and chiasm hypoplasia as well as to detect the presence of associated intracranial abnormalities such as posterior pituitary ectopia or neuronal migration anomalies that may indicate neuroendocrine or neurological dysfunction.[1,2]

Further Reading

1. Brodsky MC, Glasier CM, Pollock SC, Angtuaco EJ. Optic nerve hypoplasia: identification by magnetic resonance imaging. *Arch Ophthalmol* 108:1562–1567, 1990.
2. Brodsky MC, Glasier CM. Optic nerve hypoplasia: clinical significance of associated central nervous system abnormalities on magnetic resonance imaging. *Arch Ophthalmol* 111:66–74, 1993.

Case 5

Clinical Presentation

A 2-year-old boy with growth failure.

Radiographic Studies

Axial noncontrast cranial CT shows a fluid-filled suprasellar mass with rim calcification (black arrows, Fig. 5A). Sagittal T1-weighted MRI demonstrates a hyperintense egg-shaped mass arising in the sella, extending into the suprasellar cistern (Fig. 5B). Axial T2-weighted MRI (Fig. 5C) shows that the fluid-containing central cystic portion of the mass is hyperintense to gray matter. The arciform low-intensity region on the posterior wall of the mass corresponds to the dense calcific wall seen on CT (black arrows, Fig. 5C).

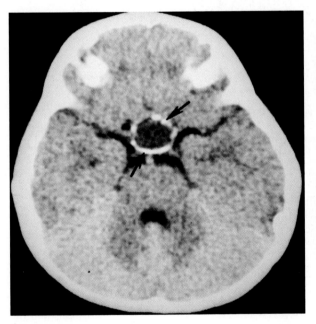

A

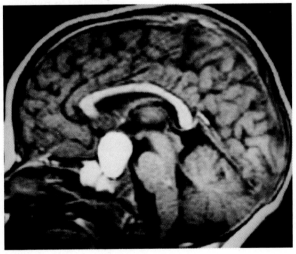

B

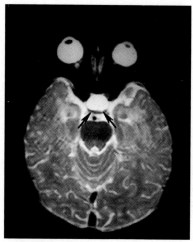

C

Diagnosis Craniopharyngioma

Discussion and Differential Diagnosis

Craniopharyngioma is the most common suprasellar mass in children. Other masses include optic or hypothalamic glioma and various germ cell tumors. Arachnoid and Rathke cleft cysts may also occupy the suprasellar cistern. Langerhans' cell histiocytosis may present as a mass in the pituitary infundibulum that rarely enlarges to fill the suprasellar cistern. Unusual suprasellar masses include "ectopic posterior pituitary" tissue in patients with growth hormone deficiency and lipomas and hamartomas of the tuber cinereum, which are typically found in children with precocious puberty. Pituitary macroadenomas, meningiomas, and aneurysms are much less common in children than in adults. Imaging diagnosis of craniopharyngioma is usually not difficult when a mixed cystic and solid suprasellar mass containing calcium is present.

The vast majority of craniopharyngiomas are calcified, with either floccular or rim calcification. The cystic portion of the tumor may be low attenuation (simulating CSF) or high attenuation on CT. CT is important for postsurgical follow-up to detect the presence of residual or recurrent calcification, which is indicative of tumor. High-resolution MR prior to surgical resection is performed to demonstrate the relationship of the tumor to the optic chiasm, hypothalamus, and adjacent circle of Willis vasculature. The tumor has variable signal intensity on T1- and T2-weighted images. Gadolinium administration frequently shows enhancement of the solid portion of the tumor and variable rim enhancement of the cyst.

Further Reading

1. Pfleger MJ, Gerson LP. Supratentorial tumors in children. *Neuroimaging Clin N Am* 3(4):671–687, 1993.

Case 6

Clinical Presentation

A 16-year-old girl with progressive back pain.

Radiographic Studies

Initial lateral thoracolumbar radiograph (Fig. 6A) shows destruction of the antero-superior portion of the first lumbar vertebral body with T12-L1 disc space narrowing. Subsequent lateral film (Fig. 6B) demonstrates near-complete destruction of L1 with gibbus formation. Sagittal T2*-weighted gradient echo MRI of the thoracolumbar spine (Fig. 6C) confirms obliteration of the T12-L1 disc space, retropulsion of the body of L1 with compression of the conus medullaris.

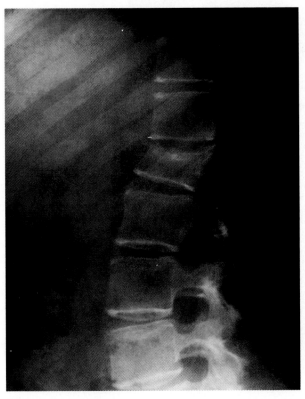

A

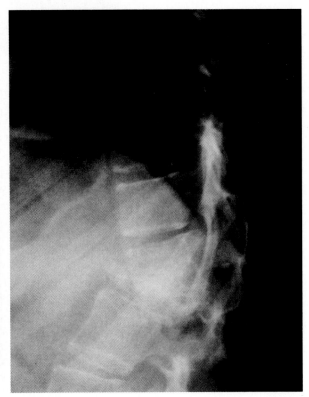

B

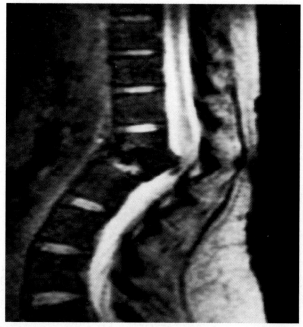

C

Diagnosis Tuberculous Spondylitis

Discussion and Differential Diagnosis

Primary and metastatic tumors, Langerhans' cell histiocytosis, and, conceivably, severe Scheuermann disease are noninfectious conditions that could simulate radiographic findings of tuberculous spondylitis. Infectious conditions simulating tuberculous spondylitis include various bacterial and fungal agents. Brucellosis affecting the spine has been reported to closely simulate tuberculosis.[1,2] Typical radiographic findings in tuberculous spondylitis include vertebral endplate erosion with associated disc space narrowing. Disc space narrowing in granulomatous spondylitis occurs later than in typical bacterial disco-vertebral infection. Paravertebral fluid collections (cold abscesses), although not present in this case, are frequently found in association with tuberculous spondylitis. MR imaging may show high signal in involved vertebral bodies on T1- or T2-weighted imaging.

Further Reading

1. de Castro CC, Hesselink JR. Tuberculosis. *Neuroimaging Clin N Am* 1(1):119–139, 1991.
2. Smith AS, Weinstein MA, Mizushima A, et al. MR imaging characteristics of tuberculous spondylitis vs. vertebral osteomyelitis. *AJNR Am J Neuroradiol* 10:619–625, 1989.

Case 7

Clinical Presentation

A 3-month-old girl with flattening of the left forehead.

Radiographic Studies

Frontal skull radiograph (Fig. 7A) shows asymmetric frontal skull deformity (plagio-cephaly) with elevation of the left sphenoid wing and orbital roof, forming the "Harlequin eye" deformity (black arrows, Fig. 7A). Axial "bone window" CT slice (Fig. 7B) demonstrates a small left anterior cranial fossa, elevation of the left orbital roof and sphenoid wing and sclerosis of the left coronal suture (black arrow, Fig. 7B).

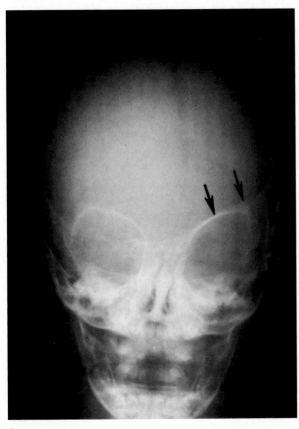

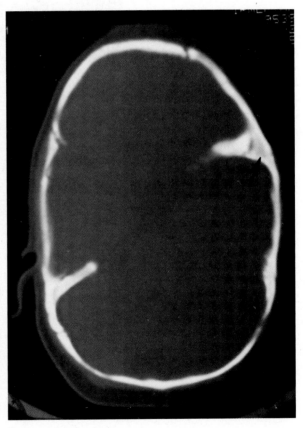

A

B

Diagnosis Coronal Craniosynostosis

Discussion and Differential Diagnosis

Unilateral primary coronal synostosis should be distinguished from bilateral coronal synostosis, which is frequently associated with various craniofacial syndromes. Unilateral coronal synostosis is sporadic, in contrast to the craniofacial syndromes associated with bilateral coronal synostoses, which are hereditary. The two most well known craniofacial syndromes associated with bilateral coronal synostosis are Crouzon (craniofacial dysostosis) and Apert (acrocephalosyndactyly). Patients with Crouzon syndrome may be developmentally normal whereas patients with Apert syndrome are usually developmentally delayed. In Apert syndrome, the severe syndactyly of the hands and feet is characteristic and a plastic surgery challenge.

Premature closure of the coronal suture results in loss of the normal serrated appearance of the suture as well as sclerosis of the sutural margins. There may be compensatory bulging of the contralateral posterior parieto-occipital skull.

Further Reading

1. Harwood-Nash DC, Fitz CR. *Neuroradiology in Infants and Children.* St. Louis: CV Mosby; 1976:71–90.

Case 8

Clinical Presentation

A 16-year-old boy with neck pain following an automobile accident in which he had not been belted in.

Radiographic Studies

Lateral radiograph of the cervical spine (Fig. 8A) shows the characteristic fracture of the posterior elements of C2 (black arrow, Fig. 8A) with anterior subluxation of C2 on C3. CT in another patient (Fig. 8B) illustrates the bilateral posterior element fractures. This patient has retropharyngeal air from an associated laryngeal injury. This fracture by definition involves the posterior elements of C2 bilaterally and, as in Figure 8A, passes from the superoposterior to the anteroinferior aspect of the neural arches.

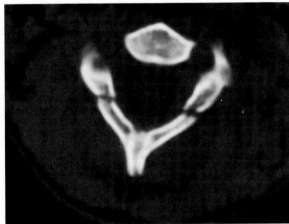

B

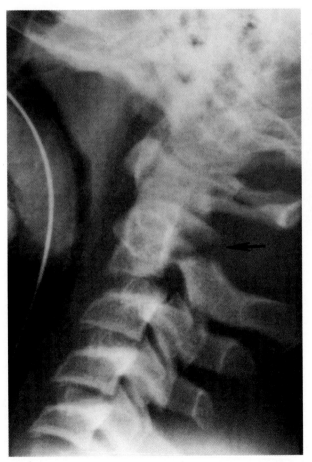

A

Diagnosis Hangman Fracture

PEARLS

- Oblique views and lateral radiographs with cephalad angulation may be helpful in demonstrating the fracture on plain films.

- Spinal CT is the most helpful.

Discussion and Differential Diagnosis

Findings on plain lateral radiographs are usually unequivocal in patients with this injury. Fortunately, the patients are usually neurologically normal because of the large size of the spinal canal at C2, which allows significant movement without cord compromise. The mechanism of injury is probably hyperextension.[1,2] Subluxation of C2 on C3 is usually present secondary to disruption of the anterior longitudinal ligament.[1,2]

PITFALLS

- The fracture may be impossible to visualize on the frontal projection, so an optimal lateral radiograph is essential for diagnosis.

Further Reading

1. Elliott JM Jr, Rogers LF, Wissinger JP, Lee JF. The hangman's fracture: fractures of the neural arch of the axis. *Radiology* 104:303–307, 1972.
2. Rogers LF. The spine. In: *Radiology of Skeletal Trauma.* New York: Churchill Livingstone; 1982:287.

Case 9

Clinical Presentation

A 1-month-old infant with congestive heart failure and a cranial bruit.

Radiographic Studies

Initial chest radiograph (Fig. 9A) shows cardiomegaly and vascular congestion compatible with congestive heart failure. Axial contrast-enhanced CT (Fig. 9B) demonstrates massive enlargement of the vein of Galen but no evidence of hydrocephalus. Sagittal midline ultrasound image (Fig. 9C, anterior to the right) shows dilatation of the vein of Galen, draining venous sinus, and torcular (black arrows, Fig. 9C). Color Doppler sagittal image (Fig. 9D, anterior to the right) confirms high flow away from the transducer in the enlarged venous structures (Fig. 9D, Color Plate 1). Three-dimensional phase-contrast magnetic resonance angiography (MRA) with 30 cm/sec flow encoding (Fig. 9E) confirms the dilated vein of Galen/falcine sinus dilatation and clearly shows a small vascular malformation (white arrows, Fig. 9E) draining into the dilated venous structures. Vertebral artery injection from a digital cerebral angiogram prior to embolization documents the noninvasive imaging findings (Fig. 9F).

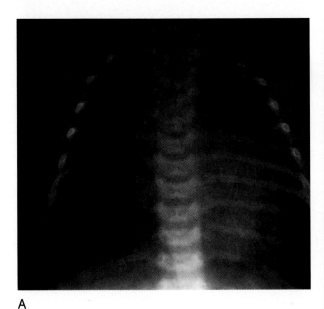

A

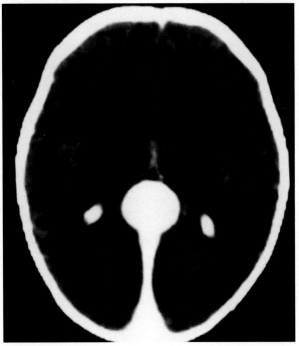

B

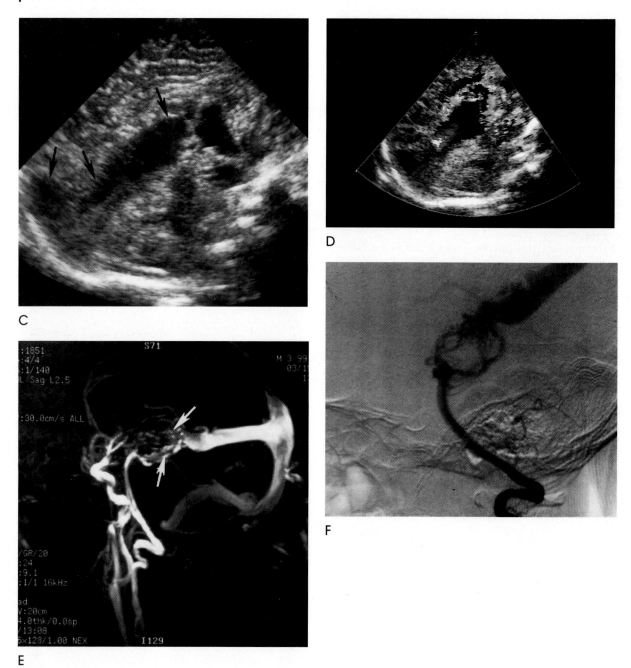

Diagnosis Vein of Galen Aneurysm

PEARLS

● Extracardiac arteriovenous
shunting should be
considered in the differential
diagnosis of infants with high-
output cardiac failure.

Discussion and Differential Diagnosis

Galenic malformations can be simply divided into direct fistulae between cerebral arteries and the vein of Galen and arteriovenous malformations that have venous drainage into the galenic system. Many patients have persistence of fetal drainage such as the persistent falcine vein seen in this case. Patients with galenic malformations usually present in infancy with high output heart failure and a cranial bruit. Older infants and children may present because of hydrocephalus secondary to occlusion of the aqueduct of Sylvius. Current therapy consists of neurointerventional procedures, including arterial and/or venous embolization. Noninvasive imaging—including cranial sonography with Doppler and MRI/MRA—is used to establish the diagnosis, and digital angiography is performed for planning and during performance of neurointerventional procedures.

PITFALLS

● Duplex Doppler quickly
separates congenital cystic
masses such as cyst of the
superior vermian cistern from
high-flow galenic
malformations.

Further Reading

1. Horowitz MB, Jungreis CA, Quisling RG, Pollack I. Vein of Galen aneurysms: a review and current perspective. AJNR *Am J Neuroradiol* 15:1486–1496, 1994.

Case 10

Clinical Presentation

A 2-year-old girl with seizures.

Radiographic Studies

T1-weighted axial (Fig. 10A) and coronal (Fig. 10B) images show lumpy gray matter intensity nodules protruding into the posterior horns of the lateral ventricles (black arrows, Figs. 10A, 10B). The nodules were also isointense to gray matter on proton density and T2-weighted images (not shown).

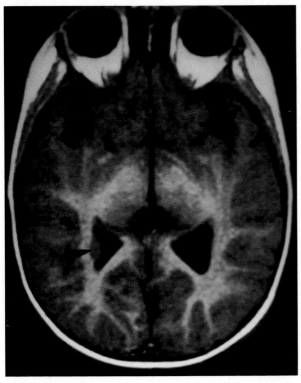

A

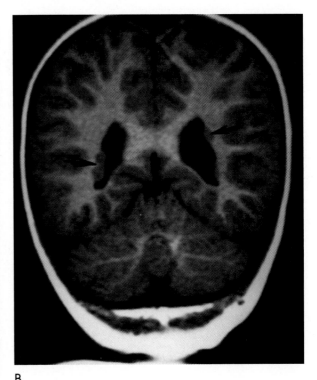

B

Diagnosis Gray Matter Subependymal Heterotopias

Discussion and Differential Diagnosis

According to Barkovich, gray matter heterotopias are most usefully categorized on imaging as subependymal (as in this case), focal subcortical, and diffuse heterotopias such as band heterotopias. The etiology of abnormalities of neuronal migration leading to the various heterotopias is not known. Heterotopic gray matter is typically isodense to orthotopic gray matter on CT and isointense to normal gray matter on all pulse sequences on MRI without evidence of contrast enhancement. Other lesions that should not be confused with subependymal heterotopias include subependymal tubers of tuberous sclerosis and the periventricular calcifications of the various TORCH infections. Prominent dependent glomus of the choroid plexus or hemorrhage into the occipital horns of the lateral ventricles are other entities that could simulate subependymal lesions.

Further Reading

1. Barkovich AJ, Gressens P, Evrard P. Formation, maturation, and disorders of brain neocortex. *AJNR Am J Neuroradiol* 13:423–446, 1992.

Case 11

Clinical Presentation

Newborn infant with poor feeding and abnormal temperature control.

Radiographic Studies

Axial T2-weighted image (Fig. 11A) shows fusion of the thalami (black arrows) and of the frontal lobes. Note formation of a rudimentary straight sinus posteriorly in Figure 11A. Coronal T1-weighted image (Fig. 11B) demonstrates partial formation of an interhemispheric fissure (black arrows, Fig. 11B, also seen posteriorly in Fig. 11A) and the presence of a relatively large volume of brain parenchyma. The hippocampus appears to be absent.

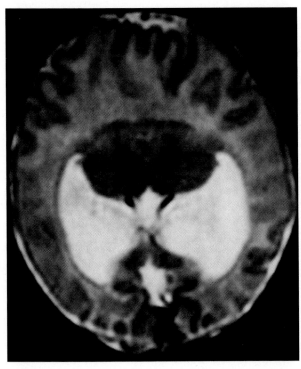

A

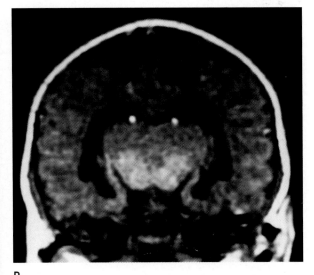

B

Diagnosis Holoprosencephaly

Discussion and Differential Diagnosis

Holoprosencephaly represents a failure of normal formation and separation of the cerebral hemispheres and diencephalon. The more severe forms are often, but not always, associated with facial malformations, especially with prominent midline facial clefts and hypotelorism. The condition is frequently lethal, often related to neuroendocrine dysfunction. Chromosomal abnormalities, especially trisomy 13, may be associated with holoprosencephaly. This malformation develops during the first weeks of embryogenesis and may be diagnosed on fetal sonography in the second or third trimester. The most severe (alobar) form is associated with a thin "pancake" of cerebral cortex anteriorly with a large monoventricle and dorsal cyst. The less severe semilobar and lobar forms have better (but still abnormal) development and lack of normal separation of the cerebral hemispheres.[1]

Further Reading

1. Fitz CR. Holoprosencephaly and septo-optic dysplasia. *Neuroimaging Clin N Am* 4(2):263–281, 1994.

Case 12

Clinical Presentation

A 2-month-old infant with suspected seizures.

Radiographic Studies

Midline sagittal cranial ultrasound (Fig. 12A) shows characteristic lack of parallelism of the paramedian gyri and central radiation of the echogenic sulci toward the midline (black arrows, Fig. 12A). Axial cranial CT (Fig. 12B) demonstrates parallel lateral ventricles with dilatation of the occipital horns (colpocephaly). Coronal T1-weighted MRI (Fig. 12C) illustrates the "candelabra" appearance of the lateral ventricles and low-riding interhemispheric fissure. The temporal horns are dilated secondary to hypoplasia of mesial temporal lobe structures. "Probst bundles" (black arrows, Fig. 12C) are present bilaterally.

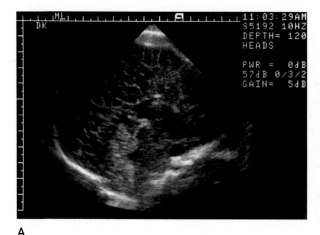

A

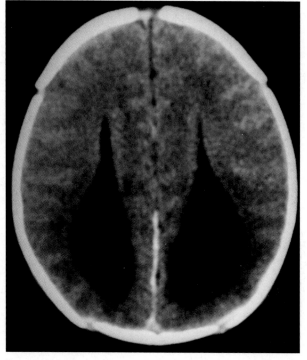

B

PEARLS

● Isolated callosal agenesis is often diagnosed as an incidental finding.

PITFALLS

● "Colpocephaly" simply indicates dilatation of the occipital horns, and alone is not specific for agenesis. Colpocephaly is frequently seen in infants with posthemorrhagic hydrocephalus.

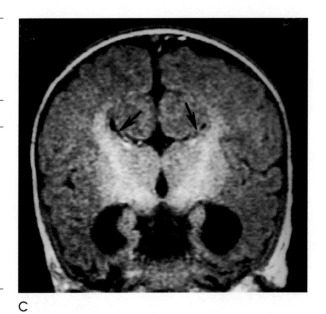

C

Diagnosis   Absent Corpus Callosum

Discussion and Differential Diagnosis

Callosal absence may be partial or complete. When partially absent, the splenium is most frequently involved, especially in patients with Chiari II malformation. Partial absence of the anterior corpus callosum is seen only in patients with holoprosencephaly.[1] Callosal agenesis is frequently an isolated anomaly but may be associated with intracranial lipomas, neuronal migration anomalies, and large interhemispheric cysts. Patients with isolated agenesis may be neurologically normal. Absence of the corpus callosum is occasionally found in infants with sagittal synostosis. Neonatal or even prenatal sonography is frequently diagnostic, but MRI is preferred to detect associated cerebral malformations.

Further Reading

1. Barkovich AJ. Apparent atypical callosal dysgenesis: analysis of MR findings in six cases and their relationship to holoprosencephaly. *AJNR Am J Neuroradiol* 11:333–339, 1990.

Case 13

Clinical Presentation

A newborn infant with bulging, skin-covered frontal mass.

Radiographic Studies

Axial noncontrast computed tomography (CT) (Fig. 13A) shows a midline frontal bilobed mass containing soft tissue (brain) centrally and surrounding fluid attenuation CSF (black arrows, Fig. 13A). Hypertelorism is present but there is no herniation of brain tissue into the orbits. Sagittal T1-weighted MRI demonstrates frontal lobe tissue herniating anteriorly at the level of the nasion with surrounding CSF (black arrows, Fig. 13B). The corpus callosum is absent.

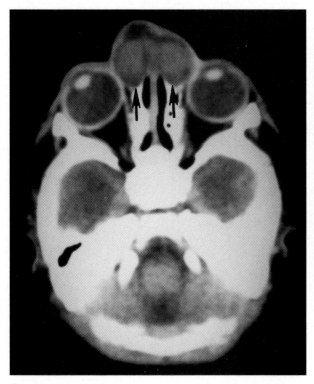

A

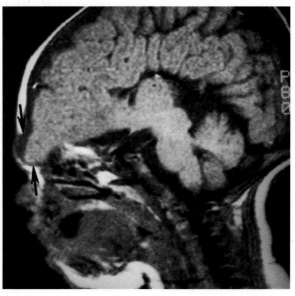

B

Diagnosis Nasofrontal Cephalocele

Discussion and Differential Diagnosis

The majority of cephaloceles in the Western hemisphere are located in the occipital region. The second most common location is anteriorly, including nasofrontal (as in this case), nasoethmoidal, or nasoorbital lesions.[1,2] Cephaloceles may contain meninges only; meninges and CSF; or meninges, CSF, and brain. Basal cephaloceles also occur anteriorly and may protrude into the sphenoid sinus or pharynx. Other intracranial anomalies are frequently present and the majority of the patients are neurodevelopmentally abnormal. Other masses, such as capillary hemangiomas of infancy and dermoid lesions, may simulate cephaloceles. Preoperative neuroimaging is crucial to define intracranial extent of congenital facial lesions because craniotomy is required for definitive treatment of cephaloceles.

Further Reading

1. Naidich TP, Altman NR, Braffman BH, McLone DG, Zimmerman RA. Cephaloceles and related malformations. *AJNR Am J Neuroradiol* 13:655–690, 1992.
2. Naidich TP, Bauer B. *Neuroradiology Test and Syllabus,* part 1. Reston, VA: American College of Radiology; 1990:274–291.

PEARLS

- Any midline calvarial, facial, or oropharyngeal mass in an infant may have an intracranial connection.

PITFALLS

- Cephaloceles may present within the sphenoid sinus or pharynx. Imaging of such lesions should include sagittal and coronal planes to determine the relationship between basal and pharyngeal masses and the intracranial contents.

Case 14

Clinical Presentation

A 15-year-old boy with developmental delay and seizures.

Radiographic Studies

Sagittal T1-weighted (Fig. 14A) and axial T2-weighted images (Fig. 14B) demonstrate extensive lack of normal sulcation and gray matter cortical thickening (black arrows, Fig. 14A) in the posterior frontal and parieto-occipital cortex bilaterally. Note the small cluster of cortical veins overlying the right parietal cortex (black arrows, Fig. 14B).

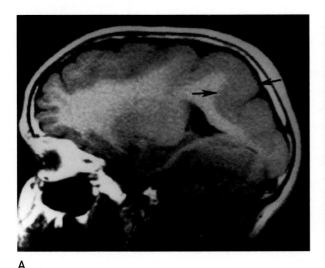

A

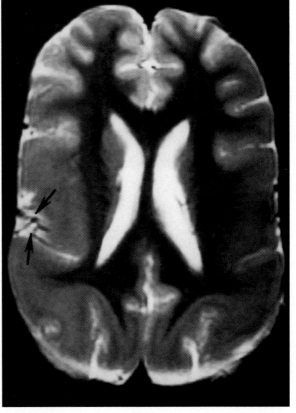

B

Diagnosis Pachygyria

Discussion and Differential Diagnosis

Neuronal migration disorders are characterized by dysmorphic gray matter with signal generally isointense to more normal appearing gray matter.[1] Increased thickness of otherwise normal-appearing gray matter distinguishes a focal area of pachygyria from a tumor. Neuronal migration anomalies do not enhance after administration of intravenous contrast material. Areas of pachygyria may be interspersed with areas of agyria (lissencephaly) in the same brain. Patients with pachygyria frequently present with chronic seizure disorders. Because of the relatively poor visualization of the superficial cortex with ultrasound, CT—or preferably MRI—is optimal for the detection of neuronal migrational anomalies.

Further Reading

1. Barkovich AJ, Gressens P, Evrard P. Formation, maturation, and disorders of neocortex. *AJNR Am J Neuroradiol* 13:423–446, 1992.
2. Barkovich AJ. Abnormal vascular drainage in anomalies of neuronal migration. *AJNR Am J Neuroradiol* 9:939–942, 1988.

Case 15

Clinical Presentation

A 6-month-old girl presented with constipation.

Radiographic Studies

Sagittal T2-weighted MR image (Fig. 15A) demonstrates hypoplasia of the sacrum and a hyperintense lobulated presacral mass with a wide communication into the thecal sac (black arrowheads, Fig. 15A). The linear area of hyperintensity between the bladder and the mass (black arrow, Fig. 15A) is a tuberculin syringe filled with chloral hydrate in the rectum. The mass is isointense to bladder urine on an axial T1-weighted image (Fig. 15B). The rectal syringe is seen as an area of focal hyperintensity behind the bladder (black arrow, Fig. 15B). Postsurgical plain film of the pelvis shows a "sickle deformity" of the sacrum (Fig. 15C). Barium enema (Fig. 15D) shows rectal stenosis.

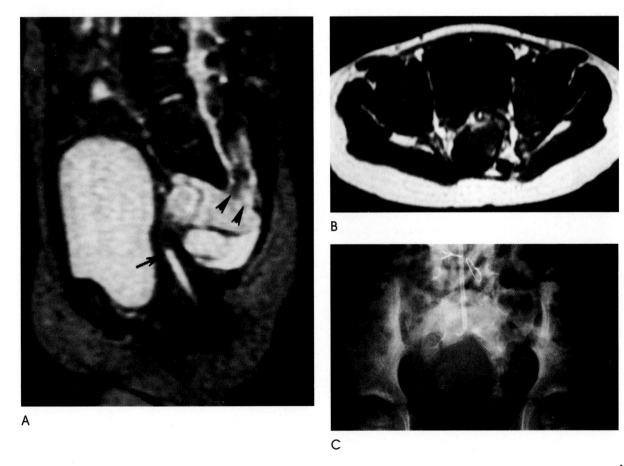

A

B

C

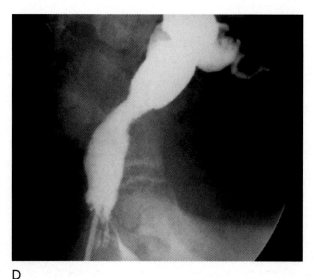

D

Diagnosis Currarino Triad

Discussion and Differential Diagnosis

The classic "triad" of anomalies includes anorectal malformation, presacral mass, and bony deformity of the sacrum. Vesicoureteral reflux is another abnormality commonly seen in these patients. Infants with anorectal anomalies should undergo screening neuroimaging of the spine in the neonatal period. Screening should include plain radiography of the spine and pelvis and spinal sonography. If a sacral defect is seen or if spinal sonography suggests intraspinal pathology, MRI evaluation of the spine is necessary. The presence of sacral deformity in an infant with anorectal malformation suggests the presence of a presacral mass that may represent a simple presacral meningocele or a teratoma. Mixed lesions also occur.[1,2] High-resolution MR imaging provides adequate preoperative information concerning intrathecal extension of the presacral mass.

Further Reading

1. Hunt PT, Davidson KC, Ashcraft KW, Holder TM. Radiography of hereditary presacral teratoma. *Radiology* 122:187–191, 1977.
2. Cohn J, Bay-Nielsen E. Hereditary defect of the sacrum and coccyx with anterior sacral meningocele. *Acta Pediatr Scand* 58:268–274, 1969.

Case 16

Clinical Presentation

A 6-year-old girl with multiple café au lait spots and a family history of tumors.

Radiographic Studies

Axial T2-weighted images (Fig. 16A, 16B) show multiple areas of high signal in the globus pallidus, thalamus, pons, and middle cerebellar peduncles (black arrows, Fig. 16A, 16B).

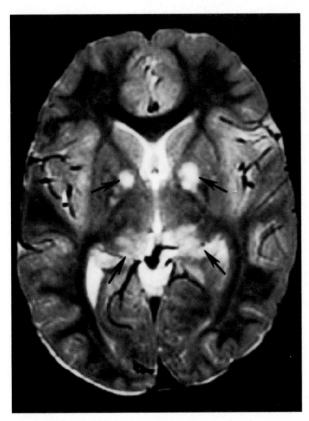

A

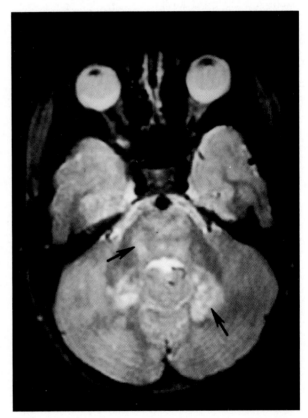

B

Diagnosis Neurofibromatosis Type 1 (NF-1): Brain

Discussion and Differential Diagnosis

Neurofibromatosis type I is the most common of the phakomatoses. It is inherited in an autosomal dominant pattern but there is a high rate of spontaneous mutation. The defect is carried on chromosome 17. Characteristic skin lesions include café au lait spots and axillary freckling. Lisch nodules in the iris, osseous lesions, family history, and the presence of neurofibromas or optic glioma are diagnostic criteria for diagnosis of NF-1. There is little pathological material to indicate the nature of the characteristic high-signal lesions seen on MRI in the basal ganglia, brainstem, and cerebellum in patients with NF-1. These signal abnormalities are present in most children between age 1 year and adulthood but are less commonly seen in infants and adults with NF-1. Brain tumors occur commonly in patients with NF-1. In addition to optic gliomas, astrocytomas of the hypothalamus, cerebellum, and brainstem are seen with increased frequency in patients with NF-1.

Further Reading

1. Braffman B, Naidich TP. The phakomatoses: part 1; neurofibromatosis and tuberous sclerosis. *Neuroimaging Clin N Am* 4(2):299–324, 1994.

Case 17

Clinical Presentation

A term newborn with hepatosplenomegaly and petechial skin rash.

Radiographic Studies

Anterior coronal cranial ultrasound image shows punctate and linear areas of increased echogenicity in the periventricular white matter and basal ganglia compatible with calcification (black arrows, Fig. 17A). Axial noncontrast CT (Fig. 17B) confirms the periventricular and basal ganglia calcifications. Axial T2-weighted MRI demonstrates abnormally increased signal intensity in the white matter with subtle low signal foci in the white matter and basal ganglia (black arrows, Fig. 17C) corresponding to areas of calcification. Pronounced low signal is seen in the areas of calcification on an axial T2*-weighted gradient echo image (Fig. 17D).

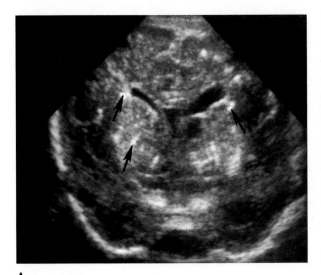

A

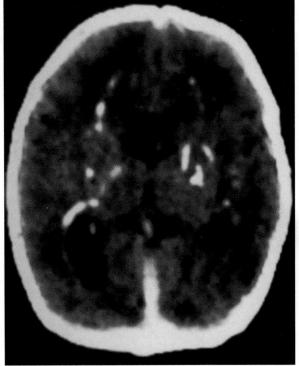

B

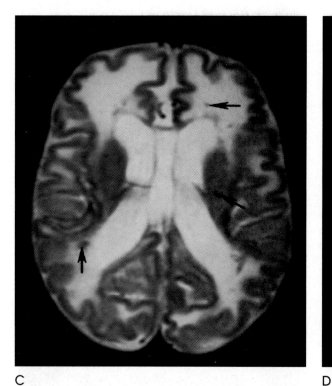

C

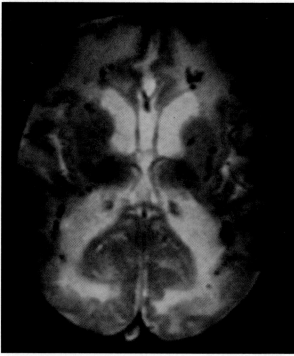

D

Diagnosis   Cytomegalovirus (CMV) Encephalitis

Discussion and Differential Diagnosis

Cytomegalovirus infection is the most common of the TORCH group of congenital infections. Classically, infants with CMV infection present with hepatosplenomegaly and petechiae. Central nervous system manifestations of CMV disease are thought to depend on the stage at which the fetus is infected. Fetuses with infection during the first two trimesters, when neuronal migration is active, may demonstrate extensive polymicrogyria or lissencephaly. Affected infants are frequently microcephalic. Extensive encephalomalacia, delayed myelination, ventriculomegaly, and periventricular calcifications may be present. Of the other TORCH infections, toxoplasmosis most closely mimics the findings of CMV because both may have leukoencephalopathy and extensive calcification associated with microcephaly. It is important to attempt to identify infants with lissencephaly secondary to CMV disease because noninfectious lissencephaly is often associated with chromosomal abnormalities and various syndromes with genetic implications.

Further Reading

1. Barkovich AJ, Lindan CE. Congenital cytomegalovirus infection of the brain: imaging analysis and embryologic considerations. *AJNR Am J Neuroradiol* 15:703–715, 1994.

PEARLS

• For congenital infections, remember "TORCH": *T,* toxoplasmosis; *O,* other (i.e., syphilis); *R,* rubella; *C,* cytomegalovirus; and *H,* herpes type 2 or HIV.

PITFALLS

• The periventricular calcifications of TORCH infections should not be confused with calcified subependymal tubers of tuberous sclerosis.

Case 18

Clinical Presentation

A 5-year-old boy with persistent neck pain, multiple café au lait spots, and a family history of tumors.

Radiographic Studies

Lateral cervical spine radiograph (Fig. 18A) shows widening of multiple neural foramina, anterior and posterior vertebral body scalloping, and upper prevertebral thickening. Sagittal T1-weighted contrast-enhanced MR of the cervical spine demonstrates round, enhancing masses at the foramen magnum, C1, and C2 as well as enhancing masses in the prevertebral (black arrows, Fig. 18B) and suboccipital (black arrowheads, Fig. 18B) soft tissues. Axial T1-weighted contrast-enhanced MR shows the dumbbell lesion at C2 (black arrows, Fig. 18C) and the right prevertebral and extensive right subcutaneous and intermuscular enhancing masses.

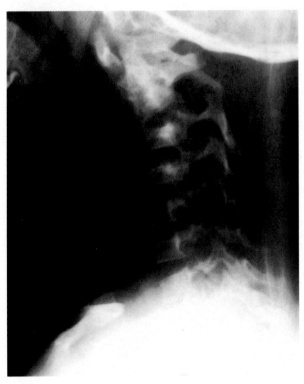

A

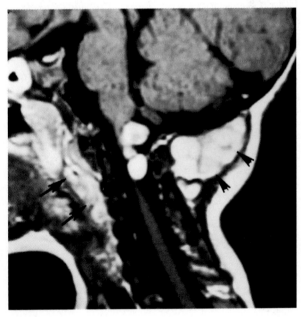

B

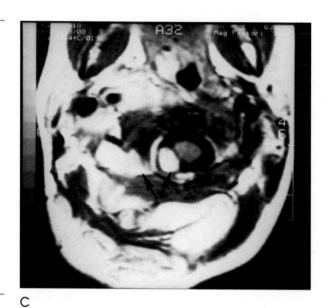

C

Diagnosis Neurofibromatosis Type 1 (NF-1): Spine Involvement

Discussion and Differential Diagnosis

Spinal involvement is commonly seen in patients with both NF-1 and NF-2. In patients with NF-1, most spinal tumors are neurofibromas, although intramedullary tumors are uncommonly seen. Intramedullary tumors, especially ependymomas as well as intradural extramedullary meningiomas and schwannomas, are seen most commonly in NF-2. In NF-1, massive extraspinal tumors may be associated with either minimal or extensive intraspinal involvement. Dural ectasia without soft tissue mass may be associated with extensive bony deformity similar to that seen with intraspinal tumor. Contrast-enhanced MR is necessary to separate patients with dural ectasia from those with bony changes secondary to soft tissue tumors.

Further Reading

1. Egelhoff JC, Bates DJ, Ross JS, Rothner AD, Cohen BH. Spinal MR findings in neurofibromatosis types 1 and 2. *Am J Neuroradiol* 13:1071–1077, 1992.

Case 19

Clinical Presentation

A 10-year-old girl with known chronic polyarticular arthritis with worsening neck pain.

Radiographic Studies

Anteroposterior view of the hands (Fig. 19A) demonstrates periarticular swelling with joint space–centered erosions and variable-sized phalanges. There is particularly severe erosive destruction of the carpal bones with "carpal crowding." Lateral cervical spine radiograph (Fig. 19B) shows fusion of the posterior elements of C5-C7 with decreased size of the C4-C6 vertebral bodies. Sagittal T1-weighted midline MR image of the spine (Fig. 19C) is unremarkable. After the administration of intravenous contrast material (Fig. 19D), there is intense enhancement of the predental space (black arrows, Fig. 19D) and of the interspinous ligaments between C1 and C2 (black arrowheads, Fig. 19D). Sagittal T2*-weighted image (Fig 19E) demonstrates high signal fluid/hypervascular pannus in the predental space (black arrow, Fig. 19E) and interspinous ligaments between C1 and C2 (black arrowhead, Fig. 19E).

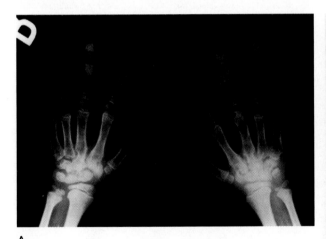

A

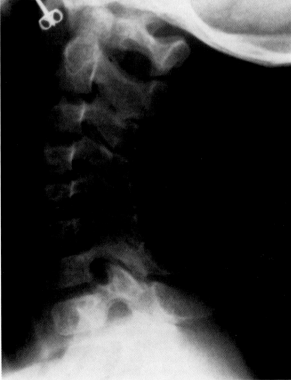

B

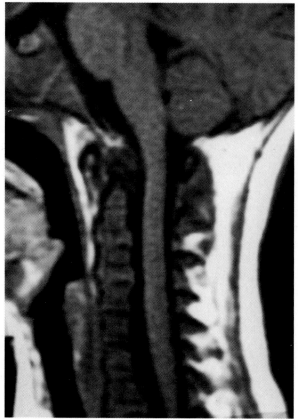

C

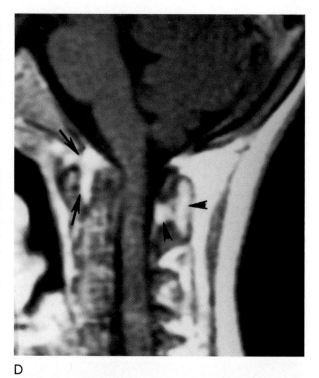

D

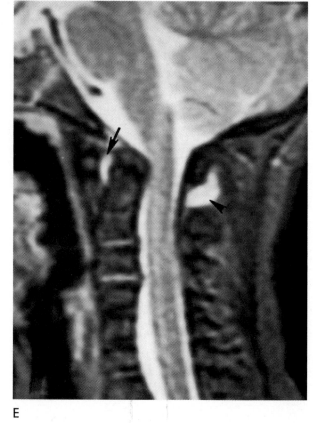

E

Diagnosis Juvenile Rheumatoid Arthritis (JRA): Spine

- Different size and asymmetry of shape of phalanges and cervical vertebral bodies are characteristic of JRA.

- Erosive periarticular changes in the large joints are similar to those seen in hemophilia.

Discussion and Differential Diagnosis

Juvenile rheumatoid arthritis may be polyarticular or pauciarticular and can involve both small and large joints. Erosive changes occur relatively late in the disease. Because the disease affects young children during the years of active skeletal growth and maturation, radiographic manifestations of skeletal growth disturbance are common. These manifestations include apparently advanced bone age, overgrowth and undergrowth of bones, and actual bony ankylosis, which is most dramatically seen in the facet joints of the cervical spine.[1] Atlanto-axial subluxation may occur in children as in adults. Periosteal reaction may be seen in the tubular bones during active phases of the disease. MRI with contrast enhancement can be used to assess disease activity. Hypervascular pannus is hyperintense on T2-weighted images and shows intense contrast enhancement. Hypovascular and fibrotic tissue typically does not enhance.[2] MRI is used to assess possible spinal cord compression in patients with known or suspected atlanto-axial subluxation.

Further Reading

1. Wilkinson RH, Weissman BN. Arthritis in children. *Radiol Clin North Am* 26(6):1247–1265, 1988.
2. Stiskal MA, Neuhold A, Szolar DH, et al. Rhematoid arthritis of the craniocervical region by MR imaging: detection and characterization. *AJR Am J Roentgenol* 165:585–592, 1995.

Case 20

Clinical Presentation

A 10-year-old boy with quadriparesis following motor vehicle accident in which he was not belted in.

Radiographic Studies

Lateral cervical spine radiograph (Fig. 20A) shows greater than 1.5 cm distance between the basion (black arrow, Fig. 20A) and the tip of the odontoid (black arrowhead, Fig. 20A). This measurement is called the DB (dens-basion) distance. There is massive retropharyngeal soft tissue swelling. Sagittal reconstruction to the left of midline of high-resolution cervical spine CT demonstrates posterior subluxation of the superior articulating surface of the atlas (black arrows, Fig. 20B) from the left occipital condyle (black arrowheads, Fig. 20B). Midline sagittal T2*-weighted MR image shows high-signal retropharyngeal edema and impingement of the upper cervical spinal cord by the odontoid. The tectorial membrane is stripped from the clivus and the torn distal end is buckled inferiorly (black arrow, Fig. 20C). The apical ligament of the odontoid is torn and there is edema in the posterior atlanto-occipital membrane (black arrowhead, Fig. 20C).

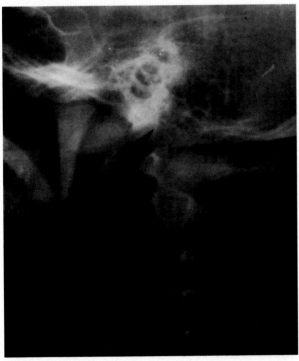

A

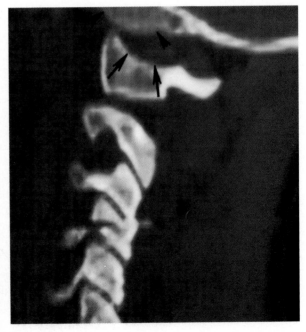

B

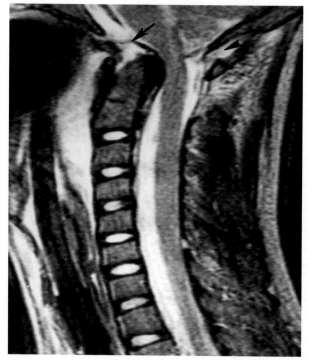

C

Diagnosis Traumatic Atlanto-occipital Dislocation (AOD)

Discussion and Differential Diagnosis

Traumatic AOD is seen most commonly in children who have been hit by a motor vehicle. Survival is not rare but is usually accompanied by severe neurologic abnormality caused by spinal cord and lower cranial nerve injury. The patients may be neurologically intact at the scene of the accident. Prompt neck immobilization and correct interpretation of properly exposed and positioned lateral neck radiographs are essential in the care of these patients. Careful attention to the relationship between the basion and the apical portion of the odontoid process (DB distance) is essential in the interpretation of all posttrauma lateral cervical spine radiographs. Widening of this distance and associated retropharyngeal swelling is seen in most children with traumatic AOD. Although CT can show subluxation more clearly and define associated fractures, and MRI can demonstrate cord compression, edema, and ligamentous injury, the keystone for initial diagnosis of traumatic AOD is still the lateral cervical spine radiograph.

Further Reading

1. Bulas DI, Fitz CR, Johnson DL. Traumatic atlanto-occipital dislocation in children. *Radiology* 188:155–158, 1993.

Case 21

Clinical Presentation

A 7-year-old girl with café au lait spots and left-sided proptosis.

Radiographic Studies

Water's view of the skull shows an "empty orbit" sign with apparent orbital enlargement on the left with elevation of the sphenoid wing (black arrows, Fig. 21A). Axial T1-weighted (Fig. 21B) and T2-weighted (Fig. 21C) MR images demonstrate hypoplasia of the left sphenoid wing, a tortuous, enlarged left optic nerve and nerve sheath (black arrowheads, Fig. 21B), and a left middle cranial fossa arachnoid cyst.

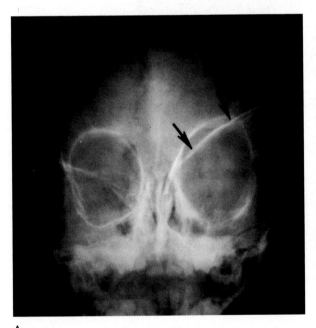

A

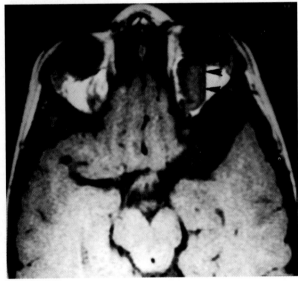

B

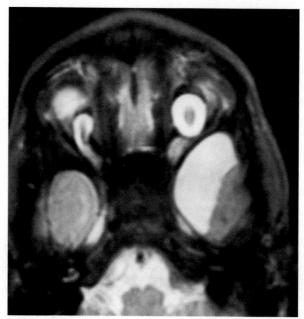

C

Diagnosis Neurofibromatosis Type 1 (NF-1): Sphenoid Wing Dysplasia

Discussion and Differential Diagnosis

The "empty orbit" sign in patients with NF-1 is usually the result of hypoplasia of the ipsilateral sphenoid bone and may be associated with herniation of middle cranial fossa contents into the orbit. The "empty orbit" sign in NF-1 is rarely caused by tumor with bony destruction of the sphenoid, although there is an association of sphenoid wing hypoplasia and plexiform neurofibromas of the orbit.[1] Sphenoid hypoplasia is one of the characteristic bony dysplasias that are used as diagnostic criteria in the diagnosis of NF-1. Other characteristic bony findings in NF-1 include lambdoid sutural defects, pseudarthrosis of the clavicle and tibia, and "ribbon ribs." Optic gliomas are seen in 5 to 15% of children with NF-1 and usually present prior to age 7 years.[2] Optic nerve tumors in NF-1 range from benign hamartomatous lesions to glioblastoma multiforme.

Further Reading

1. Pont MS, Elster AD. Lesions of skin and brain: modern imaging of the neurocutaneous syndromes. *AJR Am J Roentgenol* 158:1193–1203, 1992.
2. Lott IT, Richardson EP Jr. Neuropathological findings and the biology of neurofibromatosis. *Adv Neurol* 29:23–31, 1981.

Case 22

Clinical Presentation

An 18-month-old infant with hypotonia and ophthalmoplegia.

Radiographic Studies

T2-weighted axial MR images show abnormal high signal in the lentiform nuclei and medial thalamus (Fig. 22A) and in the dorsal midbrain and cerebral peduncles (Fig. 22B).

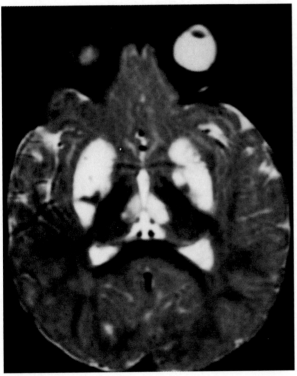

A

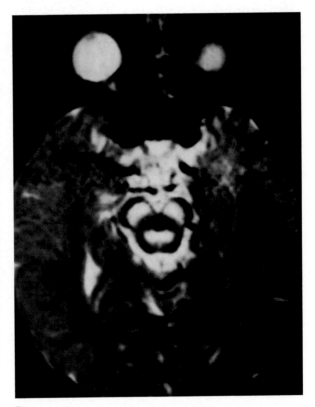

B

Diagnosis Leigh Disease (Subacute Necrotizing Encephalomyelopathy)

PEARLS

- Low attenuation changes on CT and long T1 and T2 signal in the basal ganglia and brainstem on MRI are characteristic findings in infants with Leigh disease.

PITFALLS

- The other mitochondrial encephalopathies as well as profound asphyxia may demonstrate similar imaging findings on CT and MRI.

Discussion and Differential Diagnosis

Leigh disease is actually not one disorder but the manifestation of one of several metabolic abnormalities caused by various enzyme deficiencies. Patients with Leigh disease tend to present in infancy with hypotonia, cranial nerve abnormalities, and seizures. Elevated lactate levels can be found in the serum and in the spinal fluid. The characteristic signal abnormalities on MRI and low attenuation findings on CT in the basal ganglia and brainstem suggest the diagnosis in infants with characteristic clinical abnormalities.[1] MRI proton spectroscopy may provide a more precise diagnostic tool by demonstrating abnormally elevated lactate in areas of brain showing abnormal signal intensity change on imaging.[2]

Further Reading

1. Greenberg SB, Faerber EN, Riviello JJ, et al. Subacute necrotizing encephalomyelopathy (Leigh disease): CT and MRI appearances. *Pediatr Radiol* 21:5–8, 1990.
2. Barkovich AJ, Good WV, Koch TK, Berg BO. Mitochondrial disorders: analysis of their clinical and imaging characteristics. *AJNR Am J Neuroradiol* 14:1119–1137, 1993.

Case 23

Clinical Presentation

A 2-month-old infant with pneumococcal meningitis, bulging fontanelle, and seizures.

Radiographic Studies

Axial noncontrast CT demonstrates ventriculomegaly with focal edema in the right posterior parietal cortex (black arrows, Fig. 23). A septation is present in the left lateral ventricle.

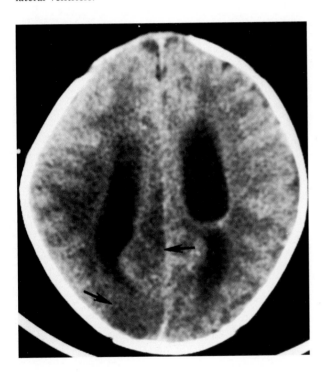

Diagnosis Bacterial Meningitis with Infarction

- Infarction with meningitis may be secondary to either arterial or venous occlusion.

- Tuberculosis or other opportunistic organisms should be considered if basilar enhancement and hydrocephalus are present.

Discussion and Differential Diagnosis

Bacterial meningitis continues to be a common problem in infants and children. Bacteria usually gain access to the brain through seeding of the choroid plexus due to sepsis. Other sources of infection include congenital dermal sinuses and other midline defects, skull fractures, and infected ventricular catheters. In newborn infants with meningitis, ventriculitis is virtually always present and complications such as brain abscess, hydrocephalus, vascular occlusion, and encephalomalacia are more common than in the older infant and child. Subdural effusions are seen more commonly in older infants.

Further Reading

1. Barnes PD, Poussaint TY, Burrows PE. Imaging of pediatric central nervous system infections. *Neuroimaging Clin N Am* 4(2):367–391, 1994.

Case 24

Clinical Presentation

A 2-year-old boy with hyperactivity, pallor, and emaciation (diencephalic syndrome). Extensive workup for gastrointestinal disease was normal.

Radiographic Studies

Sagittal T1-weighted image shows low-signal lobulated mass in the suprasellar and inter-peduncular cistern displacing the midbrain and pons posteriorly (black arrows, Fig. 24A). Axial T2-weighted image shows the tumor to be markedly hyperintense (Fig. 24B). There is intense tumor enhancement on the coronal T1-weighted image (Fig. 24C) following administration of contrast.

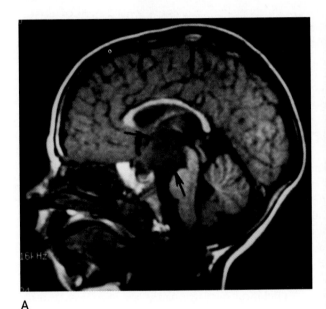

A

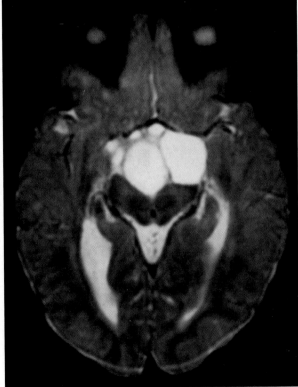

B

PEARLS

● Hypothalamic/optic chiasm gliomas occur with an increased incidence in patients with neurofibromatosis type 1.

PITFALLS

● To distinguish craniopharyngioma from hypothalamic/optic pathway glioma, look for hyperintensity in the tumor on T1-weighted images as well as focal low signal suggestive of calcification, findings frequently present in craniopharyngioma but uncommonly in gliomas.

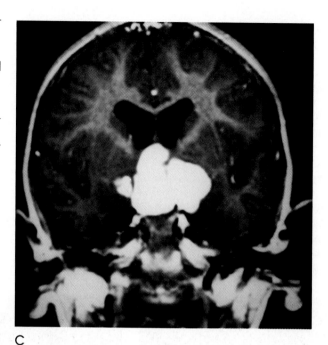

C

Diagnosis Hypothalamic Astrocytoma

Discussion and Differential Diagnosis

Suprasellar masses in children include craniopharyngioma, hypothalamic/optic pathway glioma, germ cell tumors, Langerhans' cell histiocytosis, and tuber cinereum hamartoma. Gliomas tend to be bulky lesions, are hypointense to gray matter on T1-weighted images and hyperintense on T2-weighted images, and show variable enhancement. The optic nerves and visual pathways are frequently enlarged. Children with both germ cell tumors and histiocytosis frequently present with diabetes insipidus. Germ cell tumors tend to be large and may have associated masses in the pineal region as well as leptomeningeal spread of tumor. In histiocytosis, the pituitary infundibulum is abnormally prominent but large masses are infrequent. Patients with histiocytosis often have lytic lesions in the calvarium, skull base, or elsewhere in the skeleton. Children with hamartoma of the tuber cinereum present with precocious puberty. Hamartomas are isointense to gray matter on all pulse sequences and rarely enhance.

Further Reading

1. Edwards-Brown MK. Supratentorial brain tumors. *Neuroimaging Clin N Am* 4(2):437–455, 1994.

Case 25

Clinical Presentation

A 5-year-old girl with diabetes insipidus.

Radiographic Studies

Axial (Fig. 25A) and coronal (Fig. 25B) CT images of the face and skull base acquired with bone algorithm reconstruction show multiple "punched out" lesions (black arrows, Fig. 25A, 25B). Axial contrast-enhanced CT of the brain at the level of the suprasellar cistern demonstrates an enlarged pituitary infundibulum (black arrows, Fig. 25C). The normal pituitary infundibulum should be the same size or smaller than the adjacent basilar artery. The mastoid air cells are under-pneumatized and sclerotic bilaterally (black arrowheads, Fig. 25A).

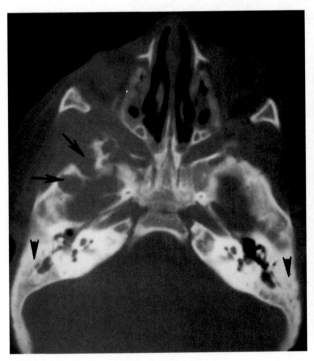

A

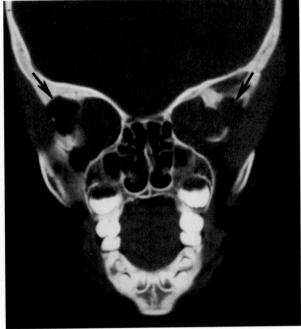

B

PEARLS

- "Punched out" bony lesions with well-defined but nonsclerotic margins in a child involving any portion of the bony skeleton but especially the skull are typical of Langerhans' cell histiocytosis.

- Solitary lytic lesions with discrete sclerotic margins in the calvarium are most commonly epidermoidomas.

PITFALLS

- Radionuclide skeletal scintigraphy may be negative in patients with histiocytosis[2] and thus radiographic skeletal survey is recommended for evaluation of multifocal skeletal involvement.

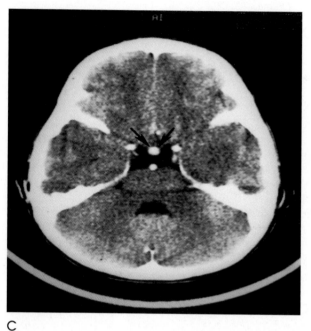

C

Diagnosis   Langerhans' Cell Histiocytosis

Discussion and Differential Diagnosis

Histiocytosis may involve both soft tissue and bone, but bony lesions are most common. Bony lesions may involve any portion of the skeleton and may be either solitary or disseminated.[1] Classically, bone lesions of histiocytosis have very well defined margins with beveled edges. Soft tissue masses may be associated with the bone lesions. When soft tissue involvement with bone destruction is present, imaging findings are not specific for histiocytosis, although thickening of the pituitary infundibulum in a child with diabetes insipidus even without bony lesions should suggest the diagnosis. When histiocytosis involves the mandible, the teeth may become loose and a radiographic "floating tooth" sign may be present. Involvement of the spine typically causes loss of height of one or more vertebral bodies and the appearance of vertebra plana. A button sequestrum may be seen in radiographs of histiocytosis bone lesions. Osteomyelitis, primary bone and soft tissue tumors, and metastases from neuroblastoma, leukemia, and lymphoma may simulate findings of aggressive histiocytosis bone and soft tissue lesions.

Further Reading

1. Meyer JS, Harty MP, Mahboubi S, et al. Langerhans cell histiocytosis: presentation and evolution of radiologic findings with clinical correlation. *Radiographics* 15:1135–1146, 1995.
2. Treves ST. *Pediatric Nuclear Medicine.* New York: Springer-Verlag; 1985:37–38.

Case 26

Clinical Presentation

A newborn infant with large mass on her back.

Radiographic Studies

Thoracolumbar spine radiograph (Fig. 26A) shows marked widening of the spinal canal from the midthoracic region into the sacrum (black arrows, Fig. 26A). The soft tissue mass is seen lateral to the dysraphic spine (black arrowheads, Fig. 26A). Thoracic spinal segmentation anomalies are present. Lateral skull radiograph demonstrates the typical whorled irregular ossification of lacunar skull (Luckenschadel). The craniofacial ratio is enlarged, suggestive of hydrocephalus (Fig. 26B). Coronal cranial ultrasound shows marked ventriculomegaly, absence of the septum pellucidum, and inferior pointing of the frontal horns of the lateral ventricles (black arrows, Fig. 26C). Midline sagittal T1-weighted MRI in another patient shows a dysplastic body and splenium of the corpus callosum, marked tectal beaking (black arrowhead, Fig. 26D), enlarged massa intermedia, and an elongated cerebellum with cerebellar tissue present inferiorly in the posterior fossa and upper spinal canal (black arrows, Fig. 26D).

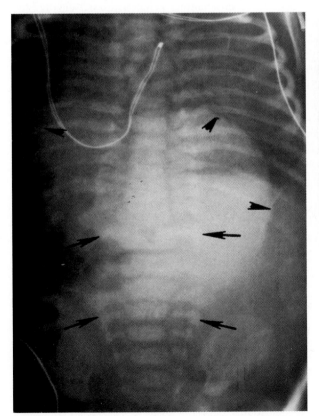

A

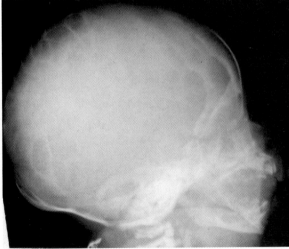

B

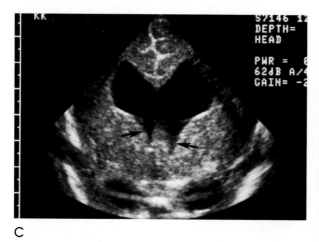

C

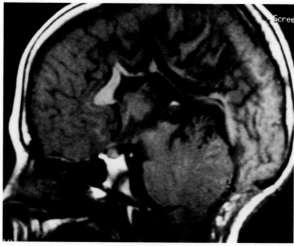

D

Diagnosis   Myelomeningocele/Chiari II Malformation

Discussion and Differential Diagnosis

The Chiari II malformation is a group of neuroanatomic abnormalities seen in patients with myelomeningocele. Multiplanar MRI best shows the extensive neuropathology found in these patients. Intracranial findings include hydrocephalus, dysgenesis of corpus callosum, fenestration of the falx with gyral interdigitation, enlarged massa intermedia, midbrain tectal beaking, and both superior extension of the cerebellum through a dysplastic tentorium and inferior displacement of the fourth ventricle and cerebellum into the foramen magnum and cervical spinal canal.[1] Syringohydromyelia is frequently found in association with hydrocephalus and shunt malfunction. Chiari I malformation refers to inferior displacement of the cerebellar tonsils in patients without myelomeningoceles. Patients with Chiari I malformation have an increased incidence of syringohydromyelia.[2] Chiari III malformation includes patients with occipital or high cervical cephaloceles containing posterior fossa structures in conjunction with intracranial findings of Chiari II malformation.[3]

Further Reading

1. Barkovich AJ. *Pediatric Neuroimaging.* New York: Raven Press; 1995:238–246.
2. Elster AD, Chen MY. Chiari I malformations: clinical and radiologic reappraisal. *Radiology* 183:347–353, 1992.
3. Castillo M, Quencer RM, Dominguez R. Chiari III malformation: imaging features. *AJNR Am J Neuroradiol* 13:107–113, 1992.

PEARLS

- The vast majority of infants with myelomeningocele have hydrocephalus and intracranial findings of Chiari II malformation.

- Lacunar skull is thought to be a mesodermal bone dysplasia that disappears by 3 to 6 months of age.

PITFALLS

- Newborn infants with Chiari II malformation may not have hydrocephalus at birth but develop ventriculomegaly later. Serial measurement of head circumference and cranial sonography should be performed in infants with myelomeningocele who have normal or minimally enlarged ventricular size at birth.

Case 27

Clinical Presentation

A 10-month-old boy with recent pseudomonas sepsis, persistent fever, and a stiff neck.

Radiographic Studies

Lateral cervical spine radiograph shows marked demineralization of C6 and C7, no evident disc space at that level, and extrusion of a fragment of bone into the prevertebral space (black arrows, Fig. 27A). Midline sagittal T2*-weighted gradient echo scan (Fig. 27B) demonstrates increased signal in the C6-C7 vertebral bodies/disc space with prevertebral high signal compatible with edema. Parasagittal T2*-weighted gradient echo scan to the right of Figure 27B shows the high signal at the C6-C7 level and, in addition, the extruded bone fragment adjacent to the vertebral bodies appears as a low-signal abnormality (black arrow, Fig. 27C).

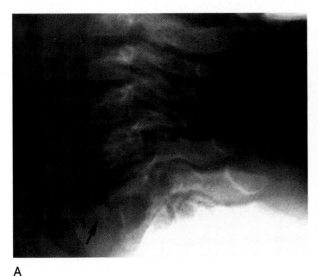

A

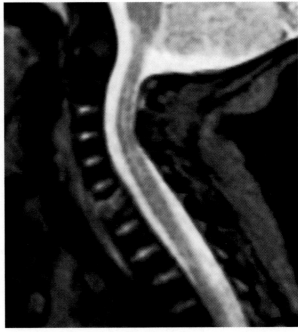

B

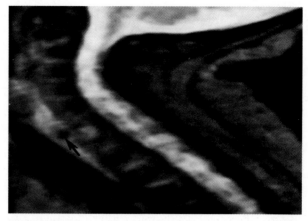

C

Diagnosis Vertebral Osteomyelitis

Discussion and Differential Diagnosis

Vertebral osteomyelitis is frequently associated with bacteremia. Bacteria may gain access to the vertebral column via Batson's plexus. Retropharyngeal infection, penetrating trauma and recent surgery[1] may also be associated with cervical spondylitis. In the neonatal period, spondylitis may be associated with multifocal osteomyelitis, and nuclear scintigraphy or radiographic skeletal survey should be considered to exclude multiple sites of infection. Conventional radiographs show demineralization, frank bony destruction, kyphosis, and, as in this case, extruded bone fragments into adjacent soft tissue. MR imaging in vertebral osteomyelitis shows replacement of normal marrow signal in the involved vertebral body with lengthening of T1 and T2 relaxation times. Contrast enhancement may be seen in the disc space or vertebral body or in the epidural space or spinal cord in cases of intraspinal spread of infection.[2,3] Paravertebral collections may be seen in pyogenic or tuberculous spondylitis. Other entities that can mimic vertebral osteomyelitis include primary neoplasms, metastatic disease (particularly from neuroblastoma or leukemia), and vertebral involvement with Langerhans' cell histiocytosis. Neoplastic involvement of the vertebral body classically spares the disc space, which is usually involved early in infectious spondylitis.

Further Reading

1. Baker LL, Bower CM, Glasier CM. Atlanto-axial subluxation and cervical osteomyelitis: two unusual complications of adenoidectomy. *Ann Otol Rhinol Laryngol* 105(4):295–299, 1996.
2. Ruiz A, Post JD, Ganz WI. Inflammatory and infectious processes of the cervical spine. *Neuroimaging Clin N Am* 5(3):401–425, 1995.
3. Thrush A, Enzmann D. MR imaging of infectious spondylitis. *AJNR Am J Neuroradiol* 11:1171–1180, 1990.

Case 28

Clinical Presentation

A 4-year-old girl with severe back and abdominal pain. She was in the back seat of the family car wearing a lap belt at the time of a frontal collision.

Radiographic Studies

Anteroposterior (Fig. 28A) and lateral (Fig. 28B) views of the thoracolumbar spine show subluxation of the L1-L2 facet joints (white arrows, Fig. 28B) with a fracture involving the posterosuperior portion of the L2 vertebral body and posterior elements (black arrows, Fig. 28A, 28B). The L1-L2 disc space is widened secondary to disruption of the intervertebral disc. Sagittal reconstruction from thin section spine CT (Fig. 28C) demonstrates the facet dislocation as well as some retropulsion of the L2 vertebral body into the spinal canal. Axial CT scan at the level of L2 shows an "empty facet" sign resulting from facet subluxation (black arrows, Fig. 28D). There is extensive subcutaneous edema dorsally (at tails of black arrows, Fig. 28D). There is free fluid in the right paracolic gutter (white arrow, Fig. 28D) as well as mesenteric edema. At surgery, the superior mesenteric artery was found to be partially avulsed.

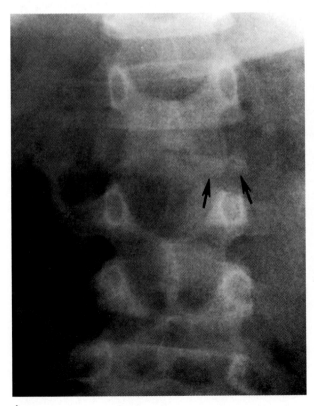

A

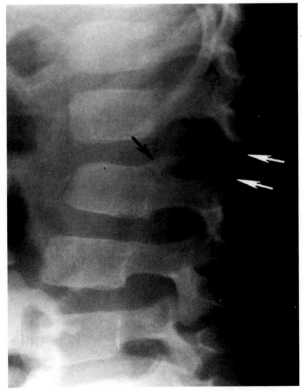

B

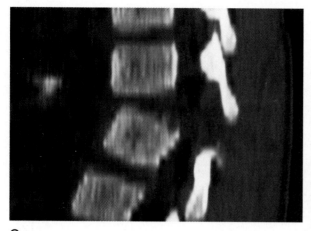

C

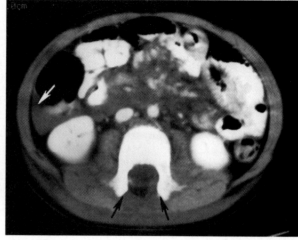

D

Diagnosis Chance Fracture

Discussion and Differential Diagnosis

The Chance fracture was first described in 1948.[1] The use of seat belts, particularly lap belts, has been associated with an increasing incidence of this injury, which is associated with extreme hyperflexion.[2] In children, Chance fractures occur in the lumbar spine, probably related to the pediatric body habitus. Severe compression forces may cause extensive injury to the soft abdominal viscera. The soft tissue component of the spinal injury includes disruption of the intervertebral disc and the posterior interspinous ligaments. There is often vertebral body subluxation that may be associated with injury to the spinal cord. Taylor and Eggli[3] have pointed out the difficulty of diagnosing lumbar flexion injuries on frontal radiographs and axial CT and recommend obtaining lateral "scout views" when performing abdominal CT in children following motor vehicle accidents. Clues to the diagnosis of the Chance fracture on AP radiographs include distraction of the facets creating an empty space between the vertebral bodies (plain film equivalent of empty or naked facet sign on CT), widening of the disrupted intervertebral disc space, and visualization of the horizontal fracture fragment as in Figure 28A.

PEARLS

- Chance fractures in children are frequently associated with injuries to the conus medullaris of the spinal cord.

PITFALLS

- Lateral spine views on a backboard may "reduce" spinal subluxation. Careful, physician-supervised flexion radiographs or MRI may be necessary to demonstrate facet subluxation and interspinous ligament disruption.

Further Reading

1. Chance GQ. Note on type of flexion fracture of spine. *Br J Radiol* 21:452, 1948.
2. Rogers LF. Transverse fractures of the spine. In: *Radiology of Skeletal Trauma.* New York: Churchill Livingstone; 1982:325–328.
3. Taylor GA, Eggli KD. Lap-belt injuries of the lumbar spine in children: a pitfall in CT diagnosis. *AJR Am J Roentgenol* 150:1355–1358, 1988.

Case 29

Clinical Presentation

A 16-year-old girl with Down syndrome was found to have hyperreflexia at the time of screening examination for Special Olympics participation.

Radiographic Studies

Neutral lateral cervical spine radiograph shows a predental interval (black arrows, Fig. 29A) of 7 mm and marked narrowing of the spinal canal (black arrowheads, Fig. 29A). Sagittal reconstruction from high-resolution spinal CT (Fig. 29B) confirms widening of the atlanto-dental interval, narrowed spinal canal, and, in addition, demonstrates fusion of the posterior arch of C1 with the occiput (black arrows, Fig. 29B). Sagittal T1-weighted cervical spine MRI shows marked compression and thinning of the upper cervical spinal cord (white arrows, Fig. 29C). Lateral cervical spine radiograph in another child with Down syndrome, who was asymptomatic, demonstrates (Fig. 29D) anterior displacement of the odontoid in relation to the clivus and an increased distance (greater than 1 cm) between the anterior lip of the foramen magnum and the tip of the odontoid (black arrows, Fig. 29D).

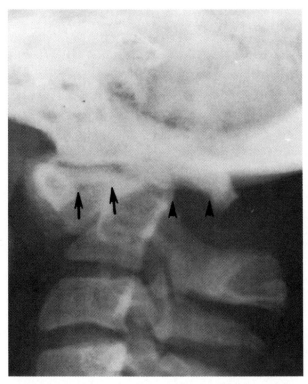

A

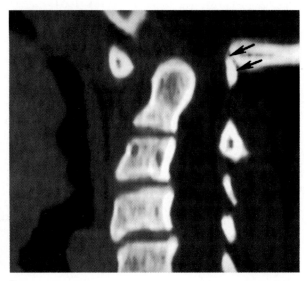

B

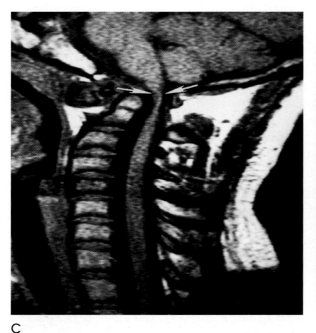

C

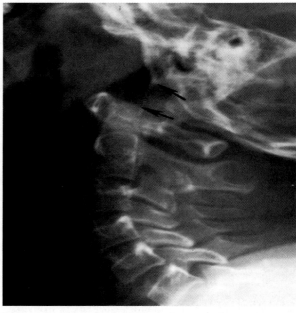

D

Diagnosis Down Syndrome: Atlanto-axial and Atlanto-occipital Subluxation

Discussion and Differential Diagnosis

Radiographic atlanto-axial subluxation without clinical symptoms is relatively common in patients with Down syndrome. Symptomatic atlanto-axial subluxation, however, is infrequent, occurring in less than 1% of these children.[1] Atlanto-occipital instability is also seen with an increased incidence. In addition to the ligamentous laxity and subluxation, bony anomalies of the craniocervical junction, especially involving the odontoid process (os odontoideum) and the ring of C1 (hypoplastic posterior arch) are found in these patients.[2] Patients with Down syndrome should undergo physical examination and lateral cervical spine radiography prior to participation in contact sports. Children with radiographic and symptomatic atlanto-axial subluxation should be examined with CT of the craniocervical junction and flexion/extension MRI of the cervical spine prior to surgical therapy. MR imaging with T1- and T2-weighted images can detect spinal canal stenosis and abnormal signal in the spinal cord related to previous injury. High-resolution CT confirms spinal canal narrowing and accurately defines associated bony anomalies.

Further Reading

1. Smoker WR. Congenital anomalies of the cervical spine. *Neuroimaging Clin N Am* 5(3):427–449, 1995.
2. Martich V, Ben-Ami T, Yousefzadeh DK, Roizen NJ. Hypoplastic posterior arch of C-1 in children with Down syndrome: a double jeopardy. *Radiology* 183:125–128, 1992.

Case 30

Clinical Presentation

A 6-month-old infant with severe developmental delay, seizures, and bilateral coloboma.

Radiographic Studies

Sagittal (Fig. 30A) and axial (Fig. 30B) T1-weighted MR images show lack of normal cortical sulcal-gyral markings with marked ventriculomegaly. A Dandy-Walker–like cystic malformation of the cerebellum and posterior fossa is noted on the sagittal image with associated hypoplasia of the cerebellum and brainstem. Multiple small islands of heterotopic gray matter are seen deep to the abnormally thickened and smooth cerebral cortex (black arrows, Fig. 30B).

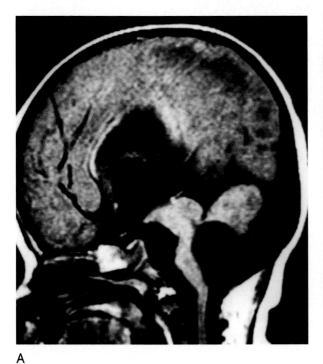

A

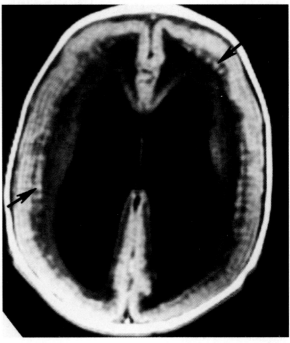

B

Diagnosis Lissencephaly (Agyria)

Discussion and Differential Diagnosis

Lissencephaly or agyria is a severe disorder of brain structure categorized as the most severe anomaly of neuronal migration. Children with lissencephaly are almost always severely developmentally delayed. There is lack of formation of normal cortical gyri and sulci. A few sulci may be present or the cortical surface may be nearly completely smooth. Lissencephaly may be localized to one area of the cortical surface. There are several different types of lissencephaly. The case presented here is an example of Walker-Warburg syndrome, which consists of various optic disc anomalies, lissencephaly, hydrocephalus, and sometimes posterior fossa malformations, as in this case. The diffuse thickening of the abnormally smooth cortex, and the underlying dysmorphic strands and nodules of heterotopic gray matter are typical of this specific form of lissencephaly.

Further Reading

1. Barkovich AJ, Gressens P, Evrard P. Formation, maturation, and disorders of brain neocortex. *AJNR Am J Neuroradiol* 13:423–446, 1992.

PEARLS

- A smooth, "agyric" cortex is a developmental normal finding in extremely premature infants and should not be confused with true lissencephaly.

PITFALLS

- Diffuse polymicrogyria/ lissencephaly with a "knobby" appearance of the cerebral cortical surface, often with associated cerebral calcifications, is seen in infants with cytomegalovirus infection. It is important to recognize this "variant" of lissencephaly because it does not carry the possible genetic implications of some of the other lissencephaly syndromes.

Case 31

Clinical Presentation

A 7-year-old boy with sickle cell disease with acute onset of left hemiparesis.

Radiographic Studies

Axial T2-weighted image at the time of presentation (Fig. 31A) shows high signal compatible with edema in the right frontotemporal cortex and insula. Axial collapsed image from three-dimensional (3-D) time-of-flight MRA at the same time as *A* demonstrates occlusion of the proximal right middle cerebral artery (white arrows, Fig. 31B). Follow-up T2-weighted image from an MR scan 2 years later shows right cerebral hemiatrophy and cystic encephalomalacia in the site of the previous infarct (Fig. 31C). Collapsed axial image from 3-D time-of-flight MRA at the same time as *C* demonstrates partial reconstitution of the right middle cerebral artery (black arrows, Fig. 31D). In addition, prominent lenticulostriate and cortical collateral vessels are seen (black arrowheads, Fig. 31D).

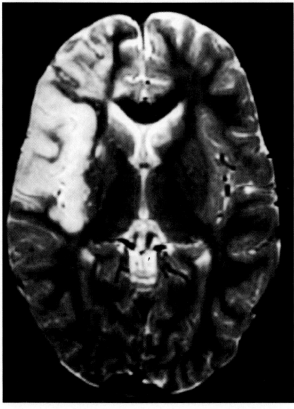

A

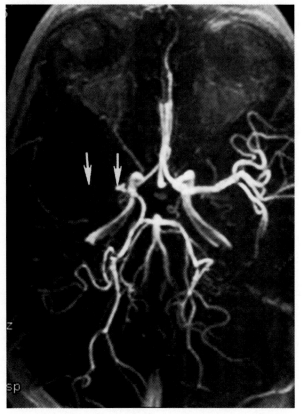

B

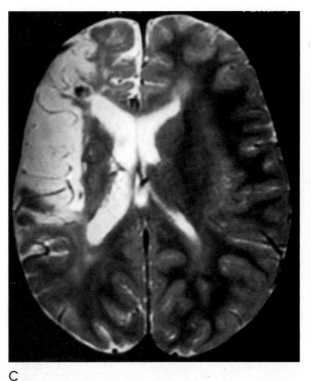

C

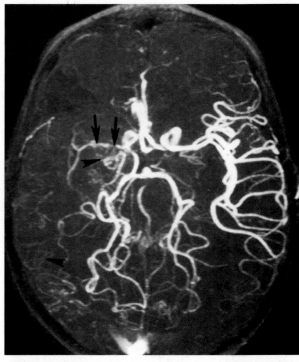

D

Diagnosis Stroke/Sickle Cell Disease

Discussion and Differential Diagnosis

Cerebral vasculopathy with stroke is a common complication of sickle cell disease. Stroke may occur in up to 17% of sickle cell patients.[1,2] Complete occlusion of the supraclinoid internal carotid arteries may lead to multiple infarcts, dementia, and radiographic findings typical of *moya-moya*. Early detection of cerebral vasculopathy in these patients using noninvasive diagnostic tools—transcranial Doppler and MRI/MRA, coupled with hypertransfusion therapy—is being studied in an attempt to prevent progressive cerebral vasculopathy and neurological deterioration in these patients.[3]

Further Reading

1. Powars D, Wilson B, Imbus C, et al. The natural history of stroke in sickle cell disease. *Am J Med* 65:461–471, 1978.
2. Wood DH. Cerebrovascular complications of sickle cell anemia. *Stroke* 9:73–75, 1978.
3. Seibert JJ, Miller SF, Kirby RS, et al. Cerebrovascular disease in symptomatic and asymptomatic patients with sickle cell anemia: screening with duplex transcranial Doppler US—correlation with MR imaging and MR angiography. *Radiology* 189:457–466, 1993.

Case 32

Clinical Presentation

A 1300-gram premature infant with hyaline membrane disease. Cranial ultrasound was performed for screening purposes. The infant had no obvious neurological abnormalities.

Radiographic Studies

Coronal (Fig. 32A) and parasagittal (Fig. 32B) transfontanelle ultrasound images show bilateral subependymal densities (single black arrows, Fig. 32A, 32B). There are densities in the left lateral ventricle (white arrowheads, Fig. 32A, 32B) and in the third ventricle (double black arrows, Fig. 32A). Note the sonolucent CSF-containing cleft (black arrowheads, Fig. 32B) separating the intraventricular density from normal choroid plexus, which is wrapping around the thalamus.

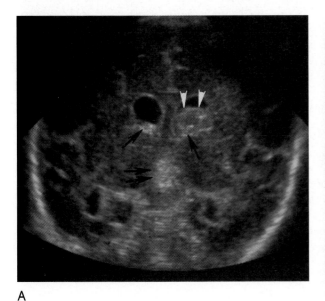

A

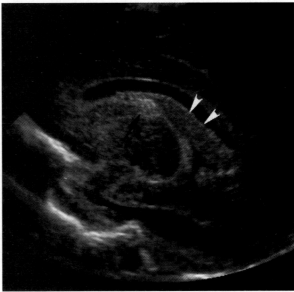

B

Diagnosis Subependymal/Intraventricular Hemorrhage

Discussion and Differential Diagnosis

Subependymal/intraventricular hemorrhage is a common problem in the neonatal intensive care unit population. The survival of ever smaller and more premature infants ensures that intracranial hemorrhage will continue to be a frequent diagnosis. In preterm infants, hemorrhage most commonly occurs within the substance of residual vascular germinal matrix tissue in the region of the caudothalamic groove as seen in Figure 32B. In older infants, hemorrhage may occur primarily within the choroid plexus. Intracranial hemorrhage is usually of increased echogenecity on ultrasound imaging. Blood (or occasionally pus) within the ventricular system may demonstrate a "snowstorm," particulate appearance on sonography.

Subependymal hemorrhage may occur as an isolated finding (grade 1 hemorrhage), with intraventricular blood but without ventricular dilatation (grade 2), with intraventricular blood and dilated ventricles (grade 3), or with intraparenchymal hemorrhage (grade 4). Post-hemorrhagic hydrocephalus and damage to periventricular white matter are the most common complications of subependymal/intraventricular hemorrhage. There is a positive correlation between the higher grades between of hemorrhage (particularly grade 4) and subsequent neurodevelopmental abnormalities. Portable cranial ultrasound is the imaging modality of choice in most premature infants with intracranial hemorrhage, with CT or MRI reserved for unusual or complicated cases.[1] The intraventricular hemorrhage in this case would be classified as a grade 3 hemorrhage because there is both intraventricular blood and mild-to-moderate ventricular dilatation.

Further Reading

1. Volpe JJ. Intracranial hemorrhage: germinal matrix-intraventricular hemorrhage of the preterm infant. In: *Neurology of the Newborn.* Philadelphia: WB Saunders; 1995:403–463.
2. Boal DK, Watterberg KL, Miles S, Gifford KL. Optimal cost-effective timing of cranial ultrasound screening in low-birth-weight infants. *Pediatr Radiol* 25:425–428, 1995.

Case 33

Clinical Presentation

A 2-year-old boy with a small pit in the skin in the midline of his nasal bridge.

Radiographic Studies

Axial high-resolution CT shows an asymmetric defect in the midline of the nasal bones (black arrowheads, Fig. 33A) with overlying soft tissue thickening and abnormality of the subcutaneous fat. Magnification view from contrast-enhanced cranial CT demonstrates a low attenuation round mass in the anteroinferior interhemispheric fissure (black arrow, Fig. 33B) compatible with fat. Sagittal T1-weighted MR image shows a focal high signal mass (black arrow, Fig. 33C) corresponding to the fatty mass seen in Figure 33B. Axial T2-weighted MR image demonstrates a high-signal, fluid-like mass just inferior to the fatty tissue noted on the other images (black arrows, Fig. 33D). At surgery, a sinus tract was resected that communicated with an intracranial cyst through a defect in the foramen cecum (white arrowheads, Fig. 33C).

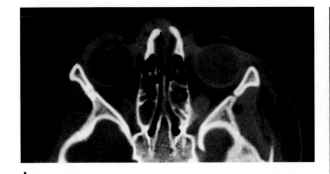

A

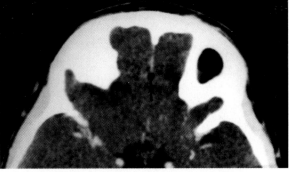

B

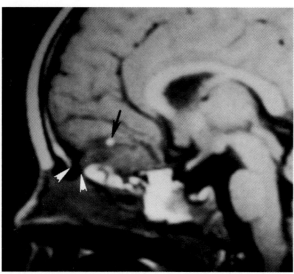

C

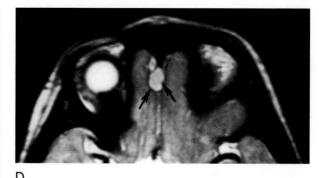

D

Diagnosis Nasal Dermal Sinus with Intracranial Dermoid Cyst

Discussion and Differential Diagnosis

The differential diagnosis of congenital nasal masses includes nasal cephalocele, nasal glioma, and nasal dermoid/dermal sinus. Infants with congenital nasal dermal sinuses present with a small pit, dimple, or soft tissue mass on the nose from the tip to the glabella. The sinus may end blindly in the soft tissues of the nose or extend intracranially through the foramen cecum. There may be an associated dermoid or epidermoid tumor in the sinus tract or in the midline intracranially. Some infants present with osteomyelitis of the frontal bone at the glabella, in which case the sinus tract may be obliterated. If CT is performed as the preoperative study, thin axial and coronal sections should be obtained through the nose and anterior cranial fossa in order to identify any defect in the anterior skull base (usually at the foramen cecum) associated with an intracranial mass or infection. Although less than ideal for definition of bony anatomy, the multiplanar capability of MRI makes it the most useful preoperative imaging modality.

Further Reading

1. Barkovich AJ, Vandermarck P, Edwards MS, Cogen PH. Congenital nasal masses: CT and MR imaging features in 16 cases. *AJNR Am J Neuroradial* 12:105–116, 1991.

Case 34

Clinical Presentation

A 2-year-old girl who refused to walk and complained of back pain. The child had a low-grade fever and an elevated erythrocyte sedimentation rate.

Radiographic Studies

Posteroanterior (PA) (Fig. 34A) and lateral (Fig. 34B) lumbar spine radiographs demonstrate narrowing of the L3–4 intervertebral disc space (black arrows, Fig. 34A, 34B). Bone scan shows increased uptake in the L3 and L4 vertebral bodies (Fig. 34C). Sagittal STIR (short T1 inversion recovery) (Fig. 34D) image demonstrates high signal compatible with edema in the L3 and L4 vertebral bodies as well as loss of normal signal in and a rounded high signal mass (black arrow, Fig. 34D) adjacent to the L3–4 disc space. Sagittal T1-weighted gadolinium-enhanced scan shows intense enhancement of a mass posterior to the L3–4 disc space (black arrow, Fig. 34E) as well as enhancement of the adjacent L3 and L4 vertebral bodies.

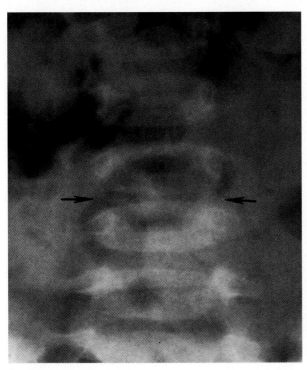

A

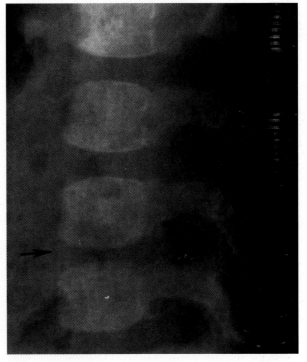

B

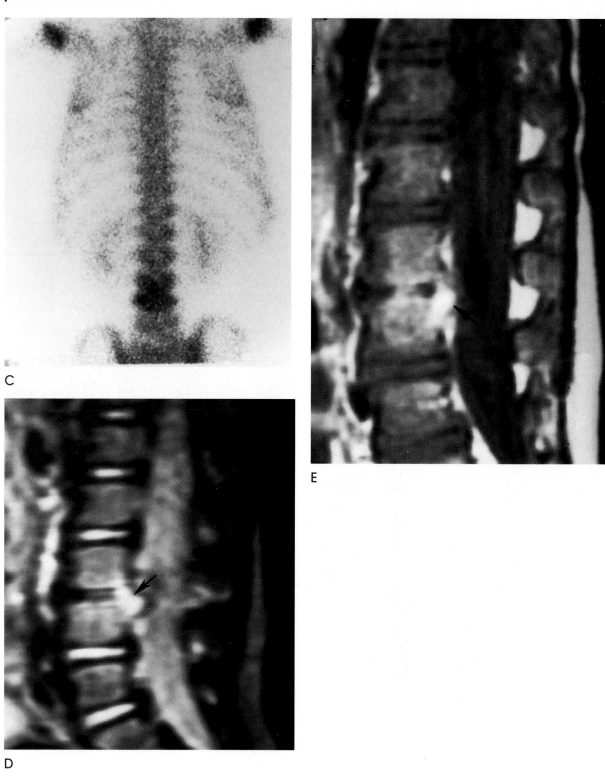

C

D

E

Diagnosis Discitis

PEARLS

- About half of all cases of childhood discitis are shown to have a bacterial cause, usually *Staphylococcus aureus.*

PITFALLS

- Plain radiographs may be normal early in the course of discitis. Bone scan is often positive prior to development of plain radiographic abnormalities.[1]

CONTROVERSY

- Some authorities believe MRI is essential in the diagnosis of discitis.

Discussion and Differential Diagnosis

In young children, discitis is usually thought to be secondary to infection of the vertebral end plates related to a blood-borne infection.[1] Discitis in children usually involves the lumbar spine. Initial radiographic findings include loss of height of the involved disc space followed by irregular erosion of the adjacent vertebral bodies. Both bone scan and MRI[2] are sensitive to early changes of discitis, perhaps within days of onset of signs and symptoms of infection. In the limping toddler or the child refusing to bear weight, bone scan has the advantage of detecting pathology remote to the spine such as the various toddler's fractures, osteoid osteomas, or osteomyelitis of the lower extremities. MRI has the advantage of high-resolution evaluation of pathology in the vertebral bodies, spinal canal, and paravertebral tissues. Contrast-enhanced CT in young children quite adequately demonstrates cortical bone destruction and paravertebral inflammation. One approach to imaging children with possible discitis is to screen with plain films and scintigraphy and reserve MRI or CT for children with negative or atypical findings on conventional imaging or for those with neurological findings suggestive of epidural mass or spinal cord tumor.

Further Reading

1. Wenger DR, Bobechko WP, Gilday DL. The spectrum of intervertebral disc-space infection in children. *J Bone Joint Surg Am* 60(1):100–108, 1978.
2. du Lac P, Panuel M, Devred P, et al. MRI of disc space infection in infants and children: report of 12 cases. *Pediatr Radiol* 20:175–178, 1990.

Case 35

Clinical Presentation

A 3-month-old infant with Erb's palsy. The baby was a 3500-gram term infant delivered vaginally with a breech presentation.

Radiographic Studies

Coronal T2*-weighted gradient echo cervical MR image (Fig. 35) shows three discrete collections of cerebrospinal fluid in the right C5, C6, and C7 neural foramina (black arrows, Fig. 35).

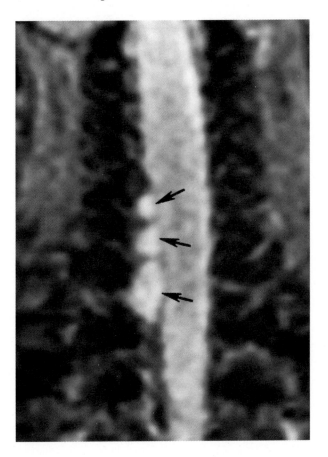

Diagnosis Brachial Plexopathy Associated with Pseudomeningocele

Discussion and Differential Diagnosis

Brachial plexopathy is seen most commonly in macrosomic term infants, especially in association with breech delivery. The injury is presumed to be caused by stretching of the neck during delivery with tears of the root sleeve or actual avulsion of the spinal nerve. The lower cervical plexus (C4–C8) is most commonly injured, leading to the clinical finding of Erb-Duchenne or Dejerine-Klumpke upper extremity paralysis. There may be an associated paresis of the ipsilateral hemidiaphragm. Plain radiographs of the upper extremity and chest should be obtained to rule out clavicular or humeral fractures. Fortunately, most infants with brachial plexopathy recover spontaneously without surgical intervention. Imaging is usually performed after 3 months of age following incomplete recovery of neurological function. MR imaging demonstrates pseudomeningoceles or damage to the cervical spinal cord associated with brachial plexopathy. If demonstration of the tiny spinal nerve roots in infants with brachial plexopathy is demanded, CT myelography with thin-section, high-resolution scanning is necessary.

Further Reading

1. Miller SF, Glasier CM, Griebel ML, Boop FA. Brachial plexopathy in infants after traumatic delivery: evaluation with MR imaging. *Radiology* 189:481–484, 1993.

PEARLS

- Brachial plexus injuries may be associated with clavicle fractures, probably related to extreme traction on the shoulder during delivery.

PITFALLS

- Pseudomeningoceles in the newborn are small lesions. High-resolution, motion-free imaging is necessary to reliably detect these abnormalities.

CONTROVERSY

- Some centers still utilize CT myelography for the evaluation of infants with brachial plexopathy in order to directly visualize injury to individual nerve rootlets.

Case 36

Clinical Presentation

A 2-month-old infant was brought to the emergency department "turning blue." The baby was in status epilepticus. There were multiple bruises on the head, trunk, and extremities as well as retinal hemorrhages.

Radiographic Studies

Axial noncontrast cranial CT images show diffuse massive cerebral edema with obliteration of the gray-white junction. There are tentorial (black arrows, Fig. 36A) and interhemispheric (black arrows, Fig. 36B) subdural hematomas. There is a left posterior scalp hematoma (white arrows, Fig. 36A) with an underlying skull fracture (not shown).

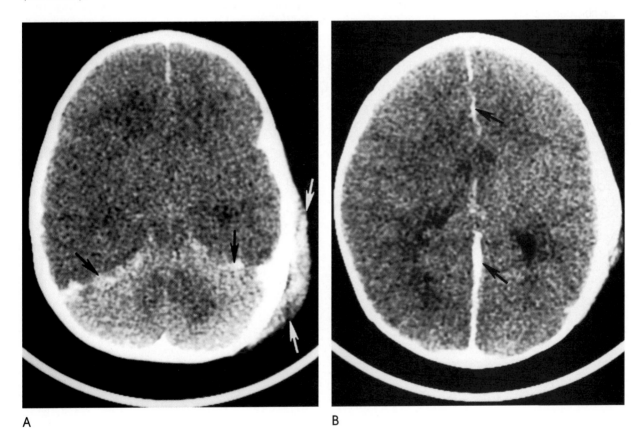

A   B

Diagnosis Child Abuse: Cerebral Injury

Discussion and Differential Diagnosis

Craniocerebral injury is the leading cause of death in abused infants. Severe shaking leads to tears of the bridging veins with subdural bleeding. Both shaking and direct blows to the head cause focal parenchymal hemorrhage and infarction. Skull fractures may or may not be associated with cerebral injury in abused infants. Asphyxia related to strangulation or to status epilepticus compounds the direct traumatic injuries found in these babies. Differential diagnosis primarily includes accidental trauma, anticoagulation therapy, and bleeding diatheses such as hemophilia and thrombocytopenia. CT is the primary diagnostic tool in the diagnosis of craniocerebral injury in abused infants. Cranial CT in infants should be performed with slice thickness no greater than 5 mm. Sedation may be necessary to allow motion-free images. Careful window and level selection at the diagnostic console is essential in order to detect small subdurals and subtle differences in attenuation between the CSF in the ventricles and the fluid in the subdural spaces. Normal subarachnoid CSF overlying the superficial gyri may be distinguished from subtle subdural hematomas with appropriate CT technique.

Further Reading

1. Harwood-Nash DC. Abuse to the pediatric central nervous system. *AJNR Am J Neuroradiol* 13:569–575, 1992.

Case 37

Clinical Presentation

A 3-year-old girl with severe failure to thrive and encephalopathy.

Radiographic Studies

Axial CT shows a diffuse atrophy pattern with mild prominence of the superficial sulci and of the ventricles (Fig. 37). There is extensive calcification in the frontal white matter and in the lentiform nuclei.

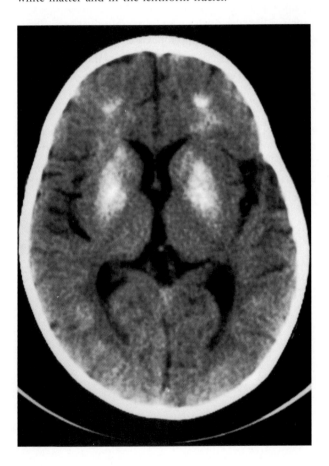

Diagnosis HIV Encephalitis: Basal Ganglia Calcification

Discussion and Differential Diagnosis

Children with HIV encephalopathy present with failure to thrive, loss of or failure to develop normal developmental milestones, and focal neurologic symptoms. Neurologic abnormalities in children with HIV disease are secondary to direct invasion of the central nervous system (CNS) with the AIDS virus. The most common neuroimaging findings in children with HIV encephalopathy include an atrophy pattern, basal ganglia and frontal white matter calcifications, and other white matter abnormalities.[1] Opportunistic CNS infections such as toxoplasmosis and CNS lymphoma are much less common in HIV-infected children than in adults. Intracranial calcifications are seen uncommonly in adults with HIV infection. Cerebral infarction may occur secondary to vascular involvement, and intracranial hemorrhage is associated with the coagulopathies and thrombocytopenia found in these patients. Inflammatory intracranial aneurysms are seen in children with HIV vasculopathy.

Further Reading

1. Kauffman WM, Sivit CJ, Fitz CR, et al. CT and MR evaluation of intracranial involvement in pediatric HIV infection: a clinical-imaging correlation. *AJNR Am J Neuroradiol* 13:949–957, 1992.
2. Haller JO, Cohen HL. Pediatric HIV infection: an imaging update. *Pediatr Radiol* 24:224–230, 1994.

Case 38

Clinical Presentation

A 6-year-old boy with neck pain.

Radiographic Studies

Sagittal (Fig. 38A) and coronal (Fig. 38B) reconstructions from a high-resolution CT of the cervical spine show dense calcification of the C4-5 intervertebral disc with mild anterior extrusion of the calcification (black arrows, Fig. 38A).

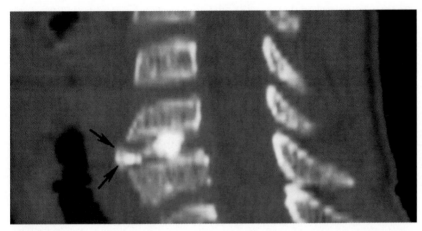

A

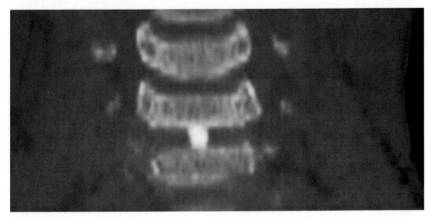

B

Diagnosis Cervical Disc Calcification

Discussion and Differential Diagnosis

Idiopathic disc space calcification may be seen in asymptomatic children. Calcification may involve single or multiple levels, usually in the cervical or thoracic spine. Children with calcified cervical discs are more likely to present with neck pain or torticollis. Rarely, a low-grade fever or an elevated sedimentation rate may be present. The calcification may be confined to the central portion of the disc or protrude anteriorly into the retropharyngeal tissues or posteriorly into the spinal canal. The disc height is generally preserved and abnormalities in the adjacent vertebral bodies are generally minimal.[1] Neurologic symptoms may be present in patients with extrusion of disc material into the spinal canal and swallowing difficulty may be present in patients with anterior herniation. Symptoms tend to subside spontaneously with conservative therapy.[2] The calcifications may persist or disappear spontaneously.

Further Reading

1. Girodias JB, Azouz EM, Marton D. Intervertebral disk space calcification: a report of 51 children with a review of the literature. *Pediatr Radiol* 21:541–546, 1991.
2. Ozonoff MB. Intervertebral disc calcification in childhood. In: *Pediatric Orthopedic Radiology.* Philadelphia: WB Saunders Co; 1992:97–98.

PEARLS

- In many cases, disc space calcification is an incidental finding.

PITFALLS

- Idiopathic disc space calcification should not be confused with infectious processes such as discitis or with tumor.

Case 39

Clinical Presentation

A 3-year-old boy who suffered an acute head injury with immediate loss of consciousness.

Radiographic Studies

Axial image from a cranial CT performed about 30 minutes after the head injury shows extensive blood (black arrows, Fig. 39A) with subfalcine herniation and left hemispheric edema. An overlying skull fracture was present. T2-weighted axial MR image 1 week later demonstrates near-complete resolution of the mass effect with high signal changes compatible with edema/infarction in the left genu and anterior forceps (black arrow, Fig. 39B) and splenium (black arrowheads, Fig. 39B) of the corpus callosum as well as in both caudate heads, putamina, and left occipital cortex.

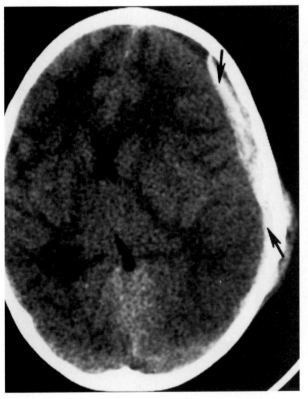

A

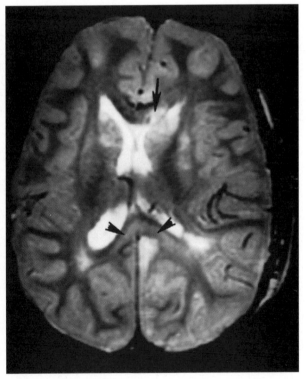

B

Diagnosis Acute Subdural Hematoma with Contusion/Shearing Injury

Discussion and Differential Diagnosis

Acute cerebral injury resulting from both accidental and nonaccidental trauma (child abuse) represents a major source of morbidity and mortality in children. Subdural hematomas are most common in infants and adolescents, and extradural hematomas are more frequent in the intervening years.[1] Brain swelling, cerebral hemorrhage, infarction, and diffuse axonal injury (DAI) are frequently found in association with subdural hematomas. CT is the imaging modality of choice for acute subdural hematomas. Appropriate CT technique includes appropriate slice thickness (5 mm or less in infants) and viewing of brain, bone, and intermediate (subdural) windows in all head-injured patients. The extraaxial fluid density should approximate that of CSF. Increase in density of this fluid should lead to suspicion of extraaxial blood. MRI is more sensitive than CT in the diagnosis of small subacute and chronic subdural hematomas and should be utilized when the diagnosis is in doubt.[2] MRI is also much more sensitive than CT for the diagnosis of DAI, which is one of the leading causes of disability in head-injured patients.

Further Reading

1. Aronyk KE. Post-traumatic hematomas. In: *Pediatric Neurosurgery.* Philadelphia: WB Saunders Co; 1994:279–296.
2. Zimmerman RA, Bilaniuk LT. Pediatric head trauma. *Neuroimaging Clin N Am* 4(2):349–366, 1994.

Case 40

Clinical Presentation

A newborn infant girl with a midline hemangioma overlying the lumbar spine. Neurologic examination is normal.

Radiographic Studies

Midline sagittal view of the lower lumbar spine from a screening spinal ultrasound examination demonstrates a low-lying conus in the lower lumbar area (white arrows identify the dorsal surface of the low-lying cord, white arrowheads identify the central echo complex, Fig. 40A) Linear increased echogenicity with some posterior acoustic shadowing compatible with a "laminar cap" (black arrows, Fig. 40A) is noted dorsally below the conus. Axial ultrasound image over the lumbar region shows two hemicords without obvious intervening spur (white arrows, Fig. 40B). Coronal T1-weighted MRI of the spine demonstrates two hemicords, thickening of the filum terminale (white arrow, Fig. 40C) and a small syrinx (black arrow, Fig. 40C). Axial T2*-gradient echo image shows two discrete hemicords without intervening spur (black arrows, Fig. 40D).

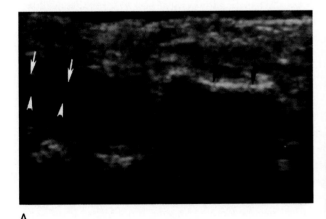

A

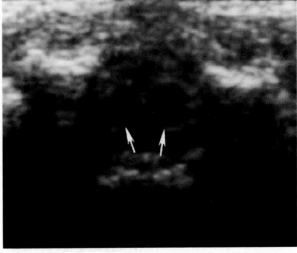

B

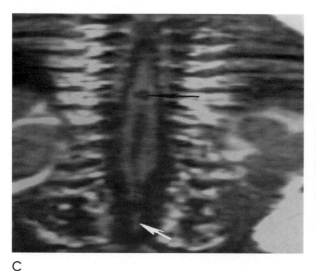

C

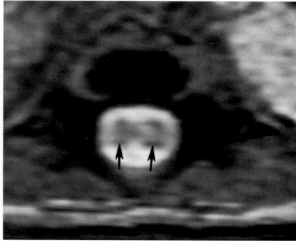

D

Diagnosis Diastematomyelia

Discussion and Differential Diagnosis

Diastematomyelia is presumed to result from splitting of the notochord. Infants with diastematomyelia are usually female, and over half have a skin lesion overlying the dysraphic abnormality. Many patients with spina bifida aperta have associated diastematomyelia. Diastematomyelia means split cord, and two hemicords are present at the level of the defect. Many patients have a fibrous, cartilaginous, or bony septum separating the hemicords. Hydromyelia is frequently present in the single cord above the split and may extend caudally into one or both hemicords.[1] Other anomalies are also common, including thickening of the filum terminale, dermal sinuses, dermoid or epidermoid tumors, and dural adhesions.[2] Plain radiographs of the spine are almost always abnormal and may show hemivertebrae, widening of the spinal canal, or a bony septum. Screening spinal ultrasound can identify the hemicords in infants with diastematomyelia[3] but is most useful during the newborn period and in patients with posterior bony dysraphism. MRI is the preferred preoperative imaging modality. MR imaging should include sagittal and axial T1-weighted images and axial T2- or T2*-weighted images. Coronal imaging is optimal to identify the length of the split cord. Axial T2-weighted images most elegantly identify or exclude a spur dividing the hemicords.

PEARLS

- Any newborn with a midline cutaneous lesion overlying the spine should undergo screening spinal ultrasound in order to determine the level of the conus and identify underlying spinal pathology.

PITFALLS

- Abnormal screening spinal ultrasound should be supplemented with MRI for complete preoperative evaluation.

- An interlaminar bar or cap, which is often present in patients with diastematomyelia, may block the ultrasound beam and make complete sonographic evaluation of the spinal canal difficult.

Further Reading

1. Schlesinger AE, Naidich TP, Quencer RM. Concurrent hydromyelia and diastematomyelia. *AJNR Am J Neuroradiol* 7(3):473–477, 1986.
2. Barkovich AJ. Congenital anomalies of the spine. In: *Pediatric Neuroimaging.* 2nd ed. New York: Raven Press; 1995:477–540.
3. Glasier CM, Chadduck WM, Burrows PE. Diagnosis of diastematomyelia with high-resolution spinal ultrasound. *Child Nerv Syst* 2(5):255–257, 1986.

Case 41

Clinical Presentation

A 1-year-old infant with seizures.

Radiographic Studies

Axial T2-weighted MR image shows symmetric bilateral CSF-filled, gray matter–lined clefts extending from the cerebral cortical surface to the ventricular lumen (Fig. 41A). Prominent vessels are seen overlying the clefts, particularly on the left (black arrows, Fig. 41A). Coronal T1-weighted inversion recovery MR image demonstrates absence of the septum pellucidum as well as unusual "diverticula" of the ventricular margins "pointing" toward the anomalous deep gray matter seams (white arrows, Fig. 41B).

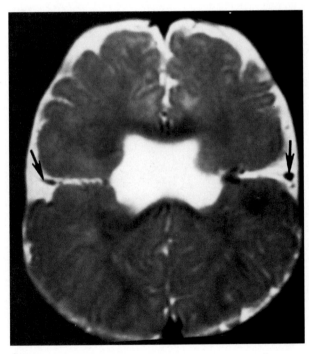

A

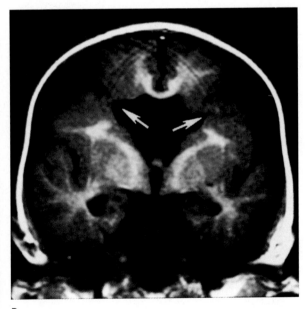

B

Diagnosis Schizencephaly

Discussion and Differential Diagnosis

Schizencephaly is usually considered a disorder of neuronal migration and refers to a cleft in the cerebral cortex that extends centrally toward the ventricle. The cleft is lined with gray matter that is dysplastic. In open-lip schizencephaly, the cleft has a definite communication with the ipsilateral lateral ventricle and is filled with CSF. In closed-lip schizencephaly, there is little CSF in the cleft, which is therefore composed entirely of dysmorphic gray matter. Schizencephaly may be unilateral or bilateral. The septum pellucidum is frequently absent. Coronal images are optimal to define the cleft, communication with the ventricular system, and associated anomalies.

Further Reading

1. Barkovich AJ, Norman D. MR imaging of schizencephaly. *AJNR Am J Neuroradiol* 9:297–302, 1988.

Case 42

Clinical Presentation

A 12-year-old boy with a right-sided facial vascular lesion and seizures.

Radiographic Studies

Lateral skull radiograph shows "tram-track" calcifications in the parieto-occipital cortex (black arrows, Fig. 42A). Axial CT of the head before (Fig. 42B) and after (Fig. 42C) the administration of contrast confirms gyriform cerebral calcification (black arrows, Fig. 42B), but no definite enhancement of the cortical lesion. There is prominent enhancement of the glomus of the right choroid plexus (black arrow, Fig. 42C). Axial gradient echo image shows profound low signal in the right parieto-occipital cortex corresponding to the calcification seen on skull radiography and CT (black arrows, Fig. 42D). Sagittal T1-weighted contrast-enhanced MR image to the right of midline shows intense serpiginous contrast enhancement in the right occipital cortex (black arrows, Fig. 42E).

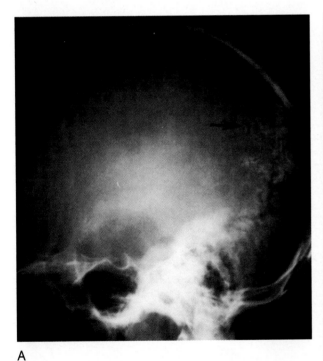

A

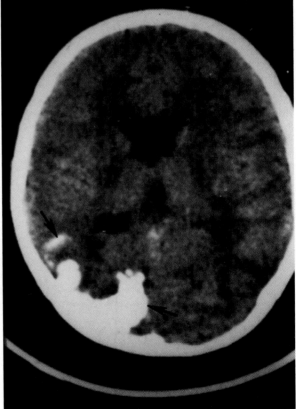

B

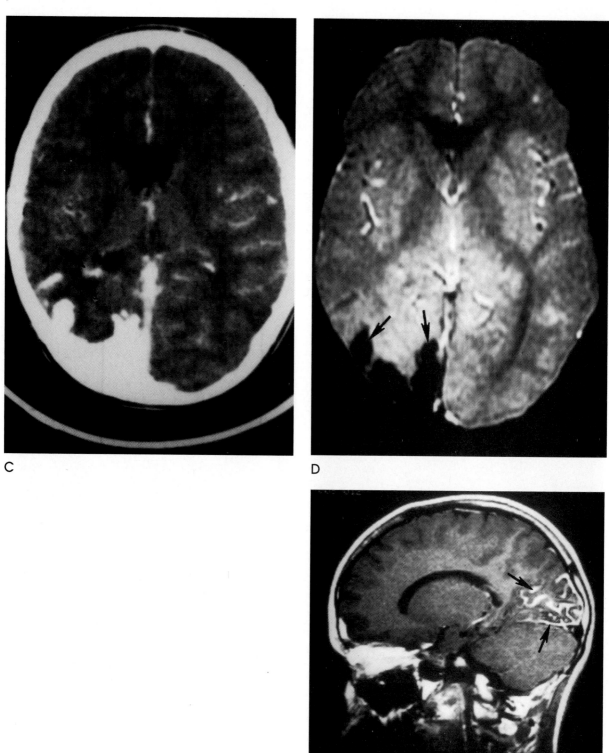

C

D

E

Diagnosis Sturge-Weber Syndrome (Encephalotrigeminal Angiomatosis)

Discussion and Differential Diagnosis

Sturge-Weber syndrome is characterized by a facial port-wine stain in association with retinal and leptomeningeal angiomatosis. The facial lesion is usually ipsilateral to the retinal and cerebral lesion. The port-wine stain is a capillary-venous malformation, as is the retinal lesion. The embryogenesis of the cerebral lesion is somewhat controversial, but the leptomeningeal angiomatosis is usually accompanied by abnormal superficial and deep cerebral venous drainage with associated dystrophic changes in the cortex.[1] Most patients present with seizures. Glaucoma is also frequently present. The neuroimaging changes reflect chronic unilateral cerebral ischemia and include cerebral hemiatrophy, cortical gyriform calcification, and gliosis. Enlarged medullary veins are frequently present as well as enlargement of the ipsilateral glomus of the choroid plexus. Leptomeningeal enhancement may be difficult to detect on CT because of associated dense calcification or because of beam-hardening artifact from the overlying calvarium.

Further Reading

1. Smirniotopoulos JG, Murphy FM. The phakomatoses. *AJNR Am J Neuroradiol* 13:725–746, 1992.
2. Brodsky MC, Baker RS, Hamed LM. Neuro-ophthalmologic manifestations of systemic and intracranial disease. In: *Pediatric Neuro-Ophthalmology.* New York: Springer; 1996:407–410.

PEARLS

- Most children with facial port-wine stains do not have ocular or leptomeningeal angiomatosis.[2]

PITFALLS

- CT is less sensitive than MRI in detecting cortical ischemic changes as well as leptomeningeal and cortical enhancement.

Case 43

Clinical Presentation

A 13-year-old girl with headaches and recent onset of seizure activity.

Radiographic Studies

Axial post-contrast CT image shows a rounded low attenuation mass with ring enhancement (black arrows, Fig. 43A) in the left frontal lobe effacing the frontal horn. Sagittal T1-weighted MR image demonstrates a low signal mass adjacent to the left frontal horn (black arrows, Fig. 43B). Axial T2-weighted image shows the left frontal mass, which is mixed hyper- and hypointense to gray matter with a low signal intensity rim (black arrows, Fig. 43C). Axial T1-weighted MRI post-gadolinium demonstrates intense rim enhancement of the periphery of the mass (Fig. 43D). Stereotactic aspiration of the left frontal lobe lesion yielded purulent material, which grew *Staphylococcus aureus*.

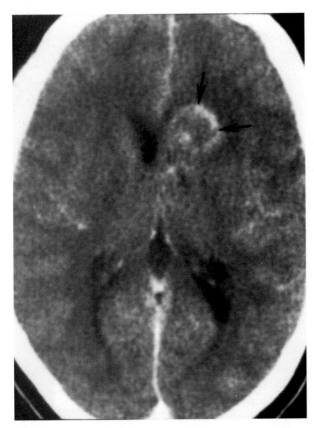

A

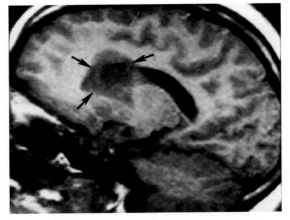

B

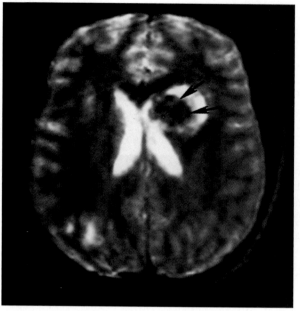

C

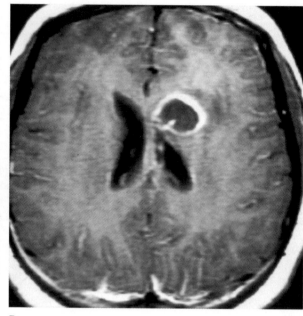

D

Diagnosis Brain Abscess

Discussion and Differential Diagnosis

Brain abscesses are more common in adolescents than in younger children. They may occur secondary to the right-to-left shunting found in children with cyanotic congenital heart disease or following episodes of sepsis. Other causes include penetrating trauma, sinusitis, mastoiditis, and infected congenital dermal sinuses. CT characteristically shows focal edema with ring enhancement after an abscess has evolved from a focal area of cerebritis. Ependymal or leptomeningeal enhancement occurs if the abscess ruptures into the ventricle or into the subarachnoid space. MRI is more sensitive than CT for early diagnosis of brain abscess. MRI typically shows edema around the abscess, which is low signal on T1-weighted images and high signal on T2-weighted images. The center of the abscess may be heterogeneous with either low or high signal on T2-weighted images. Low signal intensity rings are typically seen at the periphery of the cavity on T2-weighted or gradient echo images.[1] Ring enhancement is more easily seen on MRI than on CT.

PEARLS

- Brain abscess is a rare complication of meningitis except in newborns with gram-negative meningitis.[2]

PITFALLS

- Even appropriately treated and bacteriologically sterile brain abscesses may show ring enhancement on CT or MRI for months after diagnosis.[3]

Further Reading

1. Haimes AB, Zimmerman RD, Morgello S, et al. MR imaging of brain abscesses. *AJNR Am J Neuroradiol* 10:279–291, 1989.
2. Barnes PD, Poussaint TY, Burrows PE. Imaging of pediatric central nervous system infections. *Neuroimaging Clin N Am* 4(2):367–391, 1994.
3. Zimmerman RD, Weingarten K. Neuroimaging of cerebral abscesses. *Neuroimaging Clin N Am* 1(1):1–16, 1991.

Case 44

Clinical Presentation

A 3-year-old boy with ataxia, headaches, and papilledema.

Radiographic Studies

Sagittal T1-weighted MRI shows an isointense mass in the inferior cerebellar vermis filling the fourth ventricle (black arrows, Fig. 44A). Axial T2-weighted MRI demonstrates the mass in the region of the fourth ventricle, which is heterogeneous but predominantly isointense to gray matter (black arrows, Fig. 44B). Coronal T1-weighted gadolinium-enhanced MRI shows intense contrast enhancement in the mass (black arrow, Fig. 44C) as well as tonsillar herniation (black arrowheads, Fig. 44C). Bone scan performed as part of the metastatic workup following surgery has areas of increased activity in the L3 and L5 vertebral bodies compatible with metastases (black arrows, Fig. 44D). Axial contrast-enhanced CT in another child illustrates a heterogeneous, contrast-enhancing mass in the midline of the cerebellum with enhancing leptomeningeal tumor spread in the interpeduncular cistern (white arrow, Fig. 44E), along the tentorium and overlying the right cerebellar hemisphere (black arrow, Fig. 44E). Sagittal T1-weighted, contrast-enhanced spine MRI shows extensive, enhancing leptomeningeal masses coating the spinal cord (black arrows, Fig. 44F).

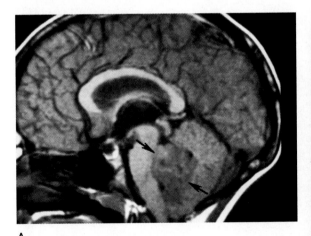

A

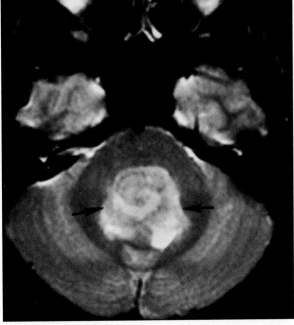

B

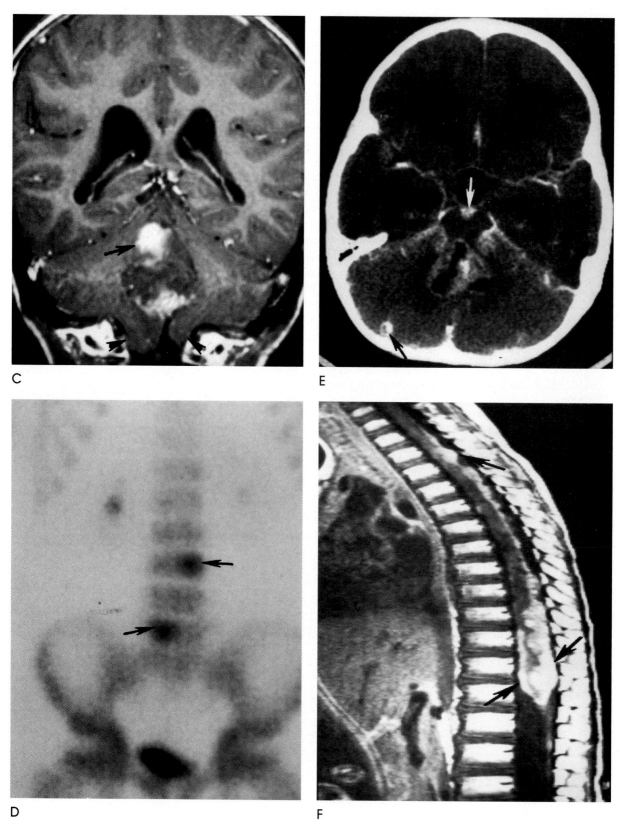

C

D

E

F

Diagnosis Medulloblastoma

Discussion and Differential Diagnosis

Medulloblastoma is the most common posterior fossa tumor in childhood. This tumor is sometimes classified as a primitive neuroectodermal tumor (PNET).[1] Medulloblastoma most commonly occurs in the first decade of life and presents after a short history of symptoms typical of posterior fossa tumors with headache, nausea, and vomiting accompanied by papilledema. In young children, medulloblastoma usually presents as a midline mass in the roof of the fourth ventricle. Hydrocephalus is usually present secondary to fourth ventricular and aqueductal obstruction. On CT, medulloblastoma is usually hyperdense to cerebellum and shows intense enhancement after contrast administration. Calcification and cyst formation may occur within the tumor. On MRI, the tumor tends to be isointense to cerebellum on both T1- and T2-weighted images and enhances postcontrast administration. Initial radiologic evaluation of children with medulloblastoma includes contrast-enhanced MRI of the head and spine as well as radionuclide skeletal scintigraphy. Contrast-enhanced MRI of the spine has replaced CT myelography in the evaluation of suspected "drop metastases."

Further Reading

1. Gusnard DA. Cerebellar neoplasms in children. *Semin Roentgenol* 25(3):263–278, 1990.
2. Vezina LG, Packer RJ. Infratentorial brain tumors of childhood. *Neuroimaging Clin N Am* 4(2):423–436, 1994.

Case 45

Clinical Presentation

A 4-year-old girl with headaches, vomiting, and papilledema.

Radiographic Studies

Axial T1-weighted MRI shows a large cyst (black arrows, Fig. 45A) with a peripheral solid nodular mass (black arrowheads, Fig. 45A) compressing the pons and displacing the fourth ventricle to the right. Axial T2-weighted image (Fig. 45B) demonstrates massively dilated temporal horns as well as the CSF intensity cyst and mural tumor nodule, which is mildly hyperintense to cerebellum. Axial (Fig. 45C) and coronal (Fig. 45D) T1-weighted contrast-enhanced MR images show intense contrast enhancement of the tumor nodule but no enhancement of the cyst wall. Figure 45D also demonstrates dilatation of the occipital horns of the lateral ventricles with adjacent low attenuation compatible with transependymal resorption of CSF (black arrows, Fig. 45D).

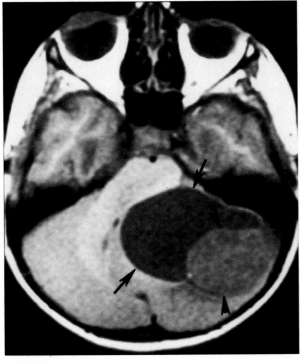

A

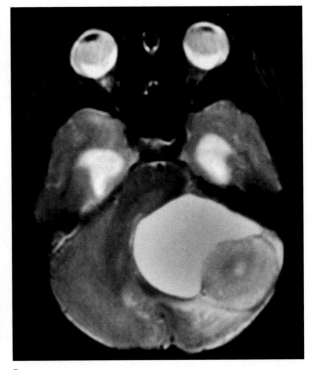

B

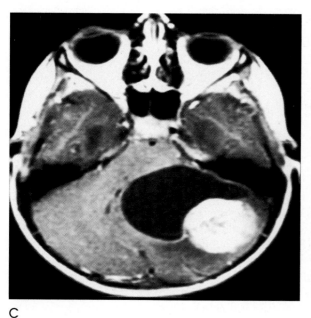

C

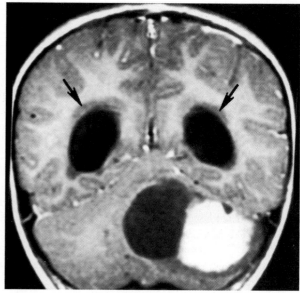

D

Diagnosis Cerebellar Juvenile Pilocytic Astrocytoma

Discussion and Differential Diagnosis

Cerebellar astrocytomas in children are commonly of the pilocytic variety, which have an excellent prognosis following complete surgical resection.[1] These tumors usually originate in the vermis and may extend into the cerebellar hemispheres. Hydrocephalus is present, associated with obstruction of the fourth ventricle and aqueduct of Sylvius. Typically, there is a large cyst that displaces the fourth ventricle associated with a prominent solid mural nodule. The mural nodule usually enhances homogeneously on CT and MRI; there is no enhancement in the cyst wall. The cyst wall is usually composed of compressed brain tissue rather than tumor.[2] Although hemangioblastomas have a similar neuroimaging appearance, they uncommonly occur during the first decade of life, when cerebellar astrocytomas are most common. On CT, the mural nodule of astrocytoma is usually isodense to brain and the cyst appears similar to CSF. On MRI, the mural nodule may be isointense or hyperintense to brain on T2-weighted images and is usually isointense to slightly hypointense on T1-weighted images. The cyst fluid, which is proteinaceous, is usually hyperintense to CSF on proton density or T2-weighted images. The tumor may less commonly consist of a solid mass with central necrosis. Calcification may occur in the solid component. Malignant degeneration is extremely uncommon in these tumors, as is leptomeningeal and systemic metastasis.

Further Reading

1. Hayostek CJ, Shaw EG, Scheithauer B, et al. Astrocytomas of the cerebellum: a comparative clinicopathologic study of pilocytic and diffuse astrocytomas. *Cancer* 72:856–869, 1993.
2. Gusnard DA. Cerebellar neoplasms in children. *Semin Roentgenol* 25(3):263–278, 1990.

Case 46

Clinical Presentation

A 12-year-old girl with bladder dysfunction and progressive spasticity in the left lower extremity associated with a left foot cavus deformity. A focal area of hypertrichosis was present overlying the sacrum.

Radiographic Studies

Sagittal T1-weighted MRI of the spine demonstrates a low-lying cord (white arrows, Fig. 46) passing into the sacral canal, which is filled with fat (black arrow, Fig. 46). At surgery, the filum terminale was thickened and infiltrated with fatty tissue.

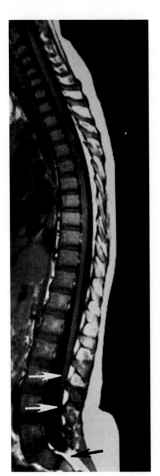

Diagnosis Tethered Spinal Cord

Discussion and Differential Diagnosis

The tethered conus syndrome is a spectrum of clinical abnormalities that may be associated with a number of neuropathological lesions. Patients may present in infancy, childhood, or adulthood with clinical symptoms of bowel and bladder dysfunction and various manifestations of motor abnormalities in the lower extremities.[1] Scoliosis may be an associated finding. Patients with tethered cord syndrome have an intraspinal lesion or lesions that are thought to prevent the normal movement of the spinal cord within the spinal canal as the vertebral column in the growing child elongates. This tethering effect results in traction on the spinal cord and roots, with subsequent neurologic abnormalities. In patients with tethered cord syndrome, the conus medullaris is usually low lying. Normally, the conus should not be present lower than the L2–3 interspace. Lesions associated with tethered cord syndrome include congenital dermal sinus, diastematomyelia, spinal lipoma, thickening of the filum terminale, and—probably most commonly—spinal bifida aperta.[2] Careful clinical examination at birth can detect many infants at risk for tethered conus syndrome. Infants at risk for tethered conus syndrome are those with spina bifida aperta (myelomeningocele, meningocele) and those with findings suggestive of spina bifida occulta (midline masses, dermal sinuses, hemangiomas, and hairy patches over the spinal column). Imaging of the spine at birth consists of screening spinal ultrasound supplemented with MRI when abnormalities are detected with ultrasound. After the neonatal period, imaging of suspected tethered conus syndrome is performed with MRI except in patients for whom MRI is contraindicated, such as those with pacemakers, aneurysm clips, or extensive non-MR compatible fixation devices. In these few patients, CT myelography is still the procedure of choice for evaluation of suspected tethered cord.

Further Reading

1. Reigel DH, McLone DG. Tethered spinal cord. In: *Pediatric Neurosurgery*. Philadelphia: WB Saunders; 1994:77–95.
2. James CA, Glasier CM. Tethered cord syndrome. In: *MRI of the Spine*. New York: Raven Press; 1994:681–686.

Case 47

Clinical Presentation

An 8-year-old boy with back pain.

Radiographic Studies

Lateral coned view from a thoracolumbar radiograph (black arrows, Fig. 47) demonstrates a wafer-thin L2 vertebral body with preservation of the adjacent disc spaces.

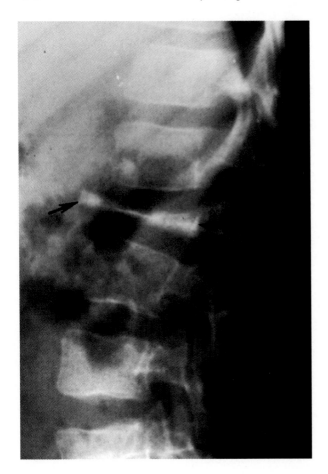

Diagnosis Vertebra Plana (Langerhans' Cell Histiocytosis)

Discussion and Differential Diagnosis

Spinal involvement is found commonly in children with Langerhans' cell histiocytosis.[1] Focal destructive lesions are seen in the vertebral bodies that may result in the characteristic vertebra plana. The posterior elements are less commonly involved than the bodies. MR imaging may show vertebral body involvement in the absence of plain film changes.[2] Typical findings on MRI in histiocytosis include lesions that are hypointense on T1-weighted images and hyperintense on T2-weighted images, with contrast-enhancing soft tissue involvement adjacent to the bony lesion.[2] CT shows focal destructive changes with or without obvious soft tissue involvement. One or multiple vertebral bodies may be involved. There may be dramatic reconstitution of height of the flattened vertebral bodies without specific therapy.

Further Reading

1. Meyer JS, Harty MP, Mahboubi S, et al. Langerhans cell histiocytosis: presentation and evolution of radiologic findings with clinical correlation. *Radiographics* 15:1135–1146, 1995.
2. George JC, Buckwalter KA, Cohen MD, et al. Langerhans histiocytosis of bone: MR imaging. *Pediatr Radiol* 24:29–32, 1994.
3. Ozonoff MB. The spine. In: *Pediatric Orthopedic Radiology.* Philadelphia: WB Saunders; 1992:109.

Case 48

Clinical Presentation

A 14-year-old girl with a long history of seizures developed progressive headaches, nausea, and vomiting over a 2-month period.

Radiographic Studies

Axial contrast-enhanced CT of the head of the patient at age 7 years shows characteristic calcified subependymal nodules at the foramen of Monro bilaterally (black arrows, Fig. 48A). Contrast-enhanced axial CT at time of presentation with headaches reveals a large enhancing mass at the right foramen of Monro with associated obstructive hydrocephalus (Fig. 48B). This mass was surgically resected and found to be a giant cell astrocytoma. Axial proton density–weighted cranial MRI of another patient shows transverse linear streaks extending from the cortex toward the ventricles (black arrows, Fig. 48C), representing the neuronal migration abnormalities seen in some patients with this disease.[1] Axial noncontrast CT scan of a 2-year-old demonstrates calcified subependymal nodules and, in addition, multiple low-attenuation white matter lesions (black arrows, Fig. 48D) with adjacent high-attenuation cortical lesions (white arrows, Fig. 48D). Axial T1-weighted inversion recovery MR image of a 2-month-old infant shows hyperintense subependymal nodules (white arrows, Fig. 48E) as well as multiple hyperintense cortical lesions.

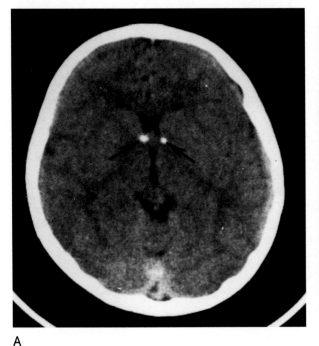

A

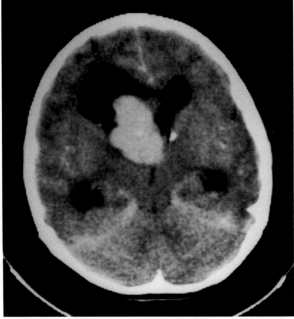

B

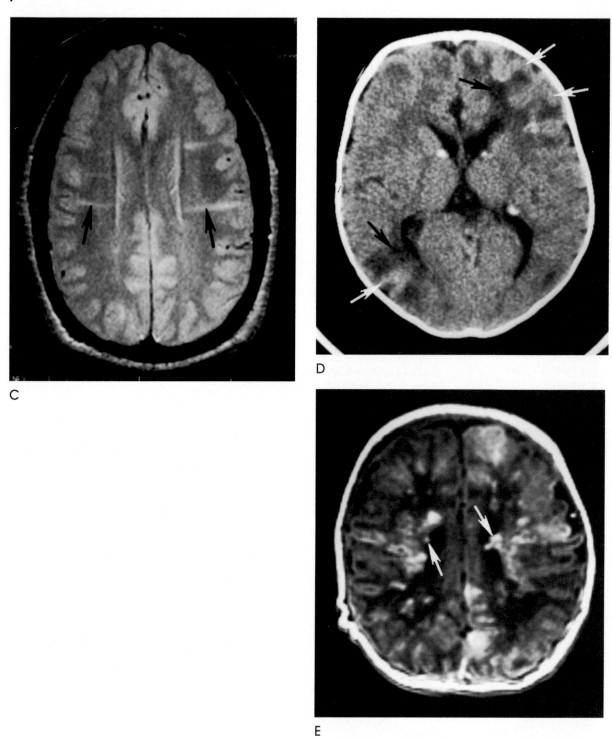

C

D

E

Diagnosis Tuberous Sclerosis

PEARLS

- The classic clinical triad found in patients with tuberous sclerosis includes mental retardation, adenoma sebaceum (cutaneous angiofibromas), and seizure disorder.

PITFALLS

- The periventricular calcifications seen in patients with TORCH infections should not be confused with the subependymal calcified tubers found in tuberous sclerosis.

CONTROVERSY

- Some authors recommend annual cranial MR scans for patients with tuberous sclerosis during the first two decades of life in order to detect subependymal giant cell astrocytomas when the tumors are small and more easily resectable.[2]

Discussion and Differential Diagnosis

Tuberous sclerosis or Bourneville's disease is a condition in which imaging is essential for diagnosis and for determining extent of disease. Infants with tuberous sclerosis may not show skin manifestations of the disease, and there may not be a family history. Three of the pathognomonic diagnostic criteria for diagnosis of tuberous sclerosis are found by imaging and include subependymal nodules, cortical tubers, and multiple unilateral or bilateral renal angiomyolipomas.[2] Other pathognomonic diagnostic criteria include retinal hamartomas, facial angiofibromas, ungual fibromas, and cutaneous fibrous plaques. Infants with tuberous sclerosis frequently have a type of seizure know as infantile spasms. Imaging of children with suspected tuberous sclerosis should include cranial MRI and abdominal ultrasound. On MRI, subependymal nodules in infants are bright on T1-weighted images but later develop low signal intensity due to calcification and changes in brain water content. Subependymal nodules frequently enhance following administration of paramagnetic contrast material. In infants, cortical tubers and white matter lesions are hyperintense to gray matter on T1-weighted images but this high signal intensity diminishes with progressive myelination. Cortical tubers and white matter lesions may enhance following gadolinium administration but enhancement is less common than in the subependymal nodules. On CT, subependymal nodules are difficult to detect in infants until the nodules calcify. White matter lesions on CT tend to be low attenuation. Subependymal nodules typically do not demonstrate contrast enhancement on contrast-enhanced CT unless a giant cell astrocytoma is present. Giant cell astrocytomas may occur in patients with tuberous sclerosis, usually at the end of the first decade or during the second decade of life.[3] These tumors are most commonly located at the foramen of Monro and present as obstructive hydrocephalus. The tumors show intense enhancement after the administration of intravenous contrast.

Further Reading

1. Braffman BH, Bilaniuk LT, Naidich TP, et al. MR imaging of tuberous sclerosis: pathogenesis of this phakomatosis, use of gadopentetate dimeglumine, and literature review. *Radiology* 183:227–238, 1992.
2. Braffman BH, Naidich TP. The phakomatoses: part 1, neurofibromatosis and tuberous sclerosis. *Neuroimaging Clin N Am* 4(2):299–324, 1994.
3. Holanda FJ, Holanda GM. Tuberous sclerosis—neurosurgical indications in intraventricular tumors. *Neurosurg Rev* 3(2):139–150, 1980.

HEAD AND NECK

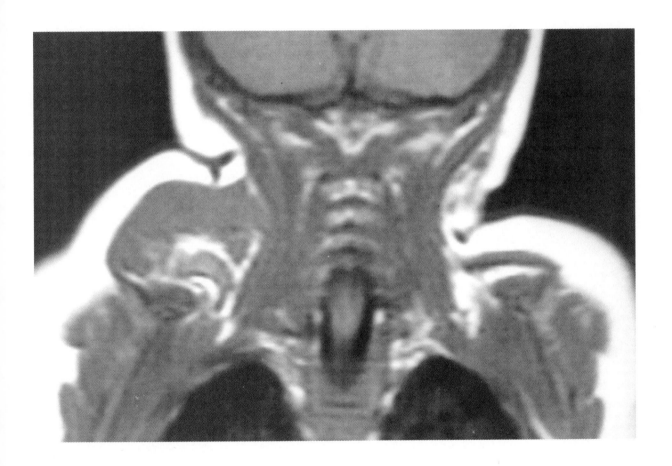

Case 1

Clinical Presentation

Penetrating injury to orbit.

Radiographic Studies

Axial CT images of the orbit with soft tissue (Fig. 1A) and bone (Fig. 1B) windows reveal a density in the right medial orbit and a collapsed globe with hemorrhage in the vitreous. Axial CT image of the orbit (Fig. 1C) from a different patient shows low-attenuation mass (white arrows, Fig. 1C) in the left medial orbit.

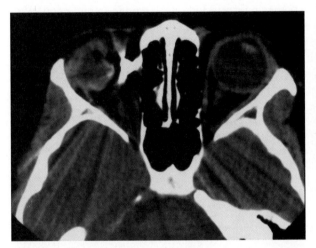

A

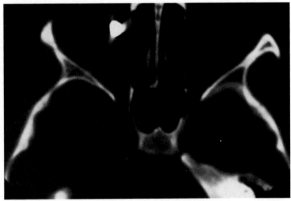

B

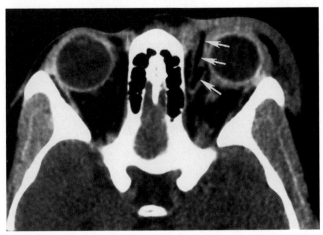

C

Diagnosis Orbital Foreign Body

Discussion and Differential Diagnosis

Penetrating wounds to the orbit account for a significant portion of all traumatic eye injuries. Skull films are relatively insensitive for detecting foreign bodies and give little information about the integrity of the globe. Ultrasound, CT, and MRI have been utilized in the workup of these patients. CT is considered the procedure of choice for the acute evaluation of a penetrating injury.[1] Associated fractures of the orbit are best seen on CT.

Metal is well seen with CT, and fragments as small as $0.06 mm^3$ can be detected.[1] Auto window glass is more difficult to detect. Intraocular wood is a special challenge, as it can be low attenuation and resemble air or fat[2] (Fig. 1C). The low attenuation is most likely the result of trapped air within the porous wood.

Complications of penetrating injuries include globe rupture and infection. With rupture, the globe will decrease in volume and may have a "wrinkled" appearance (Fig. 1A). Hemorrhage within the globe will be high attenuation acutely and may be in the aqueous or vitreous cavities or subretinal (Fig. 1A).

The differential diagnosis is limited if the appropriate history is obtained. If the foreign body is overlooked, an orbital abscess can develop.

Further Reading

1. Tate E, Cupples H. Detection of orbital foreign bodies with computed tomography: current limits. *Am J Neuroradiol* 2:363–365, 1981.
2. Roberts CF, Leehey PJ III. Intraorbital wood foreign body mimicking air at CT. *Radiology* 185:507–508, 1992.
3. Green BF, Kraft SP, Carter KD, Buncic JR, Nerad JA, Armstrong D. Intraorbital wood. Detection by magnetic resonance imaging. *Ophthalmology* 97:608–611, 1990.
4. Specht CS, Varga JH, Jalali MM, Edelstein JP. Orbitocranial wooden foreign body diagnosed by magnetic resonance imaging. Dry wood can be isodense with air and orbital fat by computed tomography. *Surv Ophthalmol* 36:341–344, 1992.

PEARLS

• With penetrating injury to the orbit, a foreign body must be searched for and ruled out.

PITFALLS

• Intraocular wood can be low attenuation and resemble air or fat. Bone window images may help distinguish wood from fat. Linear or irregular shape is key for identifying a foreign body (Fig. 1C).

CONTROVERSY

• MRI can be useful acutely if a foreign body is highly suspected but not seen on CT.[3,4] MRI should never be performed if an intraocular metallic foreign body is suspected because of the risk of further damage to the globe from movement of the foreign body in the magnetic field.

Case 2

Clinical Presentation

A 14-year-old with nasal obstruction.

Radiographic Studies

Water's view (Fig. 2A) of the maxillary sinuses reveals bilateral maxillary sinus opacification, right greater than left. Soft tissue attenuation (white arrows, Fig. 2B) is seen in the right nasopharynx projecting through the sphenoid sinus on the submental vertex view (Fig. 2B). Coronal CT reveals enlargement of the right maxillary sinus ostium (black arrows, Fig. 2C). More posteriorly, the coronal CT reveals a soft tissue density in the nasopharynx (Fig. 2D).

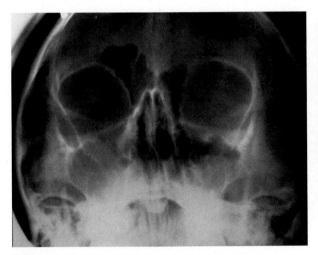

A

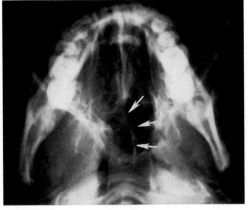

B

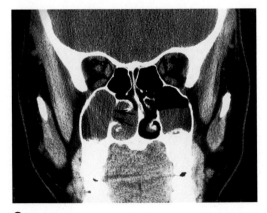

C

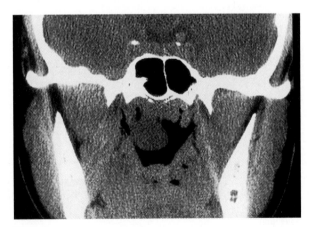

D

Diagnosis Antrochoanal Polyp

Discussion and Differential Diagnosis

The antrochoanal polyp is a benign polyp that arises in the maxillary sinus, exits through and widens the ostium, and extends into the nasal cavity.[1] Teenagers and young adults are most commonly affected.

The "polyp" has a pathologic appearance similar to intramural sinus cysts or mucous retention cysts.[2] Mucous retention cysts are caused by obstruction of mucosal gland ducts and are a fairly common incidental finding seen when imaging the sinuses. They are usually small and multiple but can be solitary and fill a sinus cavity.

This imaging appearance of antrochoanal polyp is pathognomonic and should not be confused with a more aggressive or malignant process. Complete sinus opacification can be seen with a mucocele, but the sinus itself and not the ostium is expanded with this entity. Chronic sinusitis can also cause sinus opacification but not the expansion of the ostium and extension into the nasopharynx. Nasal polyps from chronic infections or allergies are usually multiple and have an inhomogeneous appearance on CT, with high-attenuation secretions trapped between the polyps.

Further Reading

1. Yousem DM. Imaging of sinonasal inflammatory disease. *Radiology* 188:303–314, 1993.
2. Berg O, Carenfelt C, Silfverswärd C, Sobin A. Origin of the choanal polyp. *Arch Otolaryngol Head Neck Surg* 114:1270–1271, 1988.

Case 3

Clinical Presentation

An 11-day-old neonate with a neck mass.

Radiographic Studies

Anteroposterior chest X ray (Fig. 3A) reveals soft tissue asymmetry in the neck. Axial CT images of the neck (Fig. 3B) and upper mediastinum (Fig. 3C) show a well-circumscribed mass of fluid density in the left anterior neck with extension into the mediastinum.

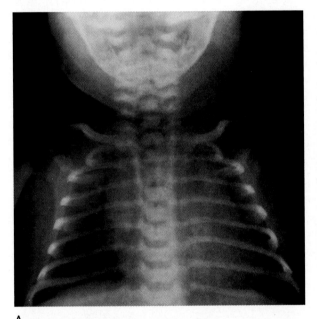

A

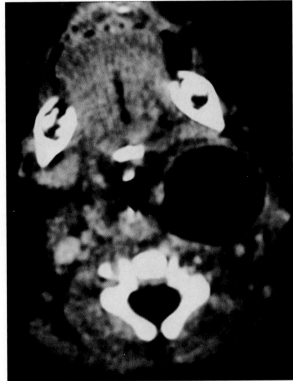

B

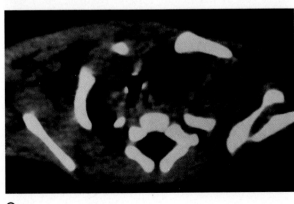

C

Diagnosis Thymic Cyst

Discussion and Differential Diagnosis

Thymic cysts in children are rare, accounting for only 3% of all superior mediastinal masses.[1] They can be unilocular or multilocular. Although the majority are found in the superior mediastinum, some are located in the base of the neck anterior to the lower third of the sternocleidomastoid muscle. Most thymic cysts are asymptomatic and incidentally found on chest X ray. Less commonly associated symptoms of dysphagia, dyspnea, cervical pain, and hoarseness occur.[2] Respiratory compromise may also be present as the result of tracheal compression.

The thymus arises from the third pharyngeal pouch. It elongates and descends to the level of the aortic arch where the two buds fuse, forming the bilobed thymus. Thymic tissue may be present anywhere along the route of descent from the posterior pharynx along the carotid sheath and into the anterior mediastinum.[3] Although the exact cause is unclear, cystic dilatation of this thymic tissue remnant occurs with a noninfective inflammatory reaction in the wall.[4] Recommended treatment is surgical excision as the cysts continue to increase in size. These lesions have no malignant potential.

The differential diagnosis of a cystic neck mass includes branchial cleft cyst, dermoid cyst, cystic hygroma (posterior triangle), and thymic and thyroglossal duct cysts (midline or near midline). Lack of septations is the key to distinguishing thymic cysts from cystic hygromas. Cystic hygromas virtually always have septations and are often hemorrhagic.

Further Reading

1. Davis RD Jr, Oldham HN Jr, Sabiston DC Jr. Primary cysts and neoplasms of the mediastinum: recent changes in clinical presentation, methods of diagnosis, management, and results. *Ann Thorac Surg* 44:229–237, 1987.
2. Wagner CW, Vinocur CD, Weintraub WH, Golladay ES. Respiratory complications in cervical thymic cysts. *J Pediatr Surg* 23(7):657–660, 1988.
3. Reiner M, Beck AR, Rybak B. Cervical thymic cysts in children. *Am J Surg* 139:704–707, 1980.
4. Samuel M, Spitz L, de Leval M, Davenport M. Mediastinal thymic cysts in children. *Pediatr Surg Int* 10:146–147, 1995.

Case 4

Clinical Presentation

A 15-year-old-boy with fever and sore throat.

Radiographic Studies

Soft tissue lateral radiograph of the neck (Fig. 4) reveals massive adenoidal and moderate palatine tonsil hypertrophy. The nasopharyngeal airway is obliterated. No bone destruction is seen.

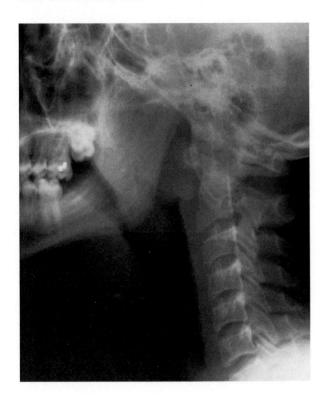

Diagnosis   Infectious Mononucleosis (IM)

Discussion and Differential Diagnosis

Infectious mononucleosis is an acute systemic self-limiting disease of children and young adults (aged 15 to 25 years) caused by the Epstein-Barr virus (EBV). Characteristic findings include fever, pharyngitis, lymphadenopathy, and splenomegaly. Imaging is rarely used in the diagnosis, which is usually made on clinical grounds based on transient serum heterophile titers and a persistent EBV antibody response.[1]

The lymphadenopathy in IM is most common in the posterior cervical chain of lymph nodes in the neck, although the anterior chain can be involved as well as hilar and mediastinal lymph nodes. Splenomegaly is present in greater than 50% of patients and hepatomegaly in 10%.[1] The lungs can be involved with a perihilar interstitial infiltrate. A small pleural effusion may be present rarely.[2]

Treatment is symptomatic and recovery is seen in 3 to 6 weeks. The differential diagnosis includes other viral exanthems and malignant diseases such as lymphoma, rhabdomyosarcoma, and lymphoepithelioma. With rhabdomyosarcoma, bone destruction is usually present.

Further Reading

1. Garten AJ, Mendelson DS, Halton KP. CT manifestations of infectious mononucleosis. *Clin Imaging* 16:114–116, 1992.
2. Silverman FN, Kuhn JP, eds. *Caffey's Pediatric X-ray Diagnosis: An Integrated Imaging Approach.* 9th ed. St. Louis: Mosby; 1985; 1:534.

Case 5

Clinical Presentation

Malformed right external ear and hearing loss.

Radiographic Studies

High-resolution 1.5-mm coronal (Fig. 5A) and axial (Fig. 5B) CT images with bone algorithm reveal bony external canal atresia with fusion of the ossicles to the atresia plate (black arrows, Figs. 5A and 5B). A vestigial cleft (white arrow, Fig. 5A) is noted that is more vertical than the normal external auditory canal.

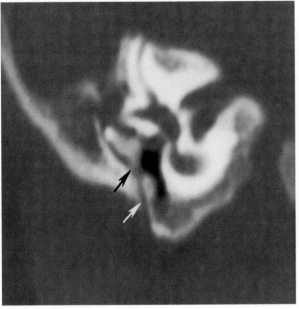

A

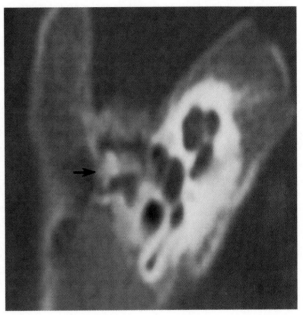

B

Diagnosis External Canal Atresia

Discussion and Differential Diagnosis

The middle and external ears develop together from the first branchial cleft.[1] Therefore, anomalies of the external ear are frequently associated with middle ear abnormalities. Anomalies of the external and middle ear are more common than inner ear anomalies,[2] with external canal atresia a common entity. Major malformations of the external canal are usually accompanied by microtia (developmentally small auricle).

The external canal can be stenotic or atretic, and the atresia may be bony or membranous. The external canal may be only a small channel through the temporal bone, which may curve inferiorly as it courses laterally.[1] With bony external canal atresia, an atresia plate replaces the tympanic membrane and forms the lateral wall of the middle ear. The ossicles are usually deformed and fused to each other and to the atresia plate.[1,2] The inner ear is usually normal but abnormalities of the oval and round windows may occur.[2]

Surgical correction can restore hearing in some cases.[1] Preoperative imaging should assess the thickness of the atresia plate, the presence of ossicular abnormalities, the size of the middle ear, the status of the inner ear, the oval and round windows, the facial nerve canal, the degree of mastoid air cell formation, and the position of the sigmoid sinus.[1,2]

Further Reading

1. Curtin HD. Congenital malformations of the ear. *Otolaryngol Clin North Am* 21(2):317–336, 1988.
2. Eelkema EA, Curtin HD. Congenital anomalies of the temporal bone. *Semin Ultrasound CT MR* 10(3):195–212, 1989.

Case 6

Clinical Presentation

Facial malformation at birth.

Radiographic Studies

Axial CT image (Fig. 6A) through the orbits reveals a small globe on the right. Coronal CT image (Fig. 6B) through the orbits shows a mass inferior to the globe on the right (black arrow, Fig. 6B). Three-dimensional image (Fig. 6C) of the face reveals a hypoplastic right orbit, maxilla, and mandible with fusion of the mandibular condyle to the maxilla (white arrow, Fig. 6C). Anteroposterior chest X ray (Fig. 6D) shows segmentation anomalies (black arrows, Fig. 6D) and rib fusions in the lower thoracic spine.

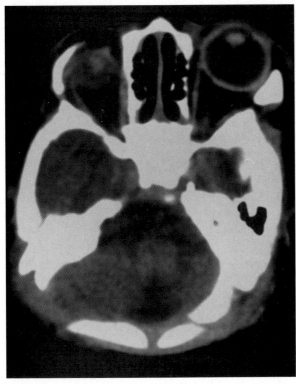

A

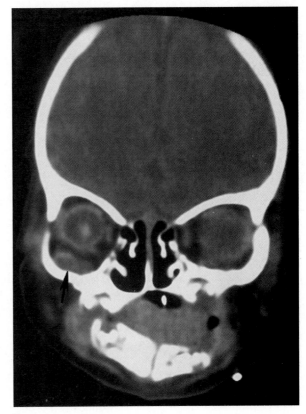

B

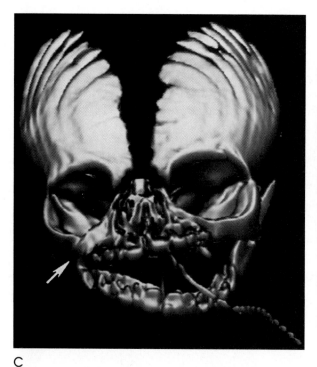

C

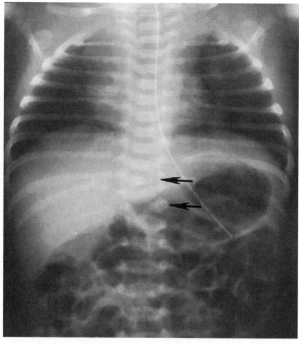

D

Diagnosis Oculoauriculovertebral Dysplasia (OAD)

Discussion and Differential Diagnosis

Hemifacial microsomia was first described in 1860 by Canton with unilateral hypoplasia of the globe, orbit, maxilla, mandibular ramus and condyle, mastoid portion of the temporal bone, and facial soft tissue.[1] Goldenhar's syndrome combines the findings of hemifacial microsomia with an epibulbar dermoid of the cornea and a coloboma of the upper eyelid. In 1963, Gorlin proposed the term oculoauriculovertebral dysplasia to combine numerous similar syndromes described by others including Goldenhar.[2] In OAD, the findings in Goldenhar's syndrome (hemifacial microsomia, epibulbar dermoid, and coloboma) are combined with auricular appendices and vertebral anomalies. The epibulbar dermoid is usually located at the limbus or corneal margin in the lower outer quadrant of the orbit[2] (Fig. 6B). A small percentage of OAD patients are mentally retarded (10%).

With hemifacial microsomia, Goldenhar's syndrome, and OAD, the structures affected are first and second branchial arch derivatives and the primordia of the temporal bone. Middle and external ear malformations are commonly associated. Infrequently, the malformation is bilateral.[1] When bilateral, differentiation from Treacher Collins' syndrome must be made. In Treacher Collins' syndrome or mandibulofacial dysostosis, bilateral hypoplasia of the maxilla and mandible are noted with bilateral malformations of the auricle and middle ear.

Further Reading

1. Aduss H. Form, function, growth, and craniofacial surgery. In: Caldarelli DD, ed. *The Otolaryngologic Clinics of North America, IV.* Philadelphia: WB Saunders; 1981:798–801, 886–887, 902–905.
2. Gorlin RJ, Jue KL, Jacobsen U, Goldschmidt E. Oculoauriculovertebral dysplasia. *J Pediatr* 63(5):991–999, 1963.

Case 7

Clinical Presentation

A 1-month-old baby with torticollis and neck mass.

Radiographic Studies

Longitudinal ultrasound views of the neck reveal fusiform enlargement of the right sternocleidomastoid muscle (black arrows, Fig. 7A) and a normal left sternocleidomastoid muscle (black arrows, Fig. 7B).

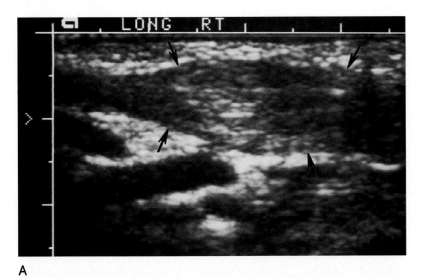

A

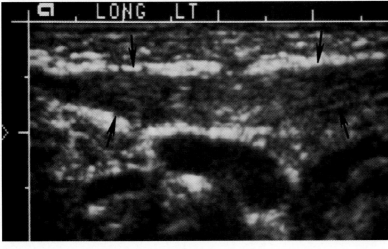

B

Diagnosis Fibromatosis Colli

Discussion and Differential Diagnosis

Fibromatosis colli (congenital muscular torticollis) presents in infants 2 weeks to 2 months of age as torticollis and a discrete mass in the neck. This condition is not present at birth but rapidly develops in the neonatal period and in some cases spontaneously disappears by 4 to 8 months.[1] It represents an injury to the sternocleidomastoid (SCM) muscle in utero or during birth, with the pathology revealing replacement of striated muscle by fibrous tissue.[1] The head is tilted toward the side of the abnormal SCM muscle but turned away from the affected side because of shortening of the muscle. Facial and skull asymmetry may be present, with the unaffected side more prominent and full.[1]

Ultrasound is the procedure of choice for examining these infants. Many clinicians are unaware of this entity and order CT or MRI for evaluation of the neck mass. CT and MRI show nonspecific enlargement of the affected SCM muscle. Ultrasound reveals the classic fusiform enlargement of the muscle on longitudinal imaging (Fig. 7A). The echogenicity of the involved muscle is variable but is usually hyperechoic to normal muscle. The muscle may be heterogeneous or homogeneous in echogenicity. A hypoechoic rim of the muscle has been described on transverse images that represents normal muscle fibers at the periphery.[2] Hyperechoic foci may be present, with distal acoustic shadowing representing focal calcification.[2]

The treatment of choice is conservative management with passive stretching of the affected SCM and strengthening exercises of the contralateral side.[3] Surgery is not indicated in most cases but may be performed if a tumor such as rhabdomyosarcoma is suspected. Surgical lengthening is done in severe cases that fail conservative management.[3]

Other causes of torticollis in the first year of life include Sprengel's deformity and Klippel-Feil syndrome.[4] These can be ruled out by scapula and cervical spine radiographs.

Further Reading

1. Kiesewetter WB, Nelson PK, Palladino VS, Koop CE. Neonatal torticollis. *JAMA* 157(15):1281–1285, 1955.
2. Chan YL, Cheng JCY, Metreweli C. Ultrasonography of congenital muscular torticollis. *Pediatr Radiol* 22:356–360, 1992.
3. Emery C. The determinants of treatment duration for congenital muscular torticollis. *Phys Ther* 74(10):921–929, 1994.
4. Ackerman J, Chau V, Gilbert-Barness E. Pathological case of the month. *Arch Pediatr Adolesc Med* 150:1101–1102, 1996.

Case 8

Clinical Presentation

A 6-month-old infant with soft neck mass.

Radiographic Studies

Coronal T1-weighted MR image of the lower neck (Fig. 8A) reveals a mass (white arrows, Fig. 8A) in the posterior triangle of the right neck with signal intensity similar to muscle. Axial T2-weighted MR image of the lower neck (Fig. 8B) shows a lesion with signal intensity similar to cerebrospinal fluid with large septa coursing through it. Axial T2-weighted MR image of the chest (Fig. 8C) in a different patient reveals a high signal lesion in the mediastinum and left axilla.

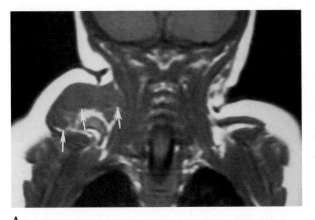

A

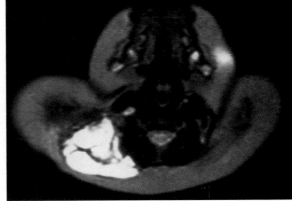

B

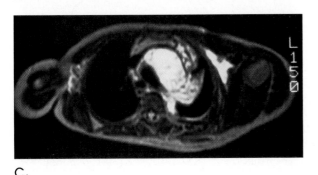

C.

Diagnosis Cystic Hygroma

Discussion and Differential Diagnosis

Cystic hygromas or lymphangiomas are dilated lymph spaces that are formed when primordial lymph sacs fail to reconnect with the central venous system from which they originated.[1] Seventy-five percent are located in the posterior triangle of the neck, with 3 to 10% extending inferiorly into the superior mediastinum.[2] Twenty percent are located in the axilla; less common locations include the retroperitoneum and bones.[2] They are usually asymptomatic except for their visible appearance.[2] Rapid growth may occur following infection or trauma, and airway obstruction may rarely occur. They are benign except for the nuchal ones identified in utero associated with Turner's syndrome and fetal hydrops, which carry a poor prognosis.[1]

Ultrasound is excellent for superficial lesions and should be the initial procedure of choice. The characteristic ultrasound appearance is a multiseptated cystic lesion, often with internal dependent echogenic hemorrhage or inflammatory debris. Doppler can reveal the absence of significant vascularity. CT or MR imaging shows the deep extent of lesions and their relationships to surrounding structures.[2] The lesions do not enhance unless a coexisting hemangioma or vascular malformation is present. MRI is superior to CT for the complete imaging evaluation. On T1-weighted images, the signal intensity varies according to the protein and hemorrhage content of the cysts. Hemorrhage-fluid levels may be present in the cysts. On T2-weighted images, the signal intensity is much greater than that of fat.[2] The cysts are thin-walled. The lesion can surround and invade normal structures.

Treatment involves surgical resection. Prior to surgery, complete delineation of the lesion by imaging should be obtained to reduce the risk of recurrence.[2] The differential diagnosis of a cystic lesion in the neck includes hemangiomas, which should enhance and have feeding arteries or draining veins; branchial cleft cysts and thyroglossal duct cysts, which should not be in the posterior triangle and are unilocular; and an abscess or necrotic lymph nodes, which should have a thick wall.[2]

Further Reading

1. Zadvinskis DP, Benson MT, Kerr HH, et al. Congenital malformations of the cervicothoracic lymphatic system: embryology and pathogenesis. *Radiographics* 12:1175–1189, 1992.
2. Siegel MJ, Glazer HS, St. Amour TE, Rosenthal DD. Lymphangiomas in children: MR imaging. *Radiology* 170:467–470, 1989.
3. Okada A, Kubota A, Fukuzawa M, Imura K, Kamata S. Injection of bleomycin as a primary therapy for cystic lymphangioma. *J Pediatr Surg* 27(4):440–443, 1992.

Case 9

Clinical Presentation

A 2-year-old child with fever, neck pain, a muffled voice, and drooling.

Radiographic Studies

Soft tissue lateral radiograph (Fig. 9A) reveals marked thickening of the retropharyngeal soft tissue. Axial CT (Fig. 9B) without contrast shows a large low-attenuation lesion (black arrows, Fig. 9B) in the retropharyngeal space. IV contrast was not given, because of a rising creatinine. Ultrasound in the axial plane (Fig. 9C) reveals a thick fluid collection with posterior acoustic enhancement (black arrows, Fig. 9C) deep to the carotid sheath. Axial contrast-enhanced CT (Fig. 9D) from a different patient shows rim-enhancing mediastinal fluid collections (black arrows, Fig. 9D) consistent with mediastinal extension.

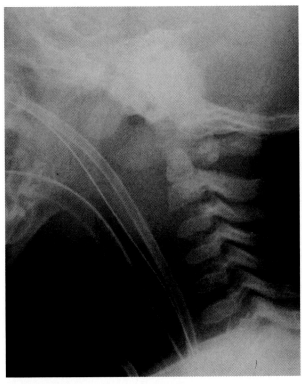

A

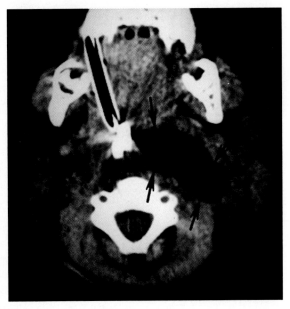

B

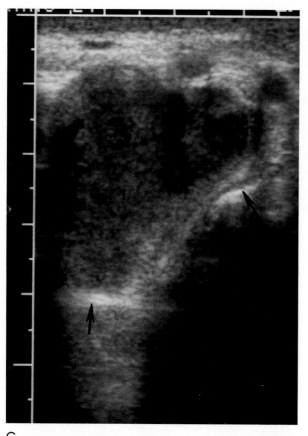

C

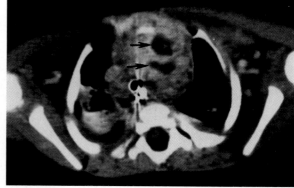

D

Diagnosis Retropharyngeal Abscess

Discussion and Differential Diagnosis

The retropharyngeal and parapharyngeal spaces are potential spaces bounded by layers of deep cervical fasciae. Acute infections of the ear, nose, and throat in children spread to lymph nodes in the retropharyngeal space with resultant lymphadenitis, suppuration, and abscess formation.[1] The inflammation and abscess can spread inferiorly into the mediastinum because of a direct continuity of the retropharyngeal space with the posterior mediastinum. Children younger than 3 or 4 years of age have a greater number of retropharyngeal lymph nodes and a greater incidence of retropharyngeal abscess: 96% occur in children under age 6 years.[1]

The lateral soft tissue neck radiograph is obtained first in the radiographic evaluation of a child with a possible retropharyngeal abscess. In children the width of the retropharyngeal space varies widely with neck position and phase of respiration. On an inspiratory film obtained in neutral or with mild neck extension, the average thickness of the normal retropharyngeal soft tissue is 3.5 mm.[1] With retropharyngeal inflammation or abscess, the retropharyngeal soft tissue will be thicker. Fluoroscopy may be helpful in better visualizing the retropharyngeal soft tissue during different

PEARLS

- Proper technique (inspiratory film with neck extension) is essential when evaluating soft tissue lateral neck radiographs for possible retropharyngeal abscess.

- Air in the retropharyngeal enlargement implies rupture of the abscess anteriorly into the esophagus. The usual organisms causing this inflammation are not gas forming.

PITFALLS

● Do not forget to look for
mediastinal extension of the
abscess.

CONTROVERSY

● The value of ultrasound in
diagnosing a drainable
(liquefied) retropharyngeal
abscess in addition to CT is not
widely known.

phases of respiration and neck position. Contrast-enhanced CT is invaluable for a comprehensive look at neck adenopathy, retropharyngeal edema or abscess, and mediastinal extension. Differentiating a phlegmon from a drainable abscess is sometimes difficult with CT as both can be low attenuation with an enhancing rim. Ultrasound is used at some institutions (Fig. 9C) after the CT to distinguish these two so appropriate medical or surgical treatment can be initiated.[2] Ultrasound is also useful in intraoperative localization of the abscess.[3]

The differential diagnosis of retropharyngeal widening in children, in addition to infection, ranges from benign tumors (cystic hygroma, hemangioma) to malignant tumors (rhabdomyosarcoma, neuroblastoma) to cervical spine trauma or osteomyelitis with adjacent hemorrhage or edema.[1]

Further Reading

1. Barratt GE, Koopmann CF Jr, Coulthard SW. Retropharyngeal abscess—a ten-year experience. *Laryngoscope* 94(4):455–463, 1984.
2. Glasier CM, Stark JE, Jacobs RF, et al. CT and ultrasound imaging of retropharyngeal abscesses in children. *Am J Neuroradiol* 13:1191–1195, 1992.
3. Seibert JJ, Lewis GJS, Seibert RW. Pediatric head and neck masses. In: Rumack CM, Wilson SR, Charboneau JW, eds. *Diagnostic Ultrasound.* St. Louis: Mosby; 1991:1086–1087.

Case 10

Clinical Presentation

Marked facial deformity at birth.

Radiographic Studies

Axial T2-weighted MR image of the brain and orbit (Fig. 10A) reveals left sphenoid dysplasia, proptosis, and diffuse infiltration of the orbital soft tissues with a high-signal soft tissue mass. Axial T2-weighted MR image of the face and posterior fossa (Fig. 10B) shows diffuse infiltration of the left face and infratemporal fossa with the characteristic "target" appearance of individual units (black arrows, Fig. 10B). Coronal T1-weighted MR image of the orbit (Fig. 10C) reveals enlargement of the orbit, which is filled with enhancing tissue. Diffuse infiltration of the left face is also seen.

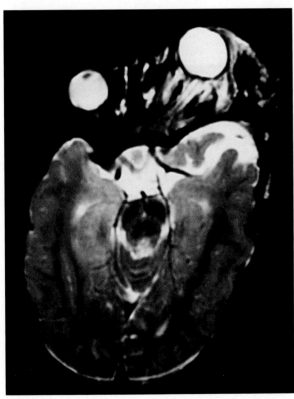

A

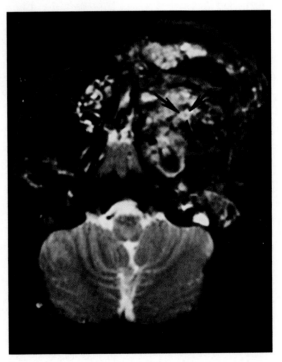

B

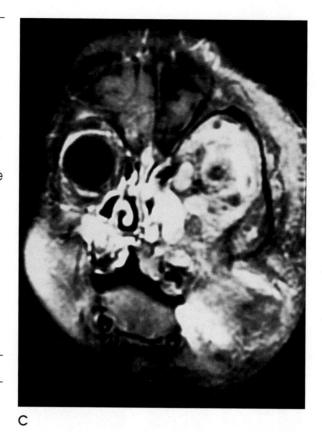

C

Diagnosis Plexiform Neurofibroma (PNF)

Discussion and Differential Diagnosis

Plexiform neurofibromas are seen exclusively in neurofibromatosis (NF) type 1 or von Recklinghausen disease. The head and neck region is the most common site of involvement, although PNF can occur in any of the spinal, cranial, or autonomic nerves.[1] Pathological examination reveals bundles of Schwann cells, axons, and endoneural fibroblasts with a cellular perineural sheath around each unit. Plexiform neurofibromas with associated thickening of the subcutaneous tissue and skin and increased deposition of fat form a bulky soft tissue mass resembling a "bag of worms."[1]

In the head and neck, the orbit is frequently involved. Bone findings in addition to sphenoid dysplasia, which is part of the spectrum of mesodermal developmental abnormalities seen with NF, include enlargement of the orbit, superior and inferior orbital fissures, and pterygopalatine fossa. A decrease in size of the ipsilateral ethmoid and maxillary sinuses is usually noted. Soft tissue findings include thickening and loss of fascial planes, enlargement of the extraocular muscles, enlargement of the ipsilateral cavernous sinus, and proptosis.[1]

CT and MRI are helpful in revealing the full extent of a PNF for possible surgical resection. Diffuse infiltration of tissues is the rule, making resection difficult to impossible in most cases. Contrast material should be administered because these lesions are vascular and enhance brightly. T1-weighted MRI with gadolinium and fat saturation in multiple imaging planes shows the lesions optimally. A characteristic target appearance has been described in benign PNF on T2-weighted MR images, with increased peripheral signal and decreased central signal intensity that corresponds with histologic findings (Fig. 10B).[2] The central portion contains fibrous and collagenous components and Schwann cells. The peripheral portion contains endoneural myxoid material with a high fluid content. Malignant degeneration can occur.

The differential diagnosis of orbital lesions in NF type 1 patients includes optic nerve gliomas, perioptic meningiomas, solitary neurofibromas, and schwannomas, which have a distinctly different appearance.[2] Optic gliomas and perioptic meningiomas enlarge the optic nerve sheath as they grow along the nerve. Solitary neurofibromas and schwannomas are typically well-defined enhancing masses that may erode bone.

Further Reading

1. Reed D, Robertson WD, Rootman J, Douglas G. Plexiform neurofibromatosis of the orbit: CT evaluation. *Am J Neuroradiol* 7:259–263, 1986.
2. Suh J-S, Abenoza P, Galloway HR, Everson LI, Griffiths HJ. Peripheral nerve tumors: correlation of MR imaging and histologic findings. *Radiology* 183:341–346, 1992.

Case 11

Clinical Presentation

A newborn with respiratory distress relieved by crying.

Radiographic Studies

Axial CT image (Fig. 11A) shows bilateral bony narrowing of the posterior choanae (black arrows, Fig. 11A) with a thickened vomer (white arrow, Fig. 11A). Right anterior bony canal stenosis is also present. Axial CT image (Fig. 11B) inferior to (A) reveals bilateral membranes occluding the posterior choanae (white arrows, Fig. 11B). Axial CT image in another patient (Fig. 11C) shows unilateral posterior choanal narrowing. Sagittal reformation (Fig. 11D) also shows the choanal narrowing.

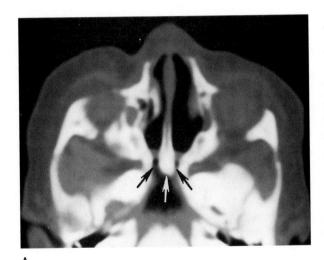

A

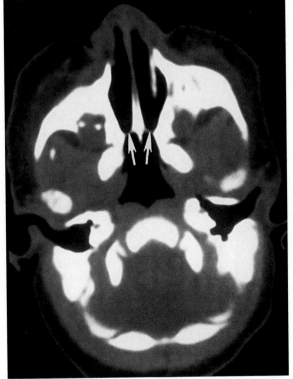

B

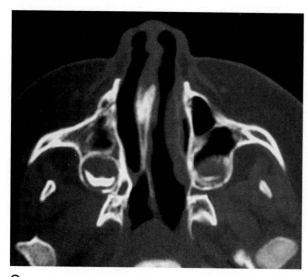

C

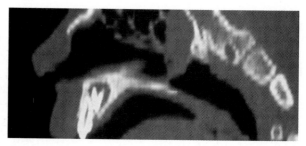

D

Diagnosis Choanal Atresia

Discussion and Differential Diagnosis

Choanal atresia occurs in 1 in 5000 births and is commonly associated with other congenital anomalies.[1,2] It can be bony (90%) or membranous (10%) and unilateral or bilateral.[1] With bilateral atresia, the infant has respiratory distress at birth, as infants are obligate nose breathers. The distress worsens with attempted feeding and is relieved by crying. With unilateral disease, the diagnosis is made much later; symptoms of chronic rhinitis and respiratory distress with rhinitis are present. The clinical diagnosis can be made by unsuccessful attempts to pass a catheter through the nasal cavity. In the past, contrast choanography was performed with lateral radiographs obtained following instillation of an oily contrast material into the nostrils.[3]

Today, CT is the procedure of choice for radiographic confirmation. Following nasal suctioning and decongestant spray, 1.5-mm axial sections are obtained with bone algorithm and cephalic angulation of the gantry 5° cephalad to a line perpendicular to the hard palate.[2] Oblique sagittal reconstructions are helpful. On axial images, the vomer is noted to be broad (Fig. 11A).[1] An atretic plate is attached to the vomer medially and the perpendicular plate of the palatine bone laterally. The lateral wall of the posterior choanae is always thickened and deviated medially.[1] Treatment is endoscopic for membranous atresia and surgical in bony atresia, with transpalatine resection of the vomer.[2]

Respiratory distress in a newborn with a normal tracheobronchial airway and lungs should suggest the diagnosis of choanal atresia. Other causes of nasal obstruction in the newborn are nasopharyngeal dermoid cysts or teratomas, nasal cephaloceles, and complex craniofacial malformations.[1]

PEARLS

- Neonates are obligate nose breathers and have respiratory distress with nasal obstruction.

- Bony inlet stenosis can also cause symptoms of nasal obstruction.[4]

PITFALLS

- Mucus in the posterior nasal cavity can simulate a membrane. Nasal suctioning and decongestant spray can help avoid this problem.

Further Reading

1. Chinwuba C, Wallman J, Strand R. Nasal airway obstruction: CT assessment. *Radiology* 159:503–506, 1986.
2. Castillo M. Congenital abnormalities of the nose: CT and MR findings. *AJR Am J Roentgenol* 162:1211–1217, 1994.
3. Capitanio MA, Kirkpatrick JA Jr. Upper respiratory tract obstruction in infants and children. *Radiol Clin North Am* 6(2):265–277, 1968.
4. Ey EH, Han BK, Towbin RB, Jaun W-K. Bony inlet stenosis as a cause of nasal airway obstruction. *Radiology* 168:477–479, 1988.

Case 12

Clinical Presentation

A 15-year-old boy with recurrent epistaxis.

Radiographic Studies

Coronal CT image of the nasopharynx (Fig. 12A) reveals an enhancing mass (white arrows, Fig. 12A) in the right nasopharynx. Axial CT image with bone windows (Fig. 12B) shows widening of the pterygopalatine fossa (black arrows, Fig. 12B) and sphenoid bone destruction. Anteroposterior digital subtraction angiogram of the external carotid artery (Fig. 12C) reveals a hypervascular mass being fed by the internal maxillary artery.

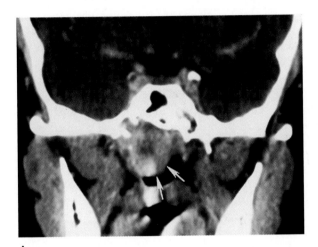

A

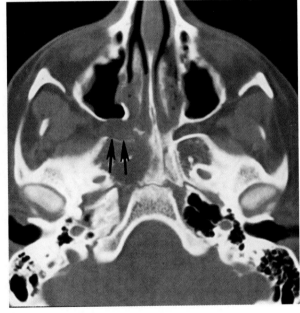

B

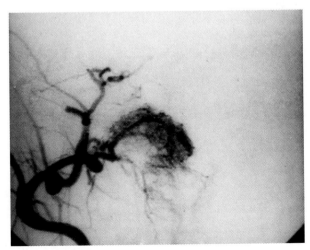

C

Diagnosis Juvenile Nasopharyngeal Angiofibroma (JNA)

Discussion and Differential Diagnosis

Juvenile nasopharyngeal angiofibromas are rare benign tumors presenting in male adolescents as nasal obstruction and epistaxis. Although these tumors are benign, they are locally aggressive and highly vascular.[1] The increased vascularity makes biopsy hazardous, and therefore it is useful to suggest the diagnosis with imaging.[2,3]

Juvenile nasopharyngeal angiofibromas usually arise in the posterior nasal cavity or nasopharynx and extend laterally through the sphenopalatine foramen into the pterygopalatine fossa. The pterygopalatine fossa is widened (Fig. 12B) with anterior bowing of the posterior wall of the maxillary sinus. This widening is highly suggestive of JNA.[3] From the pterygopalatine fossa, they can extend into the orbit through the fissures, into the sphenoid sinus, infratemporal fossa, and intracranially. They erode and/or destroy bone.

Treatment is surgical resection with preoperative embolization (usually with polyvinyl alcohol) performed to decrease operative blood loss.[2] Numerous other treatments have been employed in the past, including radiotherapy. Recurrence is common. The goal of treatment should be to control symptoms and not to make the patient tumor-free at any cost. Most deaths are treatment related.[4]

The diagnosis of JNA is highly suggested by the above CT findings and the appropriate clinical history. In a female patient the diagnosis should be in question and a chromosomal analysis may be helpful.[1] Other tumors that may mimic JNA with an enhancing soft tissue mass in the nasal cavity with bone destruction are rhabdomyosarcoma and esthesioneuroblastoma.

Further Reading

1. Sinha PP, Aziz HI. Juvenile nasopharyngeal angiofibroma: a report of seven cases. *Radiology* 127:501–505, 1978.
2. Davis KR. Embolization of epistaxis and juvenile nasopharyngeal angiofibromas. *Am J Neuroradiol* 7:953–962, 1986.
3. Weinstein MA, Levine H, Duchesneau PM, Tucker HM. Diagnosis of juvenile angiofibroma by computed tomography. *Radiology* 126:703–705, 1978.
4. Jones GC, DeSanto LW, Bremer JW, Neel HB III. Juvenile angiofibromas: behavior and treatment of extensive and residual tumors. *Arch Otolaryngol Head Neck Surg* 112:1191–1193, 1986.

- A vascular mass in the nasopharynx or nasal cavity of a male teenager with widening of the pterygopalatine fossa suggests JNA.

PITFALLS

- Biopsy or surgical resection prior to angiography and embolization may be hazardous.

Case 13

Clinical Presentation

A 15-year-old boy with acute loss of vision in the left eye.

Radiographic Studies

Axial CT of the orbits (Fig. 13A) reveals a soft tissue mass filling the sphenoid and left posterior ethmoid sinuses with extension into the left orbit (black arrows, Fig. 13A). Coronal CT with bone algorithm (Fig. 13B) shows the ethmoid and sphenoid bone destruction. Coronal T1-weighted MR image with fat saturation after gadolinium administration (Fig. 13C) reveals dural enhancement (black arrows, Fig. 13C) consistent with intracranial spread of mass.

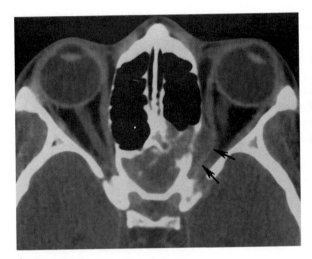

A

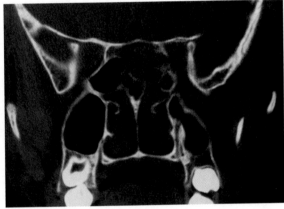

B

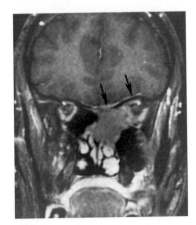

C

Diagnosis Rhabdomysarcoma

Discussion and Differential Diagnosis

Rhabdomyosarcoma is the most common soft tissue sarcoma in children. It ranks seventh in order of frequency of malignant neoplastic disease in children.[1] Two peak age ranges have been described, between 2 and 5 and 15 and 19 years, with most cases occurring in children younger than 10 years of age.[1] The most common area of origin is the head and neck region, accounting for approximately 40% of cases.[1] The next two most common areas are the genitourinary region and the extremities.

Within the head and neck region, the tumor may originate in the orbits, nasopharynx or oropharynx, nasal or oral cavity, paranasal sinuses, pterygopalatine and infratemporal fossae, middle ear, mastoid, scalp, parotid, cheek, and larynx. Lesions that originate in the head and neck have a significant propensity for intracranial extension (35%).[1] Rhabdomyosarcomas extend locally and infiltrate along fascial planes into surrounding tissues. Metastases can be spread via the lymphatic system or hematogenously, with lung and bone metastases common. CT and MRI are both useful in the imaging evaluation of head and neck tumors. CT reveals bone destruction that accompanies these tumors (Fig. 13B). MRI is particularly helpful for assessing intracranial extent (Fig. 13C) with multiple imaging planes.

The differential diagnosis of a destructive tumor in the paranasal sinuses and/or orbit includes esthesioneuroblastoma. Treatment of rhabdomyosarcoma is primarily with chemotherapy and radiation.[2] Surgery is performed only if it does not sacrifice vital structures or function.[2]

Further Reading

1. Malogolowkin MH, Ortega JA. Rhabdomyosarcoma of childhood. *Pediatr Ann* 17(4):251, 254–268, 1988.
2. Anderson GJ, Tom LWC, Womer RB, Handler SD, Wetmore RF, Potsic WP. Rhabdomyosarcoma of the head and neck in children. *Arch Otolaryngol Head Neck Surg* 116:428–431, 1990.

Case 14

Clinical Presentation

A 1-month-old boy with rapidly enlarging facial mass with overlying skin discoloration.

Radiographic Studies

Coronal T1-weighted MR image (Fig. 14A) reveals a large soft tissue mass in the right face with punctate areas of increased signal consistent with hemorrhage or calcium. Axial T2-weighted MR image (Fig. 14B) shows inhomogeneous increased signal in the mass, which diffusely infiltrates fascial planes of the face, engulfs the parotid gland, and surrounds the external ear canal. Large external carotid branches are seen with flow voids (black arrows, Fig. 14B). Axial T1-weighted image with gadolinium and fat saturation (Fig. 14C) reveals intense enhancement of the mass.

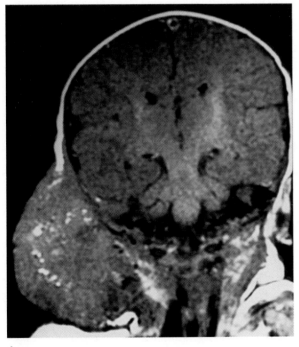

A

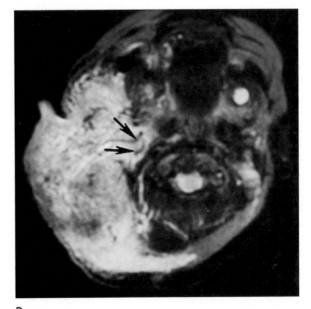

B

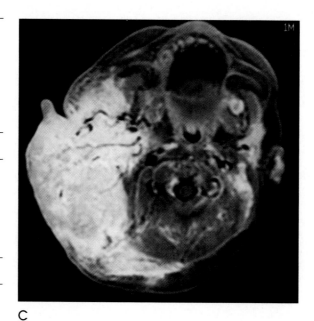

C

Diagnosis Hemangioma

Discussion and Differential Diagnosis

Vascular anomalies can be divided into hemangiomas and vascular malformations.[1–3] Hemangiomas are endothelial cell neoplasms that appear in infancy and show rapid growth throughout the first year with subsequent regression in 90% without treatment. Vascular malformations are errors of vascular morphogenesis and are present at birth and grow with the child without involution. Malformations are classified by the type of vessels present, such as arteries and veins (arteriovenous malformation), veins (venous malformation), lymphatic vessels (lymphatic malformation), and combined lymphaticovenous malformations.[1–3]

On CT, hemangiomas are usually diffusely infiltrating and have attenuation similar to muscle. Intense enhancement is noted with contrast. Detection and full extent of hemangiomas are better depicted on MRI given the high signal intensity of hemangiomas relative to muscle on T2-weighted sequences. Signs of high flow on MRI include flow voids visible in the lesion and prominent flow-related enhancement on gradient echo or time-of-flight images.[2] Post-gadolinium T1-weighted imaging with fat suppression shows the parenchymal enhancement of the lesion. On angiography, abnormal vessels and a parenchymal stain are seen.[3] Arteriovenous malformations also have flow voids on MRI and abnormal vessels/arteriovenous shunting at angiography but have no intervening enhancing soft tissue.[2] Venous malformations are slow-flow lesions with no flow voids and less intense signal in adjacent vessels on gradient echo and time-of-flight images.[2] Associated phleboliths will be obviously calcified on CT, with low signal intensity on MR imaging sequences. Lymphatic malformations are usually multiseptated, may have intrinsic hemorrhage-fluid levels, and lack imaging findings of high flow.

It is important to distinguish which vascular anomaly is present, as the treatment is different with each type. Hemangiomas are treated with watchful waiting; spontaneous regression occurs in most cases. Corticosteriods have been used with some success in symptomatic lesions.[3] More invasive treatment, such as laser therapy, is required in selected patients. Arteriovenous malformations are treated with a combination of embolization therapy and surgical resection. Percutaneous sclerotherapy has been successful in treating venous malformations. Lymphatic malformations are surgically resected if possible.

Further Reading

1. Mulliken JB, Glowacki J. Hemangiomas and vascular malformations in infants and children: a classification based on endothelial characteristics. *Plastic Reconstruct Surg* 69(3):412–420, 1982.
2. Meyer JS, Hoffer FA, Barnes PD, Mulliken JB. Biological classification of soft-tissue vascular anomalies: MR correlation. *Am J Roentgenol* 157:559–564, 1991.
3. Burrows PE, Mulliken JB, Fellows KE, Strand RD. Childhood hemangiomas and vascular malformations: angiographic differentiation. *Am J Roentgenol* 141:483–488, 1983.

Case 15

Clinical Presentation

A 2-year-old girl with left lateral orbital painless mass.

Radiographic Studies

Axial high-resolution contrast-enhanced CT shows a low-attenuation, nonenhancing mass at the left lateral canthus (white arrows, Fig. 15A). Bony notching or erosion is noted on a CT image processed using bone algorithm (black arrow, Fig. 15B).

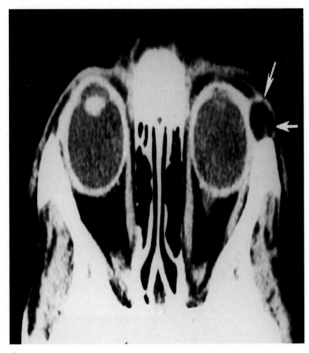

A

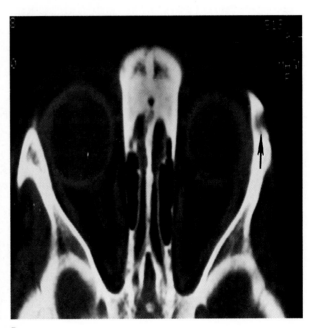

B

Diagnosis Periorbital Dermoid Cyst

Discussion and Differential Diagnosis

Orbital dermoids are congenital rests of ectodermal tissue within the periorbital bony sutures. They are painless lesions and most commonly located at the lateral margin of the orbit. When dermoids enlarge, they are often associated with scalloping or erosion of the underlying bone. These lesions are almost always extraconal but may occur both superficially or deep within the orbit. Deep lesions may occur more often in adults than in children. Dermoids are almost always low attenuation although not necessarily as low as fat on CT and do not enhance after contrast administration. A calcified wall or fat fluid levels may be present.[1] Lesions that may simulate dermoids include capillary hemangioma of infancy, cephalocele, mucocele of the nasolacrimal duct, or ectopic lacrimal gland tissue.[2] Cephaloceles typically present medially and are associated with characteristic bony defects. Lacrimal gland mucoceles are seen in conjunction with dilatation of the nasolacrimal duct. Capillary hemangiomas are soft tissue attenuation on CT and show marked contrast enhancement.

Further Reading

1. Nugent RA, LaPointe JS, Rootman J, et al. Orbital dermoids: features on CT. *Radiology* 165:475–478, 1987.
2. Barnes PD, Robson CD, Robertson RL, et al. Pediatric orbital and visual pathway lesions. *Neuroimaging Clin N Am* 6(1):179–198, 1996.

Case 16

Clinical Presentation

A 5-month-old infant with leukokoria of the right eye.

Radiographic Studies

Axial CT through the orbits without contrast (Fig. 16A) reveals a densely calcified mass filling the posterior chamber of the right globe and a small calcification (white arrow, Fig. 16A) in the region of the optic disc in the left globe. Bone windows (Fig. 16B) confirm calcification bilaterally.

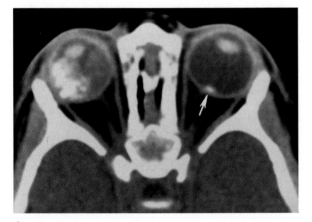

A

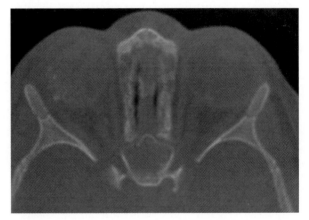

B

Diagnosis Retinoblastoma

Discussion and Differential Diagnosis

Retinoblastoma is the most common intraocular neoplasm of childhood and accounts for 1% of all pediatric malignant tumors.[1] The patient's mean age at presentation is 18 months, with 90% of these tumors occurring in children younger than 5 years.[1] Most patients are asymptomatic and present with leukokoria, which is an abnormal pupillary reflection (white light reflex). The majority of cases are sporadic; however, an inherited form accounts for one third of all cases as the result of a deletion or translocation of the long arm of chromosome 13 (13q-).[2] The inherited form tends to be bilateral, and the patients are prone to develop extraocular malignancies such as osteogenic sarcoma.[1]

CT is the procedure of choice for the initial evaluation of retinoblastoma. Images reveal an enhancing calcified mass in a normal-sized globe. Greater than 90% of all retinoblastomas are calcified. Factors that affect prognosis include choroidal invasion, optic nerve involvement, and cerebrospinal fluid (CSF) dissemination.[1] Follow-up imaging with MR may be useful, especially if CSF spread of tumor or intracranial lesions are noted.

The CT appearance of retinoblastoma is characteristic in an appropriately aged child. The differential diagnosis of leukokoria is extensive, including retinoblastoma, persistent hyperplastic primary vitreous (PHPV), Coats' disease, *Toxocara* endophthalmitis, retinopathy of prematurity (ROP), and retinal astrocytoma.[1] PHPV and ROP are associated with microphthalmos, whereas retinoblastoma occurs in a normal-sized globe. Coats' disease and toxocara endophthalmitis are not calcified. Retinal astrocytomas are associated with phakomatoses, usually tuberous sclerosis.[1]

Some patients with bilateral retinoblastoma develop a pinealoblastoma about 3 years after the ocular lesions are diagnosed. This entity is coined trilateral retinoblastoma.[3] A similar lesion can also develop in the suprasellar cistern, which some speculate is secondary to CSF spread of tumor. When all four lesions are present, the term quadrilateral retinoblastoma is used.

Further Reading

1. Smirniotopoulos JG, Bargallo N, Mafee MF. Differential diagnosis of leukokoria: radiologic-pathologic correlation. *Radiographics* 14:1059–1079, 1994.
2. Kaste SC, Pratt CB. Radiographic findings in 13q-syndrome. *Pediatr Radiol* 23:545–548, 1993.
3. Bader JL, Miller RW, Meadows AT, Zimmerman LE, Champion LAA, Voûte PA. Trilateral retinoblastoma. *Lancet* 2(8194):582–583, 1980.

Case 17

Clinical Presentation

A 10-year-old with chronic otitis media.

Radiographic Studies

Coronal high-resolution CT image of the temporal bones (Fig. 17A) with bone algorithm reveals a soft tissue mass filling the epitympanum with erosion of the scutum (black arrowhead, Fig. 17A). The soft tissue mass bulges into the external auditory canal (white arrowheads, Fig. 17A). The ossicles are surrounded by the mass and are eroded. The tegmen tympani appears intact (white arrow, Fig. 17A). Axial CT image (Fig. 17B) shows the middle ear disease and complete opacification of the mastoid air cells with erosion of the trabeculae.

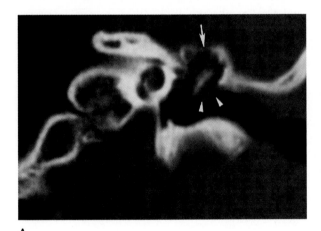

A

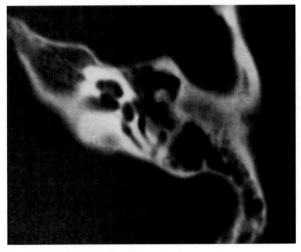

B

Diagnosis Middle Ear Cholesteatoma

Discussion and Differential Diagnosis

Cholesteatomas may be congenital or acquired. Congenital cholesteatomas are epithelial rests that can occur anywhere in or adjacent to the temporal bone.[1] Acquired cholesteatomas are more common and usually follow middle ear inflammatory disease.[1] Bone erosion occurs as these lesions grow and is the hallmark of this disease. High-resolution CT with bone algorithm is the procedure of choice in evaluating middle ear disease. Axial and direct coronal images are necessary.

With CT, cholesteatomas appear as a soft tissue mass in the epitympanic recess (Fig. 17A) with extension into the mastoid antrum. Because most cholesteatomas arise lateral to the ossicles, the lateral wall of the epitympanum and scutum are frequently eroded along with the ossicles. Bony erosion of the tegmen tympani or roof of the middle ear may occur with the risk of intracranial spread of inflammation and epidural abscess formation. Other possible areas of bone erosion include the sigmoid sinus plate, the posterior superior external auditory canal, the lateral semicircular canal, the labyrinth, and facial nerve canal.[1]

CT cannot distinguish a cholesteatoma from granulation tissue or other pathologic tissue. The CT diagnosis of a cholesteatoma is made by the characteristic bone erosion.[1] With mastoid involvement, a smooth cavity is noted with loss of the normal trabecular pattern. If the mastoids are opacified but the trabeculae are maintained or reactive bone formation is present, chronic mastoiditis is more likely than cholesteatoma.[1] MRI may be able to distinguish cholesteatoma from granulation tissue because granulation tissue enhances.

Further Reading

1. Mafee MF, Levin BC, Applebaum EL, Campos M, James CF. Cholesteatoma of the middle ear and mastoid. *Otolaryngol Clin North Am* 21(2):265–293, 1988.

Case 18

Clinical Presentation

Trauma to face with limitation of eye movement.

Radiographic Studies

Coronal CT of the orbit (Fig. 18A) reveals a disruption of the floor of the left orbit with a "hinged door" (white arrows, Fig. 18A) appearance. Coronal CT through the orbit in a different patient (Fig. 18B) shows orbital fat (white arrows, Fig. 18B) herniated through a right orbital floor disruption.

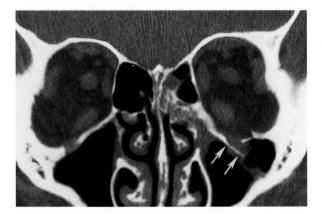

A

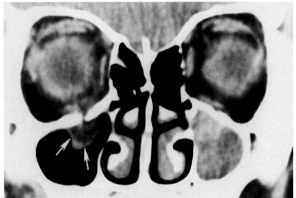

B

Diagnosis Orbital Floor Fracture

Discussion and Differential Diagnosis

Orbital blow-out fractures are the third most common fracture of the midface. Clinical findings include enophthalmos, bruising around the eye, vertical diplopia, limited upward gaze, and epistaxis.[1] The mechanism is an acute increase in intraorbital pressure from a blow to the orbit by an object slightly larger than the orbit (fist, baseball, etc.).[1] Classically, the floor of the orbit or maxillary surface is fractured as it is the weakest boundary of the orbit. The fracture usually extends through the groove of the infraorbital nerve. The orbital rim must remain intact for a pure blow-out fracture. In up to 50%, medial fractures through the lamina papyracea are present as well.[1]

Plain radiographs can suggest the diagnosis. A Caldwell projection can reveal the actual floor defect while the Waters view shows the integrity of the orbital rim.[2] CT is definitive with direct coronal imaging or coronal reconstructions. Axial CT images are not sufficient for the diagnosis. Any facial trauma CT with an air-fluid level in the maxillary sinus should prompt direct coronal imaging, if possible, or coronal reconstructions. Coronal CT findings include a discontinuous orbital floor, herniation of orbital fat (Fig. 18B) or muscle, maxillary sinus opacification or fluid, and orbital emphysema if a medial fracture is present.[1] True muscle entrapment is rare; most limitation of mobility is the result of muscle kinking associated with orbital fat herniation.[3]

The differential diagnosis is extremely limited with a history of trauma and the above CT findings. Treatment is usually conservative unless significant enophthalmos or muscle restriction is present.

Further Reading

1. Asbury CC, Castillo M, Mukherji SK. Review of computed tomographic imaging in acute orbital trauma. *Emerg Radiol* 2(6):367–375, 1995.
2. Dolan KD, Jacoby CG. Facial fractures. *Semin Roentgenol* 13(1):37–51, 1978.
3. Hammerschlag SB, Hughes S, O'Reilly GV, Naheedy MH, Rumbaugh CL. Blow-out fractures of the orbit: a comparison of computed tomography and conventional radiography with anatomical correlation. *Radiology* 143:487–492, 1982.

Case 19

Clinical Presentation

A 15-year-old with sinusitis and proptosis.

Radiographic Studies

Axial (Fig. 19A) and coronal (Fig. 19B) contrast-enhanced CT images of the orbits reveal a rim-enhancing fluid collection (white arrows, Figs. 19A and 19B) in the left medial orbit with air within it and left ethmoid and sphenoid sinusitis. Axial images with bone algorithm (Fig. 19C) show destruction of the lamina papyracea (white arrow, Fig. 19C).

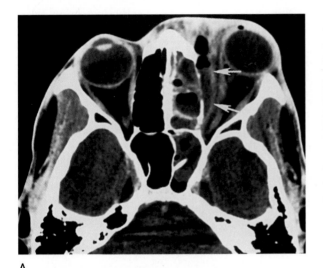

A

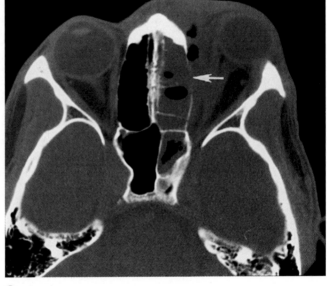

C

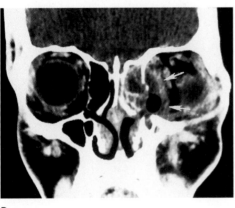

B

Diagnosis Orbital Abscess

Discussion and Differential Diagnosis

An orbital abscess is most commonly caused by adjacent sinus infection with spread through the lamina papyracea.[1] The abscess is usually located in the subperiosteal space in the postseptal portion of the medial orbit with bone destruction of the lamina papyracea. Small congenital openings in the lamina papyracea and valveless venous anastomoses between the sinus and orbit are predisposing factors.[2] Other causes of an orbital abscess include foreign body, trauma, skin infection, and bacteremia. Antibiotics have significantly lowered the mortality and morbidity of orbital abscesses.[2]

CT is the procedure of choice for evaluating the orbit for abscess. After IV contrast administration, thin sections are obtained in the axial and coronal planes. Reconstructing the images with bone algorithm is also necessary. Of prime importance is distinguishing edema or phlegmon from a rim-enhancing abscess (Figs. 19A, 19B). Abscesses are surgically drained in addition to giving patients antibiotics.[1]

A rim-enhancing fluid collection in the medial orbit with bone destruction and adjacent ethmoid sinus disease is pathognomonic for an orbital abscess. Prompt treatment is necessary to preserve vision.[1]

Further Reading

1. Krohel GB, Krauss HR, Winnick J. Orbital abscess: presentation, diagnosis, therapy, and sequelae. *Ophthalmology* 89:492–498, 1982.
2. Carter BL, Bankoff MS, Fisk JD. Computed tomographic detection of sinusitis responsible for intracranial and extracranial infections. *Radiology* 147:739–742, 1983.

PEARLS

• Most orbital abscesses are caused by adjacent ethmoid sinusitis. If sinus disease is not present, look closely for a foreign body and ask about a history of trauma.

PITFALLS

• Imaging in one plane can be misleading. In some cases, both axial and coronal images are needed. If the patient cannot tolerate direct coronal images, reformations can be obtained.

Case 20

Clinical Presentation

A 1-year-old child with cough and inspiratory stridor.

Radiographic Studies

An anteroposterior (AP) soft tissue neck radiograph (Fig. 20A) reveals the characteristic "steepling" (black arrows, Fig. 20A) of the subglottic trachea. The lateral soft tissue neck radiograph (Fig. 20B) shows indistinctness of the subglottic airway (black arrow, Fig. 20B). Marked hypopharyngeal distention is noted on the lateral view in another patient (Fig. 20C).

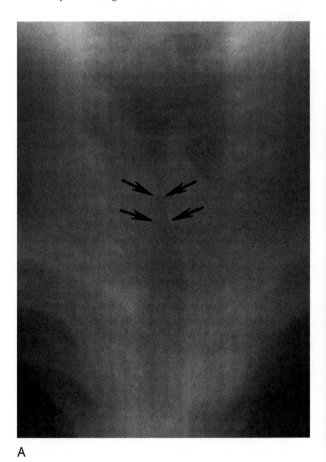

A

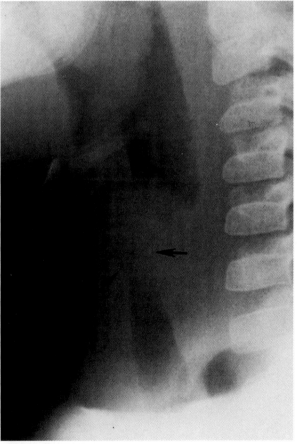

B

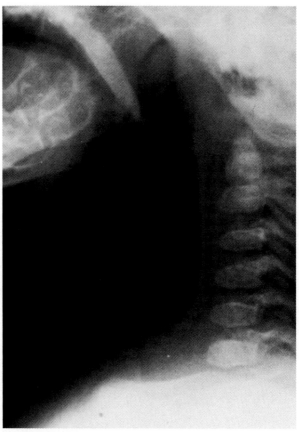

C

Diagnosis Croup

Discussion and Differential Diagnosis

Croup or laryngotracheobronchitis is an inflammation of the upper respiratory tract caused by a virus (usually parainfluenza virus). Although all of the respiratory mucosa is involved, the critical area is the subglottic region where the mucosa is loosely attached and easily elevated by edema.[1] Croup is the most common cause of acute stridor in children. The classic presentation is fever, a "brassy" cough, and acute inspiratory stridor in a child 6 months to 3 years of age.[2] It can occur in older children or adults.

The AP soft tissue radiograph reveals the classic "steepling" of the subglottic trachea (Fig. 20A) with loss of the normal shoulders. The subglottic narrowing should be symmetric. This narrowing can be seen on the lateral radiograph with indistinctness of the airway (Fig. 20B). The lateral radiograph also shows hypopharyngeal distention (Fig. 20C) and a normal epiglottis and aryepiglottic folds. Radiographs also help exclude foreign bodies in the trachea or esophagus as a cause of stridor.

The course is usually self-limited, although subglottic obstruction can occur. Cool mist is useful as a home treatment. In more severe cases with stridor at rest, aerosolized racemic epinephrine and IV or IM steroids are utilized in the emergency department.

Further Reading

1. Dunbar JS. Upper respiratory tract obstruction in infants and children. *Am J Roentgenol* 109(2):227–246, 1970.
2. Macpherson RI, Leithiser RE. Upper airway obstruction in children: an update. *Radiographics* 5(3):339–375, 1985.
3. Han BK, Dunbar JS, Striker TW. Membranous laryngotracheobronchitis (membranous croup). *Am J Roentgenol* 133:53–58, 1979.

Case 21

Clinical Presentation

A 4-year-old with abrupt onset of inspiratory stridor and fever.

Radiographic Studies

Soft tissue lateral neck radiograph (Fig. 21) reveals an enlarged epiglottis (white arrows, Fig. 21) and indistinct aryepiglottic folds (white arrowheads, Fig. 21). The hypopharynx is distended.

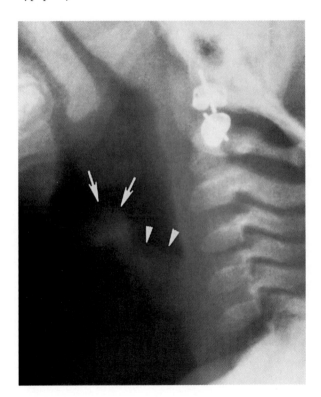

Diagnosis Epiglottitis

Discussion and Differential Diagnosis

Acute bacterial epiglottitis is a life-threatening condition, with infection and edema of the epiglottic and aryepiglottic folds. The onset of fever, dysphagia, and respiratory distress is abrupt. The age of incidence is between 18 months and 6 years of age. *Haemophilus influenzae* type B (Hib) is the etiologic agent in most cases.[1,2] With the recent introduction of the Hib vaccine in 1990, a marked decrease in incidence of epiglottitis has been noted.[1,2]

A portable lateral erect soft tissue radiograph of the neck should be obtained in the ER or OR for diagnosis. A physician skilled in endotracheal intubation or emergency tracheostomy should be present, as these patients can experience a totally obstructed airway at any time. An erect film is obtained because of the increased incidence of obstruction while the patient is lying down. The radiographs reveal an enlarged epiglottis about the size of the tip of the thumb (Fig. 21A) and indistinct aryepiglottic folds with inflammation throughout the supraglottic region. Subglottic edema can be present as well in 25% of cases.[3] The hypopharynx is distended in inspiration because of supraglottic obstruction.

The findings in epiglottitis are pathognomonic with the appropriate history. If only an enlarged epiglottis is noted, other things to consider are an omega-shaped epiglottis, a normal prominent epiglottis, hemophilia, angioneurotic edema, chronic epiglottis, Stevens-Johnson syndrome, aryepiglottic or epiglottic cyst, foreign body, trauma, caustic or chemical ingestion, thermal injury, and irradiation.[3]

Further Reading

1. Gorelick MH, Baker MD. Epiglottitis in children, 1979 through 1992. *Arch Pediatr Adolesc Med* 148:47–50, 1994.
2. Hickerson SL, Kirby RS, Wheeler JG, Schutze GE. Epiglottitis: a 9-year case review. *South Med J* 89(5):487–490, 1996.
3. McCook TA, Kirks DR. Epiglottic enlargement in infants and children: another radiologic look. *Pediatr Radiol* 12:227–234, 1982.

Case 22

Clinical Presentation

Enlarging neck mass.

Radiographic Studies

Axial post-contrast CT image (Fig. 22A) shows an oval, well-defined, near water attenuation lesion (arrowheads, Fig. 22A) in the right anterior triangle. Figure 22B is a longitudinal ultrasound scan of another patient with a clinically firm mass along the anterior margin of the sternocleidomastoid muscle. Note increased through-transmission (white arrowheads, Fig. 22B) in this echogenic lesion, which had complicated fluid at percutaneous needle aspiration (note echogenic needle tip, white arrow, Fig. 22B). Microscopic analysis revealed benign squamous epithelial cells.

Axial T1-weighted MR scan in another patient (Fig. 22C) shows a well-defined oval lesion in the right parotid gland (arrowhead, Fig. 22C). A coronal gradient echo image in this patient shows an associated sinus tract (arrows, Fig. 22D). This case is courtesy of Dr. Charles M. Bower, Little Rock, AR.

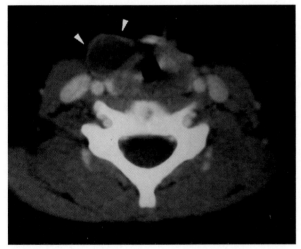

A

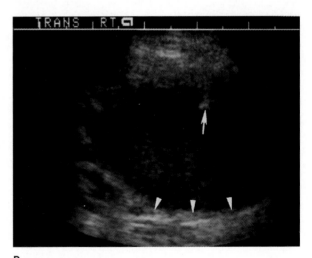

B

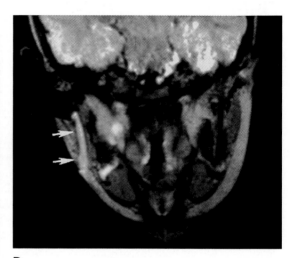

D

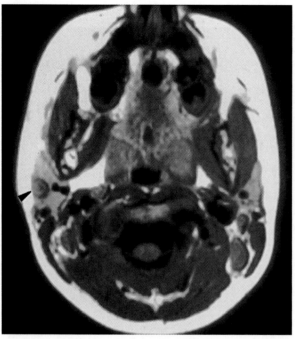

C

Diagnosis Branchial Cleft Cyst (BCC)

Discussion and Differential Diagnosis

Branchial cleft cysts are by far the most common of the anomalies of branchial cleft origin, compared with sinuses and fistulas. Ninety-five percent of all branchial cleft anomalies arise from the second branchial arch apparatus.[1] Although BCCs are of congenital origin, many do not present until young adulthood as a slowly enlarging mass at the mandibular angle. Growth of the mass is sometimes precipitated by an upper respiratory infection. The mandibular angle is a classic location, but the cysts can arise anywhere along the sinus that forms from the second branchial apparatus, which extends from the tonsillar fossa to the supraclavicular region of the neck.[1] A less common location for second branchial cleft cysts is the parapharyngeal space.[1] First branchial cleft cysts are much less common and are usually located in or around the parotid gland (Fig. 22C, 22D).

CT is the single best imaging modality for evaluation of the complex relationships these cysts have with their surrounding structures. The cysts that arise at the mandibular angle have a characteristic CT appearance. The cysts are thin-walled and fluid-filled in the absence of inflammation. Classically, the sternocleidomastoid muscle is displaced posterolateral or posterior; the carotid sheath is displaced posteromedial or medial; and the submandibular gland is displaced anteromedial or medial.[1]

The characteristic displacement of surrounding structures by CT is diagnostic. However, if the location is atypical, other cystic lesions in the neck have to be considered, such as a cystic hygroma (posterior triangle), paramedian thyroglossal duct cyst, and dermoid and epidermoid tumors.

Further Reading

1. Harnsberger HR, Mancuso AA, Muraki AS, et al. Branchial cleft anomalies and their mimics: computed tomographic evalution. *Radiology* 152:739–748, 1984.

Case 23

Clinical Presentation

A 2-year-old girl with inflamed mass in anterior neck.

Radiographic Studies

Axial ultrasound image (Fig. 23A) of the neck imaged anteriorly over the trachea (black arrowheads, Fig. 23A) reveals a mass (black arrows, Fig. 23A) in the midline with increased through-transmission but internal echoes. Axial CT (Fig. 23B) with contrast in another patient reveals a cystic mass slightly off midline with rim enhancement. Axial T1-weighted MR image (Fig. 23C) of the neck in another patient with gadolinium and fat suppression shows a fluid collection in the anterior neck in the midline with an enhancing rim and surrounding inflammatory tissue.

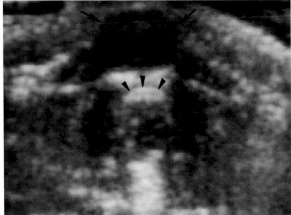

A

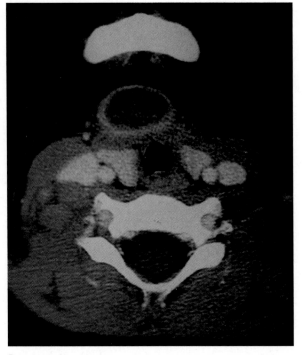

B

PEARLS

● Most thyroglossal duct cysts are cystic lesions in the midline of the anterior neck near the hyoid bone.

PITFALLS

● Do not mistake internal echoes in the cyst for a solid mass with ultrasound. Look for posterior acoustic enhancement and increased through-transmission (Fig. 23A). Be suspicious of a thyroglossal duct cyst with any midline neck mass in a child.

● Presence of thick walls and internal echoes does not always imply infection.[3]

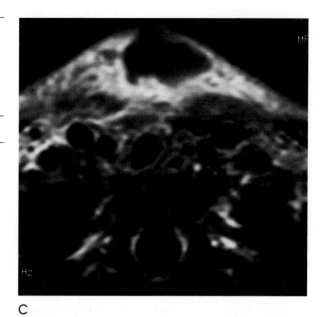

C

Diagnosis   Thyroglossal Duct Cyst

Discussion and Differential Diagnosis

Thyroglossal duct cysts are common and account for 70% of all congenital neck abnormalities.[1] The usual presentation is a mobile mass in the anterior neck in the midline or slightly off midline. The cysts commonly become symptomatic, with inflammation and infection during childhood.

During development, the thyroid primordium forms an epithelial-lined duct in the midline from the foramen cecum to the lower neck through which the thyroid gland descends to reach its final destination anterior to the trachea. The migration can be arrested anywhere along the duct, resulting in ectopic thyroid tissue. If the duct fails to involute, a cyst forms lined by secretory epithelium.[1] Sixty-five percent of all thyroglossal duct cysts are below the level of the hyoid bone in the region of the thyrohyoid membrane. Fifteen percent are at the level of the hyoid and 20% are above it.[1]

Ultrasound is frequently performed first in the evaluation of neck masses in children. If a cystic mass is seen in the midline below the level of the hyoid bone, the diagnosis of a thyroglossal duct cyst is fairly certain. These cysts have been mistaken for solid masses with ultrasound because of associated inflammation and/or infection with internal echoes (Fig. 23A).[2] The location of the thyroid gland should also be assessed when evaluating a patient with a possible thyroglossal duct cyst. Thyroid tissue can be present along the duct rather than in the normal position and can be inadvertently removed at surgery. If the thyroid gland cannot be found with ultrasound, a nuclear medicine thyroid scan is indicated.[2] CT and MRI also visualize these cysts and their relationships with surrounding structures.

The differential diagnosis of a midline cystic neck mass in a child in addition to thyroglossal duct cyst includes dermoid cyst and a liquefied submental or anterior cervical lymph node.[1] Treatment involves "radical surgery" with removal of the entire duct, midsection of the hyoid bone, and an ellipse of tissue at the base of the tongue.[1,2] This surgery—compared with simple removal of the cyst—reduces the recurrence rate from 50% to less than 20%.[2]

Further Reading

1. Reede DL, Bergeron RT, Som PM. CT of thyroglossal duct cysts. *Radiology* 157:121–125, 1985.
2. Cunningham MJ. The management of congenital neck masses. *Am J Otolaryngol* 13(2):78–92, 1992.
3. Wadsworth DT, Siegel MJ. Thyroglossal duct cysts: variability of sonographic findings. *Am J Roentgenol* 163:1475–1477, 1994.

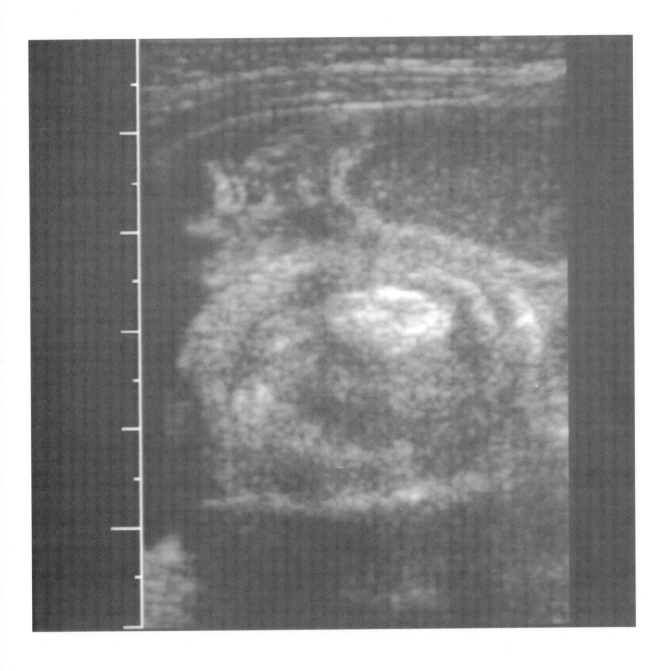

Case 1

Clinical Presentation

An asymptomatic 4-year-old boy who told his mother he swallowed a "silver thing" he found at his grandmother's house.

Radiographic Studies

Figure 1 shows a metallic density foreign body projecting over the left upper quadrant of the abdomen. It could lie in the stomach or bowel. Personal inspection of the patient ruled out artifact from clothing, monitors, and so forth.

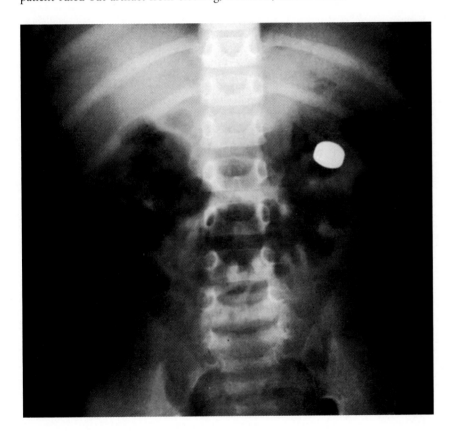

Diagnosis Button Battery Ingestion

Discussion and Differential Diagnosis

Ingestion of button batteries is a special case of foreign body ingestion that should be considered differently from ingestion of other blunt objects such as coins. Over 2000 cases occur in the United States per year. Most involve children younger than 5 years old.[1]

Button batteries are found in hearing aids, cameras, watches, hand-held games, and other devices.[1] Ingested batteries can cause damage to the GI tract by two mechanisms: (1) ulceration caused by leakage of alkali material from within the casing and (2) ulceration caused by electrolysis occurring when the battery contacts liquid, producing accumulation of extrinsic NaOH at the anode.[1]

Most battery ingestions are asymptomatic. The size of the battery and the child are important factors in determining whether the battery will impact in the esophagus. Ulceration of esophageal mucosa can occur in as little as 4 hours[2] and cause perforation leading to mediastinitis and tracheoesophageal fistula, pneumomediastinum, and pneumothorax.

Batteries larger than 15 mm in diameter may persist in the stomach. If they remain beyond 48 hours, they are unlikely to pass and should be removed. Once batteries pass the pylorus, 90% pass through the GI tract within a week. Only patients who develop perforation or obstruction require surgery.[1]

Toxic levels of mercury have been absorbed from a disintegrated mercuric oxide battery although there are no reports of development of mercury poisoning.[3] Button batteries range from 6 to 23 mm in diameter and are thicker than coins. Characteristic appearance of batteries should be familiar to radiologists.

Further Reading

1. Sheikh A. Button battery ingestions in children. *Pediatr Emerg Care* 9(4):224–229, 1993.
2. Sigalet D, Lees G. Tracheoesophageal injury secondary to disc battery ingestion. *J Pediatr Surg* 23(11):996–998, 1988.
3. Bass DH, Millar AJ. Mercury absorption following button battery ingestion. *J Pediatr Surg* 27(12):1541–1542, 1992.

Case 2

Clinical Presentation

A newborn with abdominal distention.

Radiographic Studies

Abdominal radiograph (Fig. 2A) shows dilated loops of bowel with absence of air fluid levels and a "frothy" appearance in the right lower quadrant. Contrast enema (Fig. 2B) shows a microcolon. Contrast outlines inspissated meconium in the terminal ileum.

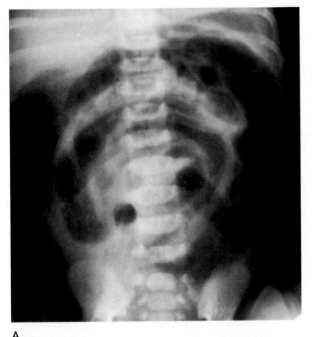

A

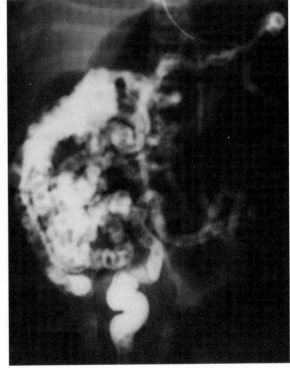

B

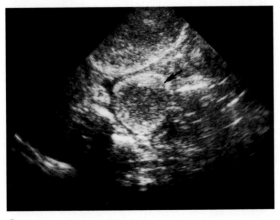

C

Diagnosis Meconium Ileus

PEARLS

- Family history of CF may be present.

- Findings of (1) few or no air-fluid levels in dilated bowel, (2) soap-bubble appearance in right lower quadrant (Neuhauser's sign), and (3) disparity in diameter of obstructed loops are helpful in diagnosing meconium ileus.

- Multiple enemas over several days may be required for complete treatment.

PITFALLS

- Use diluted water-soluble contrast to avoid hypertonic dehydration, and be sure that patient is kept well hydrated after the enema.

- In older children, strictures from oral pancreatic enzyme therapy can cause distal small bowel obstruction that appears similar to meconium ileus equivalent.

Discussion and Differential Diagnosis

Meconium ileus is the cause of 10 to 25% of cases of bowel obstruction in newborns. It occurs in 6 to 20%[2] of children with cystic fibrosis (CF). Bowel obstruction results from intraluminal obstruction by abnormally viscous meconium in the distal ileum. About half of cases are uncomplicated obstruction. The remainder have complications such as meconium peritonitis with or without cyst formation, volvulus, atresia, and intestinal gangrene.[1]

Meconium ileus is the most common cause of neonatal bowel obstruction that presents at birth as abdominal distention.[3] Abdominal radiographs may show a pattern of bowel obstruction with absence of air fluid levels and "frothy" appearance to bowel (Neuhauser's sign). The differential diagnosis includes Hirschsprung's disease, ileal atresia and stenosis, meconium plug syndrome, and small left colon syndrome. The most common major differential is between meconium ileus and ileal atresia. Both conditions present as bowel obstruction and reveal a microcolon on contrast enema. Ileal atresia is associated with air-fluid levels. Ultrasound may be helpful in differentiating the two. In meconium ileus, abdominal ultrasound shows dilated loops of bowel filled with very thick echogenic material (arrow, Fig. 2C). In ileal atresia, the dilated loops are filled with air and fluid.[4]

Contrast enema shows an unused or microcolon. Contrast refluxed into the distal ileum outlines inspissated meconium, sometimes with a "rabbit pellet" appearance. A therapeutic enema may be performed in uncomplicated cases. Gastrografin diluted to 20 to 25% solution[2] or 40% Hypaque[5] is used to outline the meconium obstruction and fill distal dilated loops. Hypertonic contrast loosens the obstruction, and causes passage of the meconium and relief of obstruction in 24 to 48 hours in 55% of cases.[2] Serial radiographs and repeat enemas may be necessary.[6] Perforation rate from enemas is reported to be in the range of from 5%[6] to 11%.[2]

Meconium ileus equivalent or distal intestinal obstruction syndrome occurs in older children with CF who develop intestinal obstruction secondary to inspissation of bowel contents in the distal ileum.[3]

Further Reading

1. Ziegler MM. Meconium ileus. *Curr Probl Surg* 31(9):736–777, 1994.
2. Rescorla FJ, Grosfeld JL. Contemporary management of meconium ileus. *World J Surg* 17(3):318–325, 1993.
3. Khoshoo V, Udall JN. Meconium ileus equivalent in children and adults. *Am J Gastroenterol* 89(2):153–157, 1994.
4. Neal MR, Seibert JJ, Wagner CW, Vanderzalm T. Use of neonatal US to distinguish between meconium ileus and ileal atresia. *J Ultrasound Med* 16:263–266, 1997.
5. Rescorla FJ, Grosfeld JL, West KJ, Vand DW. Changing patterns of treatment and survival in neonates with meconium ileus. *Arch Surg* 124(7):837–840, 1989.
6. Docherty JG, Zaki A, Coutts JA, Evans TJ, Carachi R. Meconium ileus: a review 1972–1990. *Br J Surg* 79(6):571–573, 1992.

Case 3

Clinical Presentation

A febrile 1-year-old boy with a kitten at home.

Radiographic Studies

Ultrasound (Fig. 3A) shows multiple round 1 to 3 cm hypoechoic lesions in the liver. Similar lesions were also seen in the spleen. Contrast-enhanced CT (Fig. 3B) confirms lesions in the liver and spleen but shows no adenopathy.

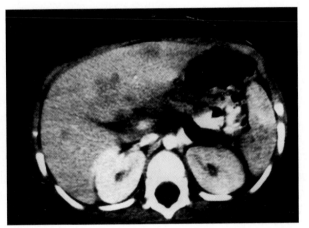

B

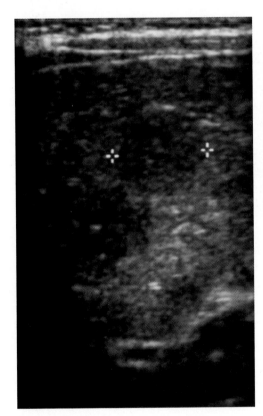

A

Diagnosis Cat-Scratch Disease (CSD)

Discussion and Differential Diagnosis

Cat-scratch disease is usually a mild self-limited disease characterized by regional lymphadenopathy following a cat scratch or inoculation of the responsible organisms into a preexisting wound.

Occasionally, CSD may involve the liver and/or spleen, with or without regional lymphadenitis. In the absence of involved peripheral nodes, the appearance of the liver and/or spleen can suggest malignant disease. In the clinical setting of a febrile child with a subacute illness and exposure to cats, CSD should be mentioned as a possible cause.

Further Reading

1. Rappaport DC, Cumming WA, Ros PR. Disseminated hepatic and splenic lesions in cat-scratch disease: imaging features. *AJR Am J Roentgenol* 156:1227–1228, 1991.
2. Dong PR, Seeger LL, Yao L, Panosian CB, Johnson BL Jr, Eckardt JJ. Uncomplicated cat-scratch disease: findings at CT, MR imaging, and radiography. *Radiology* 195:837–839, 1995.
3. Hopkins KL, Simoneaux SF, Patrick LE, Wyly JB, Dalton MJ, Snitzer JA. Imaging manifestations of cat-scratch disease. *AJR Am J Roentgenol* 166:435–438, 1996.
4. Larsen CE, Patrick LE. Abdominal (liver, spleen) and bone manifestations of cat-scratch disease. *Pediatr Radiol* 22:353–355, 1992.

PEARLS

- Appropriate clinical history may prevent expensive workup for malignancy.

- The causative agent is *Bartonella henselae*, a gram-negative bacillus usually introduced by the scratch of a cat.[3]

- Diagnosis can be made with a serum assay for *B. henselae* antibodies.[3]

PITFALLS

- May look like malignant disease.

- Rarer manifestations include lytic bone lesions, mesenteric adenitis, peritonitis, and CNS and skin lesions.[4]

Case 4

Clinical Presentation

A term newborn with a distended abdomen, vomiting, and delayed passage of meconium.

Radiographic Studies

Supine abdominal film shows dilated loops of bowel and no gas in the rectosigmoid (Fig. 4A). Contrast enema (Fig. 4B) demonstrates a small-caliber (<1 cm) left colon with a rapid transition from dilated transverse colon at the splenic flexure. Caliber of the rectum is normal. Repeat enema at age 6 months shows a normal-caliber left colon (Fig. 4C).

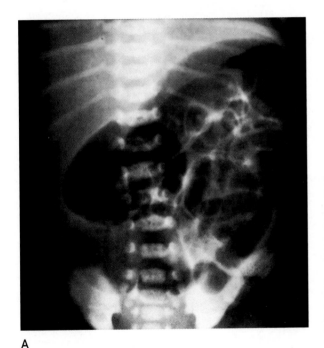

A

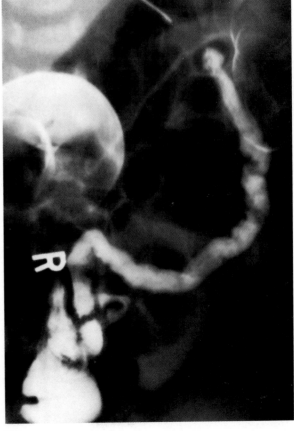

B

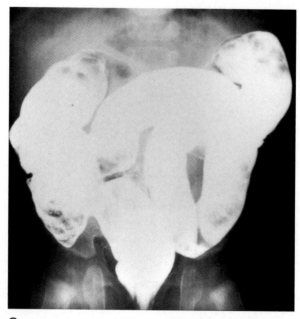

C

Diagnosis Neonatal Small Left Colon Syndrome (SLCS)

Discussion and Differential Diagnosis

Neonatal small left colon syndrome is an unusual cause of functional bowel obstruction. About half of patients are infants of diabetic mothers.[1] Maternal treatment with psychotropic drugs has also been associated with the condition.[2] On the basis of plain films, differential diagnosis includes ileal stenosis or atresia, meconium ileus (usually has no air-fluid levels whereas SLCS does), Hirschsprung's disease, and meconium plug syndrome (which may actually be an overlapping variant of SLCS).

Water-soluble contrast enema is diagnostic and therapeutic. In SLCS, the rectum dilates to 2 to 3 cm in diameter (near normal) during the enema,[3] whereas in Hirschsprung's disease, the rectum usually is more spastic and may be smaller than the sigmoid. The descending colon in SLCS is small in caliber (<1 cm) with a rapid transition to dilated colon at or near the splenic flexure.[3]

Symptoms in SLCS usually resolve after diagnostic enema and initial passage of meconium. In missed Hirschsprung's disease, symptoms persist.

Further Reading

1. Dunn V, Nixon GW, Jaffe RB, Condon VR. Infants of diabetic mothers: radiographic manifestations. *AJR Am J Roentgenol* 137:123–128, 1981.
2. Falterman CG, Richardson CJ. Small left colon syndrome associated with maternal ingestion of psychotropic drugs. *J Pediatr* 97(2):308–310, 1980.
3. Berdon WE, Slovis TL, Campbell JB, Baker DH, Haller JO. Neonatal small left colon syndrome: its relationship to aganglionosis and meconium plug syndrome. *Radiology* 125:457–462, 1977.

Case 5

Clinical Presentation

A term female newborn with a buttocks mass.

Radiographic Studies

Barium enema (Fig. 5A) demonstrates rounded widening of the presacral space with anterior displacement of the rectum. Ultrasound (US) (Fig. 5B) demonstrates an intrapelvic and external cystic mass in contiguity with the sacrum. CT (Fig. 5C) confirms the US findings.

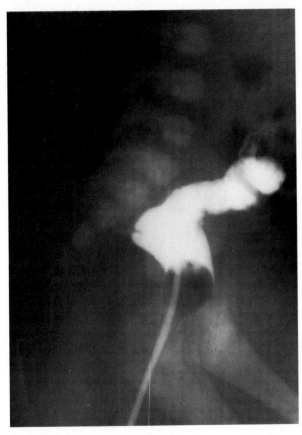

A

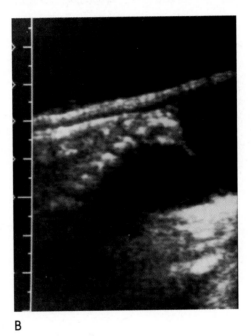

B

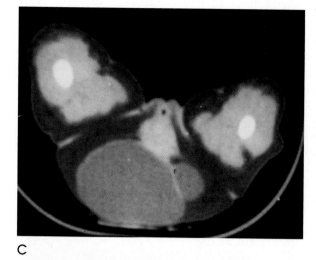

C

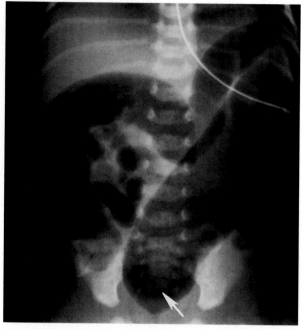

D

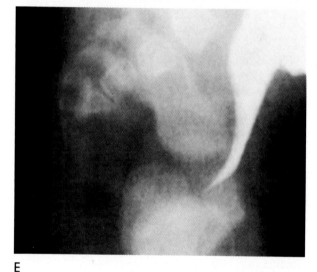

E

Diagnosis Sacrococcygeal Teratoma (SCT)

Discussion and Differential Diagnosis

Sacrococcygeal teratoma is the most common tumor in newborns. It arises from cells of Hensen's node.[1] It occurs in 1 in 40,000 births, with a marked female predominance. Other congenital anomalies are found in 18%.[2] Classification is according to location: type I is most common and predominately external, presenting as a sacral or buttock mass; type II has an external mass with definite intraabdominal extension. Figures 5A–5C illustrates a type II SCT. In type III, the mass is mostly intraabdominal with a small external component, and type IV (10%) is entirely presacral. Type is unrelated to prognosis except as it relates to time of diagnosis. Tumors may be large (as large as the entire baby) or small. Most are mixed cystic and solid. About one third show radiographic calcification.[3] Tumors are characterized histologically as mature, immature, or malignant.[4] Up to 10% are malignant at the time of birth. The rate of malignancy in nonresected tumors increases rapidly to 60% at 4 months.[5] Therefore, treatment consists of wide surgical excision including coccygectomy as soon as possible after birth.[6] Malignant tumors are treated with chemotherapy. Local recurrences may receive radiation therapy.[6]

Type IV tumors (not externally visible) are often diagnosed late and therefore have higher rates of malignancy. They may present as GI or urinary symptoms, or abdominal distention. After resection, elevated alpha-fetoprotein levels indicate a high risk of recurrence.[7] Local recurrence of benign disease or malignant recurrence of tumors originally diagnosed as benign can occur as late as 40 years[8] after resection, so continued follow-up is suggested.[4] Significant numbers of survivors have voiding dysfunction[2] or abnormal bowel habits.[9]

Occult type IV tumors may be associated with sacral anomalies and congenital anorectal abnormalities (anal stenosis).[10] This triad (Currarino triad) is more common in boys than is isolated SCT[10] and has a familial inheritance pattern in 50% of cases.[11,12] In Figure 5D, plain radiographs show rectal stenosis and a hypoplastic ("scimitar") sacrum (arrow). Barium enema (Fig. 5E) confirmed rectal stenosis and demonstrated a mass anterior to the sacrum. In 39% of cases, the mass will be a teratoma; in 48%, it will be a meningocele.[12]

Prenatal ultrasound diagnosis of SCT is now common. A fetus with SCT should be followed closely. Those who develop hydrops or placentomegaly have a poor survival rate, and the mother may develop a severe preeclampsia-type syndrome.[13] Fetal excision of SCT has been attempted.[13] Delivery of a fetus with a large tumor should be by C-section to prevent intratumoral hemorrhage and dystocia.[1] Differential diagnosis includes meningomyelocele, anterior sacral meningocele, lipoma, hemangioma, duplication cyst, and chordoma.[11]

Further Reading

1. McCurdy CM Jr, Seeds JW. Route of delivery of infants with congenital anomalies. *Clin Perinatol* 20(1):81–94, 1993.
2. Boemers TM, van Gool JD, de Jong TP, Bax KM. Lower urinary tract dysfunction in children with benign sacrococcygeal teratoma. *J Urol* 151:174–176, 1994.
3. Ein SH, Adeyemi SD, Mancer K. Benign sacrococcygeal teratomas in infants and children. A 25 year review. *Ann Surg* 191(3):382–384, 1980.
4. Lack EE, Glaun RS, Hefter LG, Seneca RP, Steigman C, Athari F. Late occurrence of malignancy following resection of a histologically mature sacrococcygeal teratoma: report of a case and literature review. *Arch Pathol Lab Med* 117:724–728, 1993.
5. Hogge WA, Thiagarajah S, Barber VG, Rodgers BM, Newman BM. Cystic sacrococcygeal teratoma: ultrasound diagnosis and perinatal management. *J Ultrasound Med* 6:707–710, 1987.
6. Schropp KP, Lobe TE, Mutabagani K, et al. Sacrococcygeal teratoma: the experience of four decades. *J Pediatr Surg* 27(8):1075–1079, 1992.

7. Bilik R, Shandling B, Pope M, Thorner P, Weitzman S, Ein SH. Malignant benign neonatal sacrococcygeal teratoma. *J Pediatr Surg* 28(9):1158–1160, 1993.

8. Lahdenne P, Heikinheimo M, Nikkanen V, Klem, P, Siimes JA, Rapola J. Neonatal benign sacrococcygeal teratoma may recur in adulthood and give rise to malignancy. *Cancer* 72(12):3727–3731, 1993.

9. Rintala R, Lahdenne P, Kindahl H, Siimes M, Heikinheimo M. Anorectal function in adults operated for a benign sacrococcygeal teratoma. *J Pediatr Surg* 28(9):1165–1167, 1993.

10. Moazam F, Talbert JL. Congenital anorectal malformations. *Arch Surg* 120:856–859, 1985.

11. Liu KK, Lee KH, Ku KW. Sacrococcygeal teratoma in children: a diagnostic challenge. *Aust N Z J Surg* 64:102–105, 1994.

12. Pfluger T, Czekalla R, Koletzko S, Münsterer O, Willemsen UF, Hahn K. MRI and radiographic findings in Currarino's triad. *Pediatr Radiol* 26:524–527, 1996.

13. Langer JC, Harrison MR, Schmidt KG, et al. Fetal hydrops and death from sacrococcygeal teratoma: rationale for fetal surgery. *Am J Obstet Gynecol* 160(5):1145–1150, 1989.

Case 6

Clinical Presentation

A 3-week-old girl with progressive vomiting over the past 3 days.

Radiographic Studies

Ultrasound (Fig. 6A) shows fluid in the gastric antrum, pyloric muscle elongation (length 22.8 mm), and thickening (single wall thickness 4.7 mm). Upper gastrointestinal series (UGI) (Fig. 6B) demonstrates an elongated narrow pylorus with a "tram track" sign and minimal passage of barium through it.

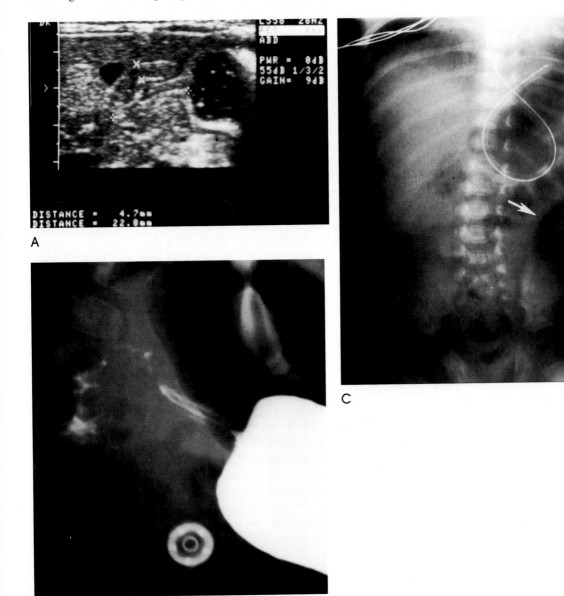

A

B

C

Diagnosis Hypertrophic Pyloric Stenosis (HPS)

Discussion and Differential Diagnosis

Hypertrophic pyloris stenosis is usually not present at birth, but develops over the first few weeks of life. It is usually seen in a term baby who presents with progressive projectile vomiting at age 2 to 6 weeks. Boys are affected more often than girls. It is occasionally seen in infants a few days old or as old as 3 months, or in premature or ill infants still in the neonatal intensive care unit (NICU). There is hypertrophy of the pyloric muscle of unknown etiology. This causes progressive gastric outlet obstruction and secondary vomiting. Commonly, the infant will have had episodes of gastroesophageal reflux since birth, so the development of projectile vomiting represents only worsening of preexisting symptoms. An experienced examiner can palpate an "olive" in 80% of cases, and imaging may not be necessary.[1] In the remainder of cases or in those with atypical history or physical findings, diagnosis can be made with either contrast UGI or ultrasound. Most experienced radiologists now prefer US. Sensitivity of US is reported at 97% with specificity of 99% and positive predictive values of 99%.[2] However, UGI may still be used at the discretion of the radiologist, a choice based on experience or equipment availability. Sometimes HPS is encountered when UGI is ordered to rule out other conditions. Vomiting from HPS is a rare cause of pneumatosis. Figure 6C (arrow) shows pneumatosis intestinalis in a premature infant in the NICU who developed vomiting at age 4 weeks and was found to have HPS.

Ultrasound criteria vary somewhat in published reports. Single muscle wall thickness in cross section, pyloric cross sectional diameter, and pyloric length should all be measured if possible. In addition, clear liquid should be given by bottle and peristalsis and emptying through the pylorus should be observed.

Ultrasound measurement criteria include a single cross sectional muscle thickness greater than 2.5 to 4.0 mm,[1-3] a cross section diameter greater than 11 mm,[2] and a length greater than 16 mm.[2] In addition, little if any liquid passes through the pylorus.

In negative cases, gastroesophageal reflux is usually responsible for symptoms. Other causes of vomiting such as pylorospasm and midgut volvulus may also be identified at UGI.[1]

Further Reading

1. Forman HP, Leonidas JC, Kronfeld GD. A rational approach to the diagnosis of hypertrophic pyloric stenosis: do the results match the claims? *J Pediatr Surg* 25(2):262–266, 1990.
2. Neilson D, Hollman AS. The ultrasonic diagnosis of infantile hypertrophic pyloric stenosis: technique and accuracy. *Clin Radiol* (49):246–247, 1994.
3. Cohen HL, Schechter S, Mestel AL, Eaton DH, Haller JO. Ultrasonic "double track" sign in hypertrophic pyloric stenosis. *J Ultrasound Med* (6):139–143, 1987.

PEARLS

- Do not forget HPS in NICU patient who develops vomiting or large gastric residuals.

- Try to obtain all three measurements, as one borderline measurement may be misleading.

- If ultrasound results are borderline, you may be imaging a very early case. A repeat study in 2 or 3 days may be conclusive.

- Be sure to tell the surgeon/anesthesiologist if liquid was administered during the US exam.

PITFALLS

- Measurements in small ex-preemies may be borderline but the "appearance" of the pylorus is that of HPS.

CONTROVERSY

- Some authors feel that UGI is indicated in negative studies to rule out other significant causes of vomiting.[1]

Case 7

Clinical Presentation

A 9-year-old boy with abdominal distention.

Radiographic Studies

Plain radiograph (Fig. 7A) shows mass effect displacing bowel loops outward. Abdominal CT (Fig. 7B) demonstrates a multiseptated mass of near water attenuation.

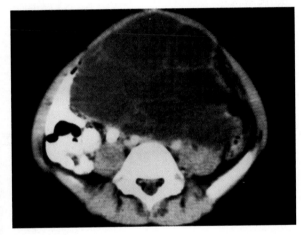

B

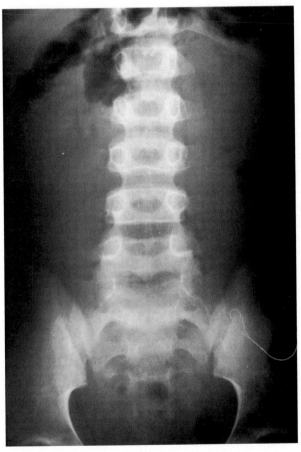

A

Diagnosis Mesenteric Cyst

Discussion and Differential Diagnosis

Mesenteric cyst represents a lymphangioma probably secondary to congenital obstruction of lymphatics. Lesions generally involve the omentum and retroperitoneum. Plain radiographs often show mass effect. Rarely, calcification is seen in the cyst wall. Obstruction can result from the cyst compressing bowel loops or from complications such as volvulus.[1] Ultrasound or CT shows a cystic mass located anywhere from the duodenum to the distal colon. Fifty percent are found in the small bowel mesentery.[1] Cysts can be single or multiple, simple or septated, and can contain echogenic or high attenuation fluid if infected or if hemorrhage has occurred. Site of origin of the cyst may not be identified by imaging, but identified only at surgery.

Appendicitis is the most frequent mistaken diagnosis.[2] Other cystic masses such as ovarian cyst, duplication cyst, and urachal cyst are often difficult to differentiate with imaging. Final diagnosis of mesenteric cyst may require pathologic confirmation of a cyst lined with endothelium or fibrous tissue.

Further Reading

1. Hebra A, Brown MF, McGeehin KM, Ross AJ III. Mesenteric, omental, and retroperitoneal cysts in children: a clinical study of 22 cases. *South Med J* 86(2):173–176, 1993.
2. Chung MA, Brandt DSV, Yazbeck S. Mesenteric cysts in children. *J Pediatr Surg* 26(11):1306–1308, 1991.

Case 8

Clinical Presentation

A 2-day-old infant with bilious vomiting and a distended abdomen (Fig. 8A).
A 3-day-old infant with bilious vomiting (Fig. 8B).

Radiographic Studies

Supine and dependent views (upright, cross-table lateral or decubitus [not shown]) of the abdomen show dilated loops with air-fluid levels (Fig. 8A). Fewer loops implies a higher level of obstruction (Fig. 8B). In Figure 8C, a contrast enema demonstrates a microcolon and incomplete rotation with dilated nonfilled proximal loops.

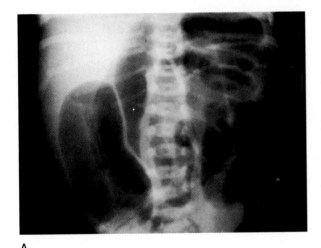

A

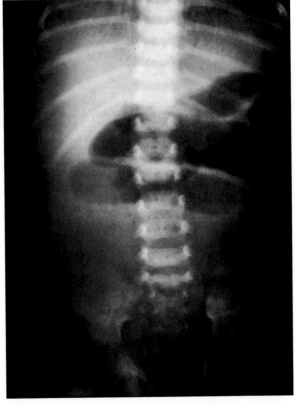

B

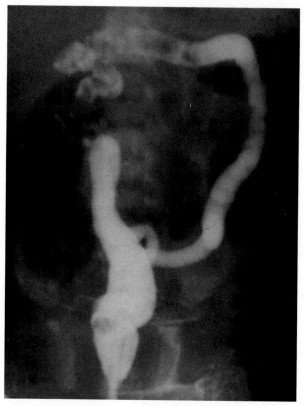

C

Diagnosis Small Bowel Atresia

Discussion and Differential Diagnosis

Small bowel atresias are fairly evenly distributed in bowel between the ligament of Trietz and the ileocecal junction.[1] Prenatal ultrasound often detects direct (dilated bowel loops) or indirect evidence (polyhydramnios, meconium peritonitis) of intestinal atresia.

Newborns present with bile-stained vomiting soon after birth (jejunal atresia) or as late as several days later (distal ileal atresia). The degree of abdominal distention is also related to the level of obstruction. Peristalsis may be visible. Twenty to 40% have indirect hyperbilirubinemia (enhanced enterohepatic circulation of bilirubin).

Dilute (15 to 40%, depending on size and condition of patient) water-soluble contrast enema is used in cases of suspected distal obstruction to distinguish between ileal atresia and other causes of distal obstruction. An enema may also be used in jejunal atresia to look for evidence of multiple atresias (microcolon) or malrotation (abnormal cecum location). Meconium ileus coexists in 20% of cases, but inability to reflux colonic contrast past the meconium suggests atresia.

- Very early films may not show characteristic abnormalities.

- Films taken of normal neonates in first few hours may show incomplete filling of bowel with air and simulate atresia.

CONTROVERSY
- Epidemiological data suggest that jejunal and ileal atresia may be different diseases.[4]

The cause of intestinal atresia distal to the duodenum is usually vascular occlusion. Possible mechanisms include abnormal formation or resorption of vessels, compression due to volvulus or herniation through an abdominal wall defect, or emboli to vessels. Multiple atresias may be familial.[2] Atresias are classified as follows:

Type I: intraluminal diaphragm

Type II: cord-like segment separating blind loops

Type IIIa: mesenteric defect with complete separation of blind loops

Type IIIb: large mesenteric defect with retrograde blood supply from ileocolic artery; volvulus and short gut may be present; this form may be hereditary and is known as "Christmas tree" or "apple peel" bowel

Type IV: multiple atresias

A similar radiographic appearance may be seen in Hirschsprung's disease, meconium plug syndrome, meconium ileus, and ileal stenosis (small to large amounts of distal air will be present). Contrast enema can usually distinguish these entities.

Further Reading

1. Touloukian RJ. Diagnosis and treatment of jejunoileal atresia. *World J Surg* 17:310–317, 1993.
2. Cragan JD, Martin ML, Moore CA, Khoury MJ. Descriptive epidemiology of small intestinal atresia, Atlanta, Georgia. *Teratology* 48:441–450, 1993.
3. Carty H, Brereton RJ. The distended neonate. *Clin Radiol* 34:367–380, 1983.
4. Heij HA, Moorman-Voestermans CG, Vos A. Atresia of jejunum and ileum: is it the same disease? *J Pediatr Surg* 25(6):635–637, 1990.

Case 9

Clinical Presentation

An 8-year-old boy with multiple congenital orthopedic anomalies had a 4-year history of solid food dysphagia.

Radiographic Studies

Barium swallow (Fig. 9A) shows a long segment stricture of the proximal half of the esophagus, a patulous esophagogastric (EG) junction, and gross gastroesophageal (GE) reflux (Fig. 9B)

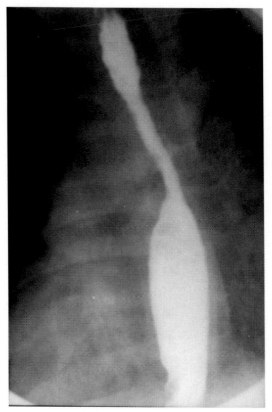

A

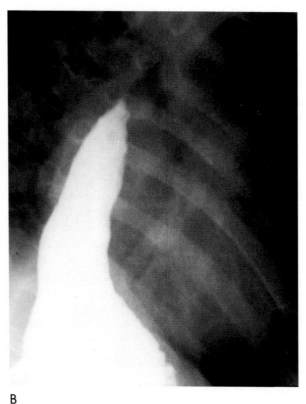

B

Diagnosis Esophageal Stricture

Discussion and Differential Diagnosis

The most common cause of stricture in children is reflux esophagitis.[1] Barrett's esophagus may develop, and adenocarcinoma, though rare, has been reported.[2] Other causes of stricture are usually obvious when an accurate history is obtained. They include stricture at the anastamotic site following esophageal atresia repair; stricture following nasogastric intubation[3]; stricture secondary to lye ingestion or foreign body impaction[4]; or caustic pill (especially tetracycline) impaction.[5] Esophageal stricture can also result from radiation and chemotherapy.[6,7]

Esophageal stricture may be associated with rare diseases such as epidermolysis bullosa dystrophica,[8] Stevens-Johnson syndrome,[9] chronic granulomatous disease of childhood,[10] and idiopathic eosinophilic esophagitis.[11] Benign tracheal remnants[1] and hamartomas[12] can also cause esophageal stricture. Symptoms of solid food dysphagia and food impaction are common to all causes.

PEARLS

- Treatment may vary according to cause.

- Look at the patient, at the history, or at other studies for clues to the etiology of stricture. For example, mitten-like hands and feet with contractures are seen in epidermolysis bullosa dystrophica.

PITFALLS

- Do not assume all cases of esophageal stricture are secondary to GE reflux.

Further Reading

1. Yeung CK, Spitz L, Brereton RJ, Kiely EM, Leake J. Congenital esophageal stenosis due to tracheobronchial remnants: a rare but important association with esophageal atresia. *J Pediatr Surg* 27(7):852–855, 1992.
2. Othersen HB Jr, Ocampo RJ, Parker EF, Smith CD, Tagge EP. Barrett's esophagus in children: diagnosis and management. *Ann Surg* 217(6):676–681, 1993.
3. Zaninotto G, Bonavina L, Pianalto S, Fassina A, Ancona E. Esophageal strictures following nasogastric intubation. *Int Surg* 71:100–103, 1986.
4. Doolin EJ. Esophageal stricture: an uncommon complication of foreign bodies. *Ann Otol Rhinol Laryngol* 102:863–866, 1993.
5. Kikendall JW. Pill-induced esophageal injury. *Gastroenterol Clin North Am* 20(4):835–846, 1991.
6. Ellenhorn JD, Lambroza A. Lindsley KL, LaQuaglia MP. Treatment-related esophageal stricture in pediatric patients with cancer. *Cancer* 71(12):4084–4090, 1993.
7. Gaspar LE, Dawson DJ, Tilley-Guilliford SA, Banerjee P. Medulloblastoma: long-term follow-up of patients treated with electron irradiation of the spinal field. *Radiology* 180(3):867–870, 1991.
8. Mauro MA, Parker LA, Hartley WS, Renner JB, Mauro PM. Epidermolysis bullosa: radiographic findings in 16 cases. *AJR Am J Roentgenol* 149:925–927, 1987.
9. Edell DS, Davidson JJ, Muelenaer AA, Majure M. Unusual manifestation of Stevens-Johnson syndrome involving the respiratory and gastrointestinal tract. *Pediatrics* 89(3):429–432, 1992.
10. Renner WR, Johnson JF, Lichtenstein JE, Kirks DR. Esophageal inflammation and stricture: complication of chronic granulomatous disease of childhood. *Radiology* 178(1):189–191, 1991.

11. Vitellas KM, Bennett WF, Bova JG, Johnston JC, Caldwell JH, Mayle JE. Idiopathic eosinophilic esophagitis. *Radiology* 186(3):789–793, 1993.
12. Smith CW, Murray GF, Wilcox BR. Intramural esophageal hamartoma: an unusual cause of progressive stricture in a child. *J Thorac Cardiovasc Surg* 72(2):315–318, 1976.

Case 10

Clinical Presentation

A 2-day-old female term newborn with a distended abdomen and vomiting.

Radiographic Studies

Supine (Fig. 10A) and cross-table lateral (Fig. 10B) radiographs show dilated bowel loops with air-fluid levels on the dependent film and no gas in the rectum. A single grossly distended loop is seen on the right. Dilute water-soluble contrast enema (Fig. 10C) shows an unused colon (microcolon) that ends just distal to the splenic flexure. Note the rounded appearance of bowel at site of obstruction.

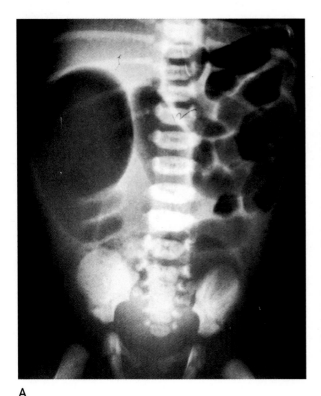

A

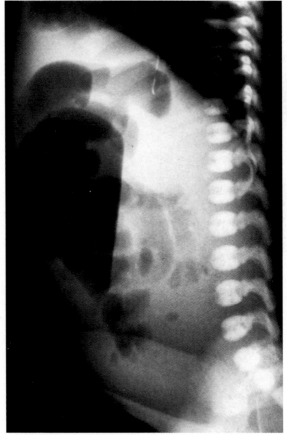

B

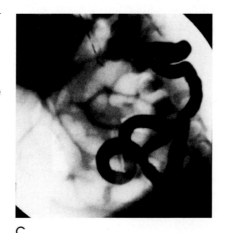

C

Diagnosis   Colon Atresia

Discussion and Differential Diagnosis

Colon atresia is the least common of all bowel atresias. It occurs in 1 in 20,000[1] to 40,000[2] live births. The cause is probably thrombotic or embolic mesenteric vascular occlusion.[3] A genetic component may be present. The condition has been reported in three members of one family.[4] The obstruction can occur anywhere in the colon and is classified as one of three types, all with a common etiology. In type I, a membrane or diaphragm occludes the lumen. Type II consists of two atretic segments of colon joined by a cord-like structure; Type III, a V-shaped mesenteric defect with the two atretic ends completely separated.[3] Clinically, the newborn presents with the same symptoms as in other cases of distal bowel obstruction: abdominal distention, vomiting, and failure to pass meconium. Symptoms may not occur until the second or third day of life.

Differential diagnosis made on the basis of clinical findings and plain films includes the more common conditions of ileal stenosis, meconium ileus, meconium plug syndrome, and Hirschsprung's disease. Contrast enema is needed to establish the diagnosis. Location of the level of obstruction may be important in planning the type of surgery (colostomy vs primary anastamosis). The association of colon atresia with other bowel atresias, Hirschsprung's disease, abdominal wall defects, and rotation abnormalities is common.[1,2]

Further Reading

1. Powell RW, Raffensperger JG. Congenital colonic atresia. *J Pediatr Surg* 17(2):166–170, 1982.
2. Landes A, Shuckett B, Skarsgard E. Non-fixation of the colon in colonic atresia: a new finding. *Pediatr Radiol* 24:167–169, 1994.

3. Pohlson EC, Hatch EI, Glick PL, Tapper D. Individualized management of colonic atresia. *Am J Surg* 155:690–692, 1988.
4. Benawra R, Puppala BL, Mangurten HH, Booth C, Bassuk A. Familial occurrence of congenital colonic atresia. *J Pediatr* 99(3):435–436, 1981.
5. Anderson N, Malpas T, Robertson R. Prenatal diagnosis of colon atresia. *Pediatr Radiol* 23:63–64, 1993.
6. Winters WD, Weinberger E, Hatch EI. Atresia of the colon in neonates: radiographic findings. *AJR Am J Roentgenol* 159:1273–1276, 1992.

Case 11

Clinical Presentation

A 36-week gestational age, 2-day-old infant with a distended abdomen and failure to pass meconium for 50 hours after birth.

Radiographic Studies

Plain radiographs (Fig. 11A, 11B) show mildly dilated bowel with air-fluid levels and a "bubbly" appearance on the left. Contrast enema (Fig. 11C) outlines a long mass that was "passed" during the procedure and measured 19 cm in length.

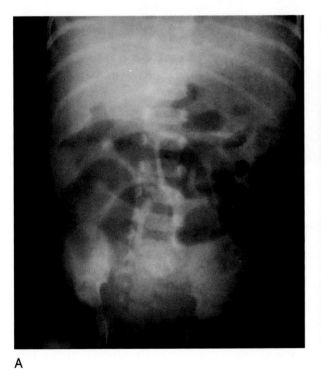

A

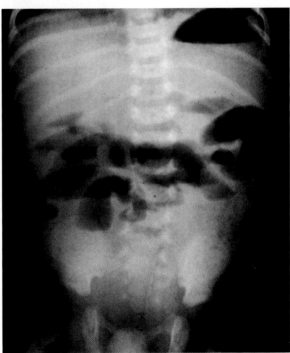

B

PEARLS

• May be secondary to hypermagnesemia caused by maternal treatment with magnesium sulfate for eclampsia.[4]

• A few cases are seen in patients with later diagnosis of cystic fibrosis and/or Hirschsprung's disease.[1] If symptoms do not resolve, sweat test and biopsy should be performed.

PITFALLS

• Perforation may occur after failure to diagnose and treat.[3]

• Air-fluid levels may develop in long-standing cases.[3]

CONTROVERSY

• MPS and SLCS may be different manifestations of the same disorder.[3]

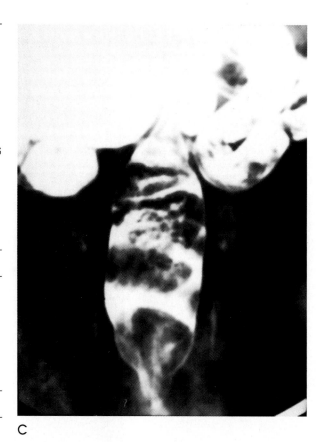

C

Diagnosis Meconium Plug Syndrome (MPS)

Discussion and Differential Diagnosis

Meconium plug syndrome is a relatively common cause (1 in 500 to 1,000 births)[1] of functional obstruction of the colon. The etiology is unknown. Suggested causes include abnormally viscous meconium and immature colonic development.[2] Meconium plug syndrome may be seen in term or premature babies or infants of diabetic mothers. Clinical presentation is usually a newborn with abdominal distention. Examination may show visible and palpable tense loops of bowel.[2] There is failure to pass normal amounts of meconium, and vomiting (often bilious) may develop.[2] Often the symptoms are indistinguishable from Hirschsprung's disease and other forms of bowel obstruction.

Plain film findings are suggestive but rarely definitive. They usually show dilated bowel with all loops of the same caliber, usually without air-fluid levels,[3] and a "soap bubble" appearance on the left.[2] Contrast enema is done to confirm the suspected diagnosis and is often therapeutic. Water-soluble contrast outlines a usually continuous collection of meconium in a normal caliber colon. Frequently, the stimulation of the enema will cause passage of a "plug" 10 to 20 cm long, and symptoms will be relieved. Sometimes, the plug is outlined proximal to the splenic flexure and the distal colon is of decreased caliber. This entity is known as small left colon syndrome (SLCS).

Meconium plug syndrome is usually self-limited, and no further symptoms occur after initial passage of meconium.

Further Reading

1. Hen J Jr, Dolan TF Jr, Touloukian RJ. Meconium plug syndrome associated with cystic fibrosis and Hirschsprung's disease. *Pediatrics* 66(3):446–467, 1980.
2. Rosenstein BJ. Cystic fibrosis presenting with the meconium plug syndrome. *Am J Dis Child* 132:167–169, 1978.
3. Hussain SM, Meradji M, Robben SG, Hop WC. Plain film diagnosis in meconium plug syndrome, meconium ileus and neonatal Hirschsprung's disease. *Pediatr Radiol* 21:556–559, 1991.
4. Cooney DR, Rosevear W, Grosfeld JL. Maternal and postnatal hypermagnesemia and the meconium plug syndrome. *J Pediatr Surg* 11(2):167–172, 1976.

Case 12

Clinical Presentation

A 6-year-old boy with bright red rectal bleeding.

Radiographic Studies

Barium enema (Fig. 12A) shows no polyps but cecum is slightly elevated. Palpation revealed a right lower quadrant (RLQ) mass. Ultrasound (Fig. 12B) shows a 3 × 5 cm circumferential mass in the distal ileum. CT (Fig. 12C) confirms the findings and shows no adenopathy.

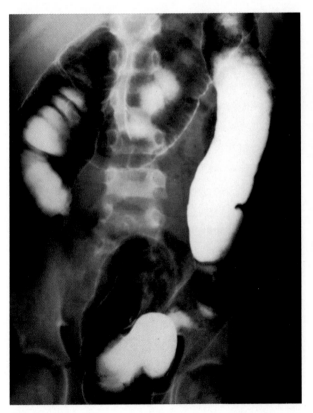

A

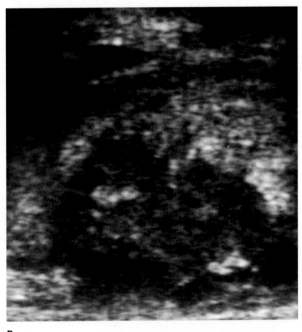

B

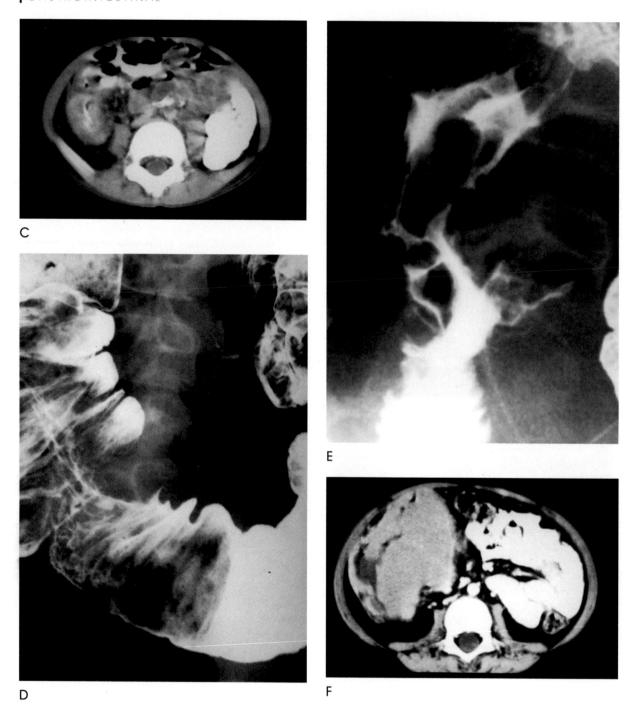

C

D

E

F

Diagnosis Burkitt's Lymphoma

Discussion and Differential Diagnosis

Burkitt's lymphoma is a type of non-Hodgkin's lymphoma that originates from undifferentiated B cell–derived lymphocytes.[1] There are two forms with identical histology. The endemic form is associated with the Epstein-Barr virus, occurs mostly in tropical climates, and usually involves the head and neck. The nonendemic or American type most commonly involves the abdomen,[1] especially the ileocecal area.[2] Urinary tract (42%), pleural (67%),[2] and gonadal (75%)[1] involvement are also common. Mean age at diagnosis is 11 years.[2] Patients may present with abdominal mass, nausea, vomiting, abdominal pain, obstruction, or rectal bleeding.[3]

In Burkitt's lymphoma, both clinical presentation and radiographic studies can be indistinguishable from those of Crohn's disease.[4] CT is most helpful in defining a large mass or involvement in areas other than bowel. Barium studies may show a large ulceration in the mass, or stricture and fistula formation similar in appearance to Crohn's disease.[4] Chemotherapy and sometimes surgery are used to treat the disease. CT is used to evaluate response to treatment and recurrence.

Further Reading

1. Rezvani L, Tully RJ, Levine C, Levine E, Rubin JM. Computed tomography in the diagnosis and follow-up of American Burkitt's lymphoma. *Gastrointest Radiol* 11:36–40, 1986.
2. Alford BA, Coccia PF, L'Heureux PR. Roentgenographic features of American Burkitt's lymphoma. *Radiology* 124:763–770, 1977.
3. Choi RE, Kopecky KK, Clark SA. Radiology clinic: 16-year-old boy with weight loss and abdominal mass. *Indiana Med* 81(7):623–624, 1988.
4. Sartoris DJ, Harell GS, Anderson MF, Zboralske PF. Small-bowel lymphoma and regional enteritis: radiographic similarities. *Radiology* 152:291–296, 1984.

PEARLS
- Burkitt's lymphoma may be the lead point for an intussusception in an older child (Fig. 12D).

PITFALLS
- Findings on barium studies, US, and CT may be indistinguishable from those of Crohn's disease. Figure 12E is a spot film from the RLQ of an 11-year-old boy who was treated for Crohn's disease but returned 6 months later with a huge abdominal mass (Fig. 12F), which proved to be Burkitt's lymphoma.
- On CT, nonopacified bowel loops may be difficult to distinguish from a mass or adenopathy. Timing of contrast administration is crucial and follow-up scans may be helpful.

Case 13

Clinical Presentation

A 17-day-old male infant presented to ER with failure to stool for 5 days. Stool was guaiac positive.

Radiographic Studies

Barium enema was ordered to rule out Hirschsprung's disease. Contrast enema (Fig. 13A) shows anterior displacement of the rectum by a smooth, rounded noncalcified presacral mass. Ultrasound (Fig. 13B) reveals the mass to be cystic (arrow) and in close proximity to the sacrum.

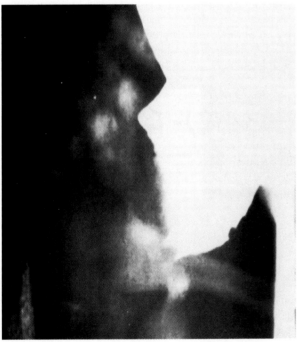

A

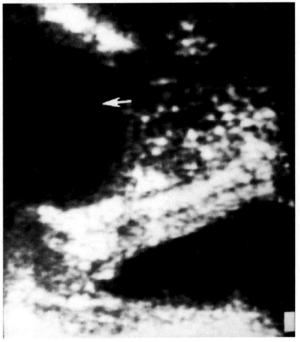

B

Diagnosis Duplication Cyst

PEARLS

- Search for multiple cysts (15%).[4]

- Look for vertebral body anomalies. They occur in 20 to 30% of cases, but these cysts are thought to be a different entity from neurenteric cysts, which also have spine anomalies.[7]

PITFALLS

- Gastric mucosa in duplication cyst (10 to 20%)[4] can cause a false-positive Meckel's scan.

Discussion and Differential Diagnosis

Duplication cysts of the GI tract are rare lesions that can occur anywhere from the base of the tongue to the anus (the ileum is the most frequent site).[1] Most are diagnosed in early childhood. Some are asymptomatic and discovered coincidentally; others present as respiratory distress (esophageal lesion), abdominal distention, pain, obstruction (from mass or intussusception), or bleeding (if cyst contains ectopic gastric mucosa). Rare cases present as hepatic cysts.[2] Clinical diagnosis is difficult. Imaging is usually needed to confirm the diagnosis. Plain films may show a mediastinal mass in esophageal lesions. In the abdomen, barium studies show mass effect, intussusception, or obstruction and, rarely, ulceration or perforation.[3] Pertechnetate scans can identify cysts containing gastric mucosa. Ultrasound can establish the diagnosis by identifying a cystic lesion with a "muscular rim" sign (echogenic inner rim and hypoechoic outer rim)[4] and peristalsis within the cyst wall.[5] Internal echoes indicate bleeding or strands of mucus in the cyst. Rarely, the lesions are solid.[4]

Duplication cysts are located on the mesenteric border of the bowel. This may help to distinguish them from Meckel's diverticulum. Duplication cysts are round and rarely communicate with bowel. Histologically, they are lined with mucosa similar to adjacent bowel.

These cysts probably are the result of failure to recanalize the lumen in fetal development,[1] though other etiological theories have also been proposed.[6]

Differential diagnosis of esophageal duplications includes other mediastinal masses. For diagnosis of duplication cysts below the diaphragm, other cystic masses such as mesenteric, omental, and ovarian cysts, anterior meningocele, giant Meckel's diverticulum, and cystic sacrococcygeal teratoma type IV must be considered. Only a giant Meckel's diverticulum will have similar characteristics on US.

Further Reading

1. Bisset GS, Towbin RB. Pedriatric case of the day. *Radiographics* 6(5):917–920, 1986.
2. Seidman JD, Yale-Loehr AJ, Beaver B, Sun C-CJ. Alimentary duplication presenting as an hepatic cyst in a neonate. *Am J Surg Pathol* 15(7):695–698, 1991.
3. Royle SG, Doig CM. Perforation of the jejunum secondary to a duplication cyst lined with ectopic gastric mucosa. *J Pediatr Surg* 23(11):1025–1026, 1988.
4. Segal SR, Sherman NH, Rosenberg HK, et al. Ultrasonographic features of gastrointestinal duplications. *J Ultrasound Med* 13:863–870, 1994.
5. Spottswood SE. Peristalsis in duplication cyst: a new diagnostic sonographic finding. *Pediatr Radiol* 24:344–345, 1994.
6. Patenaude Y, Jéquier S, Russo P. Pediatric case of the day. *Radiographics* 13:218–220, 1993.
7. Alrabeeah A, Gillis DA, Giacomantonio M, Lau H. Neurenteric cysts—a spectrum. *J Pediatr Surg* 23(8):752–754, 1988.

Case 14

Clinical Presentation

An 8-year-old girl with rectal bleeding requiring transfusion.

Radiographic Studies

Technetium scan shows faint abnormal uptake superior to the bladder on the 8-min image (Fig. 14A). The abnormality is more obvious on later image (Fig. 14B).

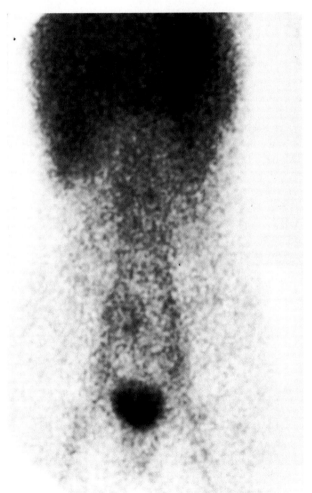

A

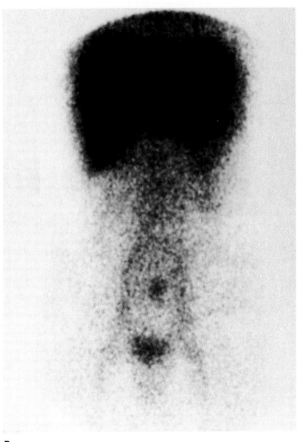

B

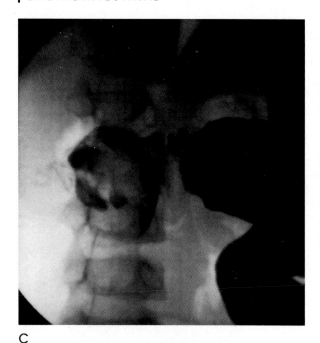

C

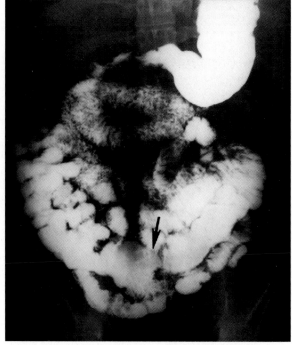

D

Diagnosis Meckel's Diverticulum

Discussion and Differential Diagnosis

Meckel's diverticulum is a true diverticulum off the antimesenteric border of the small bowel and is the most common congenital anomaly of the GI tract. Although it occurs in 2% of the population, most cases remain asymptomatic.[1] When symptoms do develop, 60% occur before age 10, and the remainder throughout childhood and into adulthood. The most common complications are obstruction due to volvulus, intussusception (Fig. 14C), internal hernia, adhesions from inflammatory reaction, and torsion.[1]

In children, hemorrhage due to peptic ulceration in ectopic gastric mucosa within the diverticulum is also an important clinical presentation. Patients present with rectal bleeding that is sometimes significant enough to require transfusion. In other cases, bleeding is occult but causes iron deficiency anemia.[2] In children, technetium-99m pertechnetate scintigraphy is 80 to 90% accurate[3] in identifying Meckel's diverticulum containing ectopic gastric mucosa; in adults accuracy is only 46%. Other imaging techniques have been tried but are not helpful in most cases.[3]

In addition to obstruction and bleeding, inflammation is the most frequently observed manifestation in children. Symptoms can mimic acute appendicitis. Other, less common, complications include foreign body impaction,[4] torsion,[5] and Meckel's diverticulum associated with omphalocele.[2]

Based on clinical findings alone, differential diagnosis includes other causes of bleeding (anal fissure, polyps, inflammatory bowel disease, etc.), obstruction (volvulus, intussusception, adhesions, hernias), or inflammation (appendicitis, inflammatory bowel disease). Technetium scanning will almost always confirm or eliminate Meckel's diverticulum as the source of bleeding. In cases of obstruction, diagnosis is made at the time of surgery.

Meckel's diverticulum is formed by incomplete regression of the proximal portion of the omphalomesenteric (or vitellointestinal) duct, which connects the embryo to the yolk sac from the third to fifth week of gestation. After that time, the placenta takes over nutritional needs and the duct atrophies. Other abnormalities of regression can result in formation of a cyst, a fistula, or fibrous band to the umbilicus.

Further Reading

1. Garretson DC, Frederich ME. Meckel's diverticulum. *Am Fam Physician* 42(1):115–119, 1990.
2. Firor HV. The many faces of Meckel's diverticulum. *South Med J* 73(11):1507–1511, 1980.
3. Kusumoto H, Yoshida M, Takahashi I, Anai H, Maehara Y, Sugimachi K. Complications and diagnosis of Meckel's diverticulum in 776 patients. *Am J Surg* 164:382–383, 1992.
4. Velanovich V, Ledbetter D, McGahren E, Nuchtern J, Schaller R. Foreign bodies within a Meckel's diverticulum. *Arch Surg* 127:864, 1992.
5. Larson J, Elliger D. Sonographic findings in torsion of a Meckel diverticulum. *AJR Am J Roentgenol* 152:1130, 1989. Letter.
6. Dutro JA, Santanello SA, Unger F, Goodwin CD. Rectal bleeding in a 4-month-old boy. *JAMA* 256(16):2239–2240, 1986.
7. Lowry PA, Carstens MC. *Meckel scan in children in with unexplained abdominal pain: is it useful?* Society for Pediatric Radiology, Boston, 1996.

PITFALLS

- False-positive technetium scans can be caused by GI duplications containing gastric mucosa.

- False-negative scans can result from only a small amount of gastric mucosa in the diverticulum; severe generalized inflammation, which may mask an area of increased uptake[1]; or a distended bladder or stomach—they should be emptied before scanning.[6]

- Abdominal pain without bleeding should not be an indication for a technetium Meckel's scan.[7]

CONTROVERSY

- Opinions differ over whether a Meckel's diverticulum discovered incidentally at small bowel follow through (Fig. 14D, arrow) or surgery should be removed (4% become symptomatic, and there is a 5 to 10% mortality rate in those).[5]

Case 15

Clinical Presentation

An 8-year-old boy with intermittent painless bright red rectal bleeding.

Radiographic Studies

Air-contrast barium enema (ACBE) (Fig. 15A, arrows) shows numerous colon masses. Fluoroscopic spot films confirm that suspected fecal material (Fig. 15B) is a mass (Fig. 15C, arrow). Another patient shows a single rectal mass (Figs. 15D, 15E, arrows).

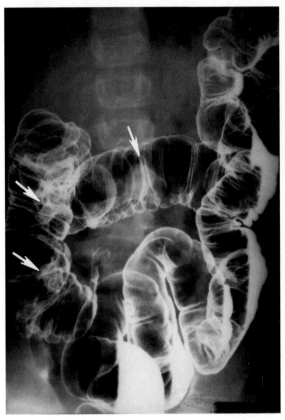

A

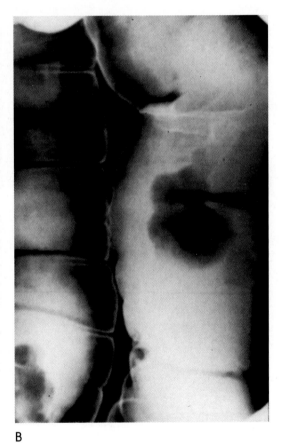

B

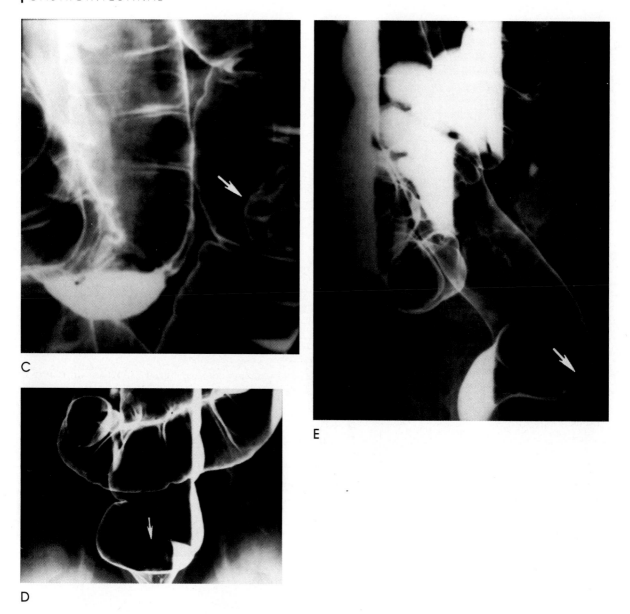

C

D

E

Diagnosis Juvenile Polyps of the Colon

Discussion and Differential Diagnosis

Juvenile colon polyps are the most common colon tumor in children,[1] occur in 1 to 2% of all children,[2] and are the most common cause of painless bright red rectal bleeding after 1 year of age.[1]

In the past, most patients had single hamartomatous or inflammatory polyps found in the rectosigmoid during proctoscopy. Sometimes multiple polyps were identified during ACBE. They were all considered benign, and it was known that the natural history included auto-amputation and spontaneous sloughing in most patients before adolescence.[1]

Most patients present with painless hematochezia. Uncommon symptoms include abdominal pain, rectal prolapse,[3] spontaneous polyp passage, or prolapse of a polyp through the rectum (10 to 30%).[1] Significant hemorrhage, diarrhea, hypoproteinemia, and failure to thrive are seen in generalized polyposis.[2]

Ninety percent of colon polyps in children are juvenile polyps. Most are 1 to 2 cm in diameter, pedunculated, with a surface of columnar epithelium that is frequently ulcerated. They contain dilated cystic spaces lined by goblet cells with inflammatory infiltrate in the stroma. They are usually considered to be hamartomas, but some experts propose inflammatory or allergic etiologies.[4]

With the common use of colonoscopy for diagnosis, it is now known that most (53%) patients have multiple polyps and most polyps (60%) are located proximal to the sigmoid colon.[3] In addition to the most frequent presentation with one to three polyps, it is now recognized that juvenile polyps may be part of three different patterns of more generalized disease that have malignant potential.

1. In infantile polyposis, there is extensive polyposis throughout the colon, terminal ileum, and, rarely, the small bowel and stomach. Patients present before 2 years of age with severe bleeding, diarrhea, hypoproteinemia, and malnutrition. One third have associated anomalies (Meckel's diverticulum, malrotation, congenital heart disease).[1] Without treatment, this form of polyposis is often fatal.[5]

2. Juvenile polyposis coli is an autosomal dominant condition in which there are numerous juvenile polyps that can undergo adenomatous—and, later, carcinomatous—change, or have simultaneous adenomatous polyps.[3] Twenty-five to 50% of these patients have a family history of juvenile polyps or various GI malignancies.

3. In diffuse juvenile polyposis, polyps may be located from the stomach to the anus, and 25% of patients have family members with GI malignancies or polyposis.[1]

In patients with the familial patterns of multiple juvenile polyps, the lifetime risk of malignancy may be greater than 50%.[5] There have been only two reported cases of malignancy arising in solitary juvenile polyps in patients without evidence of a juvenile polyposis syndrome.

PEARLS

- Colonoscopy is the diagnostic procedure of choice,[4] but polyps may be identified during barium enemas done for other reasons.

- There is a bimodal age distribution for juvenile polyps, with a second peak at age 25 years. Adults have the same symptoms.[1]

- Look for a family history of juvenile polyps or GI malignancies. This may be a clue that a patient has one of the juvenile polyposis syndromes with malignant potential. Other family members should be screened in patients with a polyposis syndrome.

- Patients with the juvenile polyposis syndromes may have digital clubbing and hypertrophic pulmonary osteoarthropathy.[5]

PITFALLS

- Patients with inflammatory bowel disease (IBD) may also have juvenile polyps that cause bleeding. Suspect juvenile polyps if a patient presents with hematochezia while IBD is quiescent.

- Not all colon polyps in children are juvenile polyps. In patients with no family history of polyps, 5.2% of solitary polyps are adenomatous polyps and therefore have malignant potential.

CONTROVERSY

- Authors disagree on how many polyps are needed to place a patient in the category of needing continued surveillance. Criteria range from 3 to 10 polyps.[6]

Further Reading

1. Heiss KF, Schaffner D, Ricketts RR, Winn K. Malignant risk in juvenile polyposis coli: increasing documentation in the pediatric age group. *J Pediatr Surg* 28(9):1188–1193, 1993.
2. Longo WE, Touloukian RJ, West AB, Ballantyne GH. Malignant potential of juvenile polyposis coli. *Dis Colon Rectum* 33(11):980–984, 1990.
3. Mestre JR. The changing pattern of juvenile polyps. *Am J Gastroenterol* 81(5):312–314, 1986.
4. Gryboski JD, Barwick KW. Juvenile polyps and ulcerative colitis. *J Pediatr Gastroenterol Nutr* 6(5):811–814, 1987.
5. Desai DC, Neale KF, Talbot IC, Hodgson SV, Phillips RKS. Juvenile polyps. *Br J Surg* 82:14–17, 1995.
6. Latt TT, Nicholl R, Domizio P, Walker-Smith JA, Williams CB. Rectal bleeding and polyps. *Arch Dis Child* 69:144–147, 1993.

Case 16

Clinical Presentation

A newborn boy with no anal opening, noted on physical exam.

Radiographic Studies

Transtabular prone radiograph shows a gas-filled blind rectal pouch ending superior to the pubococcygeal line (Fig. 16A). However, ultrasound (US) demonstrates a low pouch (Fig. 16B) inferior to the bladder. Later contrast enema per ostomy (Fig. 16C) demonstrates a fistula to the membranous urethra and confirms the intermediate type of abnormality.

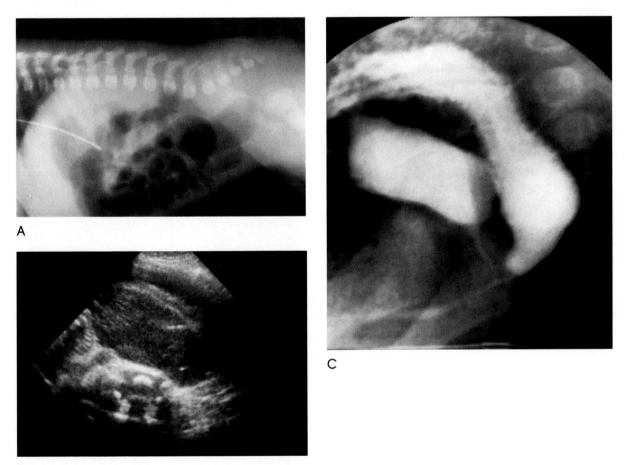

A

B

C

Diagnosis Anorectal Atresia

Discussion and Differential Diagnosis

Anorectal atresia (or imperforate anus) occurs in about 1 in 5000 births.[1] It may be an isolated malformation, but more often (72%)[1] is part of the VACTERL syndrome (vertebral, anal, cardiovascular, tracheoesophageal, renal, limb) or the caudal regression syndrome with a high incidence of associated spinal anomalies. This condition may be diagnosed by fetal US if dilated bowel and associated anomalies are identified.[1] Isolated dilated fetal bowel has many causes, including anorectal atresia.

Delineation of the level of the distal extent of the blind rectal pouch is important in determining surgical management. Three categories are described. If the rectal pouch ends in a supralevator position (above the pubococcygeal line drawn on a lateral film), the condition is considered to be *high*. If it ends at the level of the levator sling, it is placed in the *intermediate* category.[2] These two categories are the most frequent and are managed with a diverting colostomy in the newborn period, followed by a later pull-through procedure. If the blind rectal pouch ends within 1.0 cm (as measured by US) from the perineum, an anoplasty may be performed in the newborn period.

Various methods have been used to define the level of the rectal pouch. The invertogram was first described in the 1930s, but was found to give falsely high levels in many cases. Later, the prone cross-table lateral film was found to be more accurate and safer.[3] Transperineal contrast injection has also been used. Ultrasound evaluation of the blind rectal pouch is now used in many centers. Clinical evaluation of the infant's perineum is probably best to determine whether high or low lesion is present.[4] One perineal opening in a female or a smooth perineum in a male without corrugations is a sign of a high lesion. Perineal fistula and perineal pearls are external signs of a low lesion. Males with external signs of a low lesion but with a fistula into the membranous or bulbous urethra (Fig. 16C) are the intermediate type.[10]

Most (72% of males and 90% of females)[5] babies with imperforate anus will have a fistula to the genitourinary tract or the perineum. Sometimes the fistula is large enough (with or without dilatation) to allow passage of meconium, and no colostomy is needed. Identification of a fistula and delineation of its anatomy is important in surgical planning. This may require a contrast enema through the distal colostomy segment. This procedure can usually define the level of the pouch and opacify a fistula. If the bladder is allowed to fill with contrast until the patient voids, a separate voiding cystogram is not necessary.[6]

Further Reading

1. Harris RD, Nyberg DA, Mack LA, Weinberger E. Anorectal atresia: prenatal sonographic diagnosis. *AJR Am J Roentgenol* 149:395–400, 1987.
2. Stevenson RJ, Sheldon C, Ilstad ST. Percutaneous transperineal pouch localization in low imperforate anus: a new approach. *J Pediatr Surg* 25(2):273–275, 1990.

PITFALLS

- Calcified intraluminal meconium may also be seen in ileal obstruction and multiple atresias.[9]

- The invertogram may be dangerous in patients with an associated distal tracheoesophageal fistula (stomach contents empty into trachea).[12]

- False "high" appearance of the rectal pouch on invertogram can be caused by impacted meconium in the distal pouch (Fig. 16A), decompression of gas through a fistula, or contraction of the levator sling during filming.[5]

CONTROVERSY

- The value of using absolute pouch-perineal US measurements to determine early anoplasty is still being debated.

3. Narasimharao KL, Prasa GR, Katariya S, Yadav K, Mitra SK, Pathak IC. Prone cross-table lateral view: an alternative to the invertogram in imperforate anus. *AJR Am J Roentgenol* 140:227–229, 1983.
4. Seibert JJ, Golladay ES. Clinical evaluation of imperforate anus: clue to type of anal-rectal anomaly. *AJR Am J Roentgenol* 133:289–292, 1979.
5. Donaldson JS, Black CT, Reynolds M, Sherman JO, Shkolnik A. Ultrasound of the distal pouch in infants with imperforate anus. *J Pediatr Surg* 24(5):465–468, 1989.
6. Gross GW, Wolfson PJ, Pena A. Augmented-pressure colostogram in imperforate anus with fistula. *Pediatr Radiol* 21:560–562, 1991.
7. Black CT, Sherman JO. The association of low imperforate anus and Down's syndrome. *J Pediatr Surg* 24(1):92–94, 1989.
8. Currarino G, Coln D, Votteler T. Triad of anorectal, sacral and presacral anomalies. *AJR Am J Roentgenol* 137:395–398, 1981.
9. Anderson S, Savader B, Barnes J, Savader S. Enterolithiasis with imperforate anus: report of two cases with sonographic demonstration and occurrence in a female. *Pediatr Radiol* 18:130–133, 1988.
10. Glasier CM, Seibert JJ, Golladay ES. Intermediate imperforate anus: clinical and radiographic implications. *J Pediatr Surg* 22(4):351–352, 1987.
11. Karrer FM, Flannery AM, Nelson MD Jr, McLone DG, Raffensperger JG. Anorectal malformations: evaluation of associated spinal dysraphic syndromes. *J Pediatr Surg* 23(1):45–48, 1988.
12. Narasimharao KL, Pathak IC. Invertogram in a baby with imperforate anus and esophageal atresia. *AJR Am J Roentgenol* 140:833, 1983. Letter.

Case 17

Clinical Presentation

A 13-year-old boy with acute vomiting and history of 6 weeks of intermittent abdominal pain.

Radiographic Studies

Plain radiograph (Fig. 17A) is unremarkable. Because of patient's atypical history and clinical exam, ultrasound (US) was performed. Ultrasound scan of right lower-quadrant (RLQ) shows noncompressible (Fig. 17B) hyperemic (Fig. 17C, Color Plate 2) bowel measuring 8.1 mm in diameter. Transverse scan reveals a typical "target" appearance (Fig. 17D).

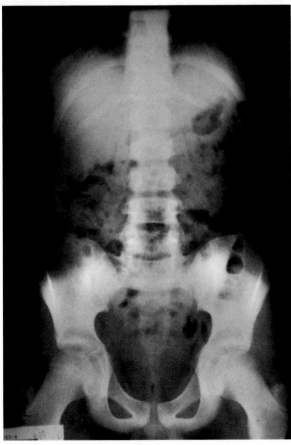

A

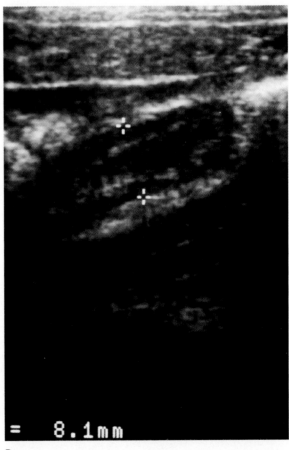

B

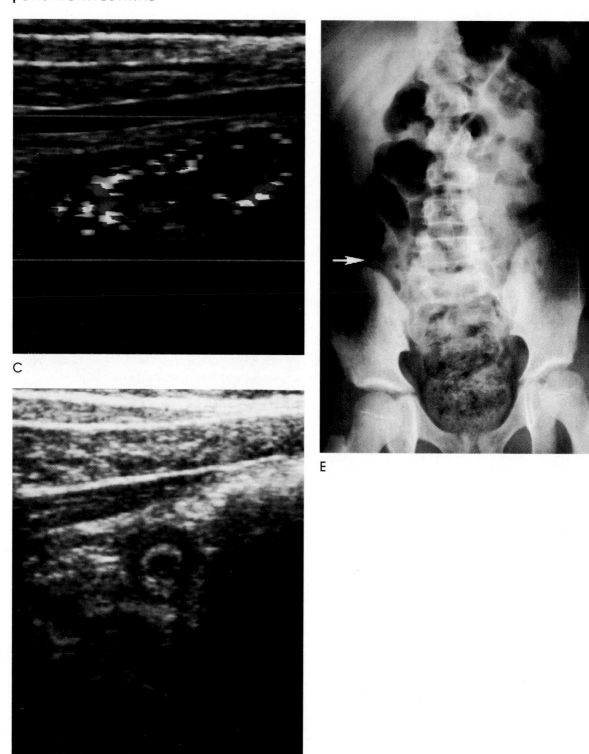

C

D

E

Diagnosis Appendicitis

Discussion and Differential Diagnosis

Acute appendicitis is a common condition in children. Appendectomy is the most common urgent abdominal surgical procedure in children (1% of all operations).[1] Diagnosis is usually made clinically with a 70 to 80% accuracy rate. In the 20 to 30% of cases that are difficult or atypical,[2] imaging procedures are often used. Plain films may be normal (Fig. 17A) or abnormal but are nonspecific unless a fecalith is seen (Fig. 17E, arrow) (10% of cases of appendicitis).[1] Helpful plain radiograph findings include lumbar scoliosis concave to the right, gas-filled small bowel loops with air-fluid levels, and paucity of RLQ gas. If rupture has occurred, a RLQ fluid or extraluminal gas collection may be seen.

In the past, barium enema was used to exclude appendicitis, if the appendix filled completely (but 10% of normal patients have nonfilling), or to confirm a periappendiceal mass. Since the mid-1980s, US has gained acceptance in both academic and community hospitals[3] as the best imaging modality to use in difficult cases. In children, US is found to be 91 to 95%[1,2,4] accurate, with a sensitivity rate of 80 to 88%[5] and specificity of 94 to 98%.[2,5] Ultrasound can decrease the negative laparotomy rate from 20 to 30% to 11 to 13%.[3,5]

The US technique involves graded compression. In appendicitis, the blind-ending appendix will measure greater than 6 mm in diameter and be noncompressible. The surrounding fat may be echogenic.[1] A "target" cross-sectional pattern is usually seen in early disease.[4] A diffusely echolucent appendix represents more advanced inflammation and a higher chance of perforation. Posterior enhancement may indicate imminent rupture.[4]

Doppler US showing hyperemic periappendiceal soft tissue and hyperemic periappendiceal or loculated pelvic fluid[6] are the best US indicators of abscess. Perforation occurs in 15 to 40% of cases.[7] Ultrasound is helpful in patient management because patients with small abscesses usually undergo immediate surgery, but those with a large phlegmon or abscess may be treated with antibiotics and percutaneous drainage followed by delayed appendectomy.[6,7] CT can be helpful to define the extent of abscess prior to drainage.

A negative US examination of the appendix may reveal other causes of symptoms, such as cholelithiasis, gynecological abnormalities, urinary obstruction, inflammatory bowel disease, Burkitt's lymphoma, or intussusception.[1,5,8]

Further Reading

1. Wong ML, Casey SO, Leonidas JC, Elkowitz SS, Becker J. Sonographic diagnosis of acute appendicitis in children. *J Pediatr Surg* 29(10):1356–1360, 1994.
2. Crady SK, Jones JS, Wyn T, Luttenton CR. Clinical validity of ultrasound in children with suspected appendicitis. *Ann Emerg Med* 22(7):1125–1129, 1993.
3. Sabra J, Roh M, Páez X, Cronan J. Use of sonography in diagnosing acute appendicitis: comparison of a teaching hospital and a community hospital. *Acad Radiol* 3:438–441, 1996.

4. Vignault F, Filiatrault D, Brandt ML, Garel L, Grignon A, Ouimet A. Acute appendicitis in children: evaluation with US. *Radiology* 176:501–504, 1990.

5. Chesbrough RM, Burkhard TK, Balsara ZN, Goff WB II, Davis DJ. Self-localization in US of appendicitis: an addition to graded compression. *Radiology* 187:349–351, 1993.

6. Borushok KF, Jeffrey RB Jr, Laing FC, Townsend RR. Sonographic diagnosis of perforation in patients with acute appendicitis. *AJR Am J Roentgenol* 154:275–278, 1990.

7. Quillin SP, Siegel MJ. Diagnosis of appendiceal abscess in children with acute appendicitis: value of color Doppler sonography. *AJR Am J Roentgenol* 164:1251–1254, 1995.

8. Frush D, Beam C, Effmann EL, reviewers. *Invest Radiol* 1992 27:489–490. Critical review of: Vignault F, et al. *Acute appendicitis in children: an evaluation with ultrasound.*

Case 18

Clinical Presentation

A 17-month-old boy presented to the emergency department with jaundice and right upper quadrant mass.

Radiographic Studies

Ultrasound shows a tubular 4 by 2 cm anechoic thick-walled mass extending from the porta hepatis to the pancreatic head. Intrahepatic ducts are not dilated (Fig. 18A). DISIDA (diisopropyl imino diacetic acid) scan demonstrates collection of tracer in both the gallbladder and the cyst at 50 min. Bowel activity is present (Fig. 18B).

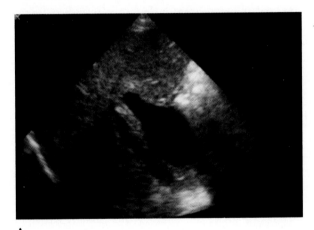

A

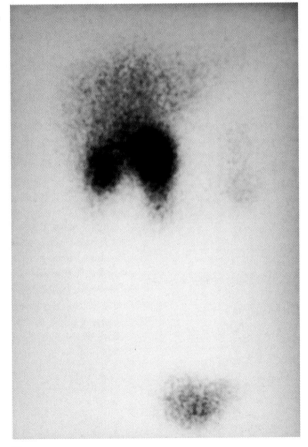

B

Diagnosis Choledochal Cyst

Discussion and Differential Diagnosis

Choledochal cyst is a rare abnormality of the biliary system, which can present at any age, but 60% of cases present before age 10 years.[1] The condition is three times more common in females and more common in Asians. In general, there is dilatation of the extrahepatic or intrahepatic biliary system or both.

The latest classification system by Todani et al[2] includes five main types with several subdivisions of some of the types. Type I, cystic or fusiform dilatation of the common bile duct, is most common (80 to 90%). Type II (2%) has a diverticulum off the common bile duct. Type III cysts (1.4 to 5%) consist of an intraduodenal choledochocele. Type IV (19%) has multiple intra- and extrahepatic cysts, and type V (also known as Caroli disease) has single or multiple intrahepatic cysts.

Choledochal cyst may be congenital (one third of cases),[3] and the remainder acquired in patients (10 to 58%)[4] in whom the junction of the pancreatic duct with the bile duct is more proximal and at a more acute angle than normal. Because the sphincter of Oddi lies distal to the junction and the pressure in the pancreatic duct is higher than in the biliary tree,[1] there is reflux of pancreatic enzymes into the biliary tree. This causes inflammation and fibrosis and results in areas of dilatation and stricture of the biliary tree. In other cases, there is no long common pancreatico-biliary channel and the cause seems to be ductal stenosis. In neonates, biliary atresia may also be present.

Different patterns of ductal dilatation cause different symptoms. In infants with associated distal bile duct atresia, the condition is congenital and commonly presents as obstructive jaundice and acholic stools.[5] Ultrasound demonstrates a cyst, DISIDA confirms cyst accumulation of tracer, and delayed GI excretion confirms the diagnosis. In fusiform dilatation, abdominal pain is the most common symptom. In cystic dilatation, palpable mass and pain are more common. Both children and adults usually have a history of intermittent fever, pain, vomiting, and jaundice related to bouts of cholangitis and pancreatitis.[1]

Ultrasound is usually performed as a screening exam for RUQ pathology. When a choledochal cyst is identified, it is important to completely map out the intra- and extrahepatic anatomy of the cyst.[6] When this is not possible, CT may be necessary. Sometimes the differential diagnosis includes other cystic masses such as duplication cysts, mesenteric, ovarian, renal, adrenal, and pancreatic cysts. In these cases, a DISIDA scan can confirm choledochal cyst by demonstrating connection with the biliary tree. If the biliary tree has not been completely visualized, percutaneous transhepatic cholangiography, endoscopic retrograde cholangiopancreatography, and intraoperative cholangiography may be necessary for surgical planning.[7]

Surgical treatment consists of excision of as much of the cyst as possible to prevent the 4 to 28%[4] incidence of malignancy and cholangitis in retained cysts. Preoperative percutaneous biliary drainage and stent placement may be indicated in some patients.[2] Following cyst resection, Roux-en-Y hepaticojejunostomy is usually performed.

PEARLS

- The classic triad of abdominal pain, jaundice, and RUQ mass is seen in fewer than 30% of patients.[1]

- Especially in infants, cysts may rupture and present with bile peritonitis.[1] Delayed scintigraphic images may show tracer leak.[8]

- Search carefully for stones, which are found in 8%.[9]

- The older the patient at diagnosis, the higher the risk of malignancy.[10]

PITFALLS

- Delayed treatment of choledochal cyst and biliary atresia can result in cirrhosis, portal hypertension, and pancreatitis.[5]

CONTROVERSY

- Some authors believe that type III cysts[11] and Caroli disease (type IV) are entirely different entities and should not be included in the classification of choledochal cysts.[1]

Further Reading

1. Kim OH, Chung HJ, Choi BG. Imaging of the choledochal cyst. *Radiographics* 15:69–88, 1995.
2. Savader SJ, Venbrux AC, Benenati JF, et al. Choledochal cysts: role of noninvasive imaging, percutaneous transhepatic cholangiography, and percutaneous biliary drainage in diagnosis and treatment. *JVIR* 2:379–385, 1991.
3. Yamashiro Y, Sato M, Shimizu T, Oguchi S, Miyano T. How great is the incidence of truly congenital common bile duct dilatation? *J Pediatr Surg* 28(4):622–625, 1993.
4. Savader SJ, Benenati JF, Venbrux AC, et al. Choledochal cysts: classification and cholangiographic appearance. *Am J Roentgenol* 156:327–331, 1991.
5. Torrisi JM, Haller JO, Velcek FT. Choledochal cyst and biliary atresia in the neonate: imaging findings in five cases. *Am J Roentgenol* 155:1273–1276, 1990.
6. Young W, Blane C, White SJ, Polley TZ. Congenital biliary dilatation: a spectrum of disease detailed by ultrasound. *Br J Radiol* 63:333–336, 1990.
7. O'Neill JA Jr. Choledochal cyst. *Curr Probl Surg* 29(6):361–410, 1992.
8. Levine GM, Sziklas JJ, Spencer RP. Bile leak from choledochal cyst in a child. *Clin Nucl Med* 16(9):678–679, 1991.
9. Akhan O, Demirkazik FB, Ozmen MN, Ariyürek M. Choledochal cysts: ultrasonographic findings and correlation with other imaging modalities. *Abdom Imaging* 19:243–247, 1994.
10. Lipsett PA, Pitt HA, Colombani PM, Boitnott JK, Cameron JL. Choledochal cyst disease: a changing pattern of presentation. *Ann Surg* 220(5):644–652, 1994.
11. Apier LN, Crystal K, Kase DJ, Fagelman D, Spier N. Choledochocele: newer concepts of origin and diagnosis. *Surgery* 117(4):476–478, 1995.

Case 19

Clinical Presentation

A 7-day-old 1800-gram male infant fed breast milk via orogastric tube had sudden onset of abdominal distention and gastric residuals.

Radiographic Studies

Abdominal film shows distended bowel loops and subtle pneumatosis in right lower quadrant (RLQ) (Fig. 19A). A left lateral decubitus film taken 4 hours later (Fig. 19B, arrow) demonstrates a large amount of free intraperitoneal air.

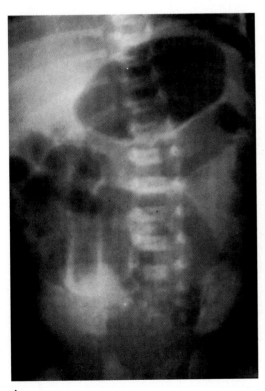

A

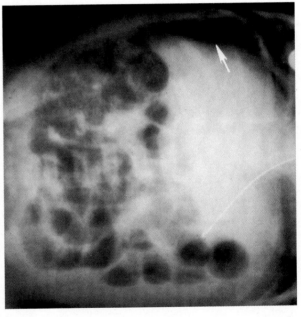

B

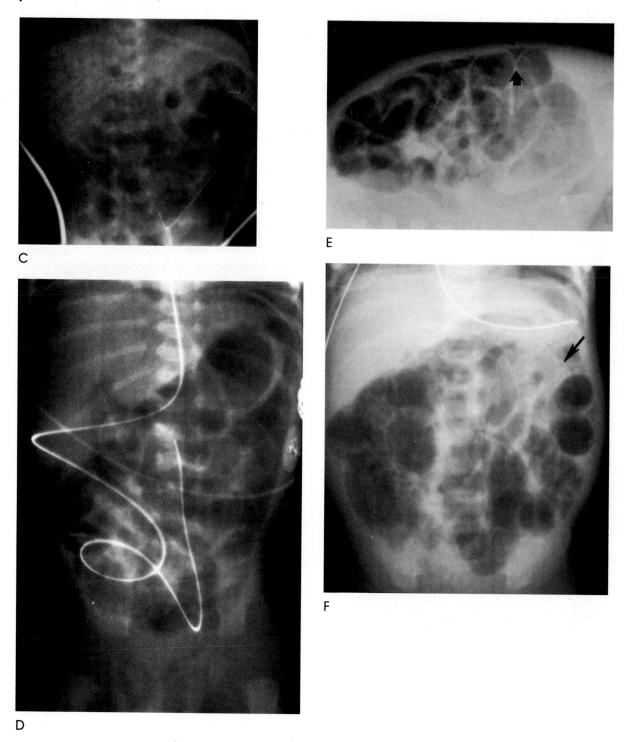

C

D

E

F

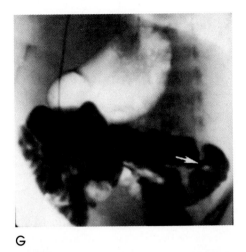

G

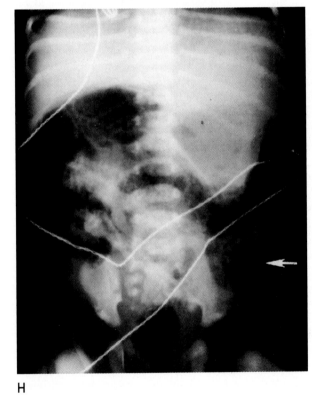

H

I

Diagnosis Necrotizing Enterocolitis (NEC)

Discussion and Differential Diagnosis

Necrotizing enterocolitis is the most common GI emergency in the neonatal intensive care unit (NICU).[1] Ten percent of infants weighing less than 1500 grams have definite NEC and another 17% have possible NEC.[2] Most patients are under 2 weeks of age and are receiving enteral feeds. Clinically, the condition presents as abdominal distention, blood in the stools, feeding residuals, and, in fulminant cases, rapid deterioration and shock. Abdominal radiographs may show a progression from nonspecific dilated bowel loops, to pneumatosis intestinalis, followed by gas in the portal venous system and perforation. However, many cases do not follow this progression, and there is sometimes poor correlation between severity of radiographic findings and clinical disease.[2] Figure 19C shows the first film taken for sudden onset of grossly bloody stools and shock in a 1700-gram infant. Distended bowel loops, pneumatosis, and a large amount of portal venous gas were all present at diagnosis.

In other cases, free air may be the first sign of the disease. Figure 19D shows a 900-gram infant with mild abdominal distention. Gross free air is obvious but no pneumatosis is seen. At surgery, findings typical of NEC were found in the distal ileum. Occasionally, free air may be difficult to confirm. A left lateral decubitus film may demonstrate air between the body wall and liver (Fig. 19B), or a cross-table lateral film may be used. A careful search for a "telltale triangle" of free air (Fig. 19E, arrow) (permission from *J Pediatr Radiol* 5:209–210, 1977) may be required.[3] Visualization of gas on both sides of bowel wall may also be helpful (Fig. 19F, arrow).

Once NEC is suspected clinically or radiographically, serial radiographs (including cross-table lateral or left lateral decubitus views) should be obtained every 4 to 8 hours or more often, until clinical improvement is well established.[4] The detection of free air is indication for surgical intervention.[2] Radiographic portal venous gas is also considered by some surgeons to be an indication for surgery because it is highly associated with bowel necrosis and may precede perforation.[1]

Rare cases may present with ascites, without other radiographic signs of NEC. Ultrasound is helpful in confirming, localizing, and characterizing fluid prior to paracentesis.[5] A fluid-debris level is a sign of occult perforation.

Surgery is required in 50% of cases.[1] The overall survival rate is 70%.[1] Necrotic bowel is resected and enterostomy is performed. Compromised but viable bowel may be left in place and completely recover, or it may heal with stricture formation in 6 to 33% of cases.[4] Contrast enema is usually performed after recovery, before takedown of the ostomy, to identify any significant strictures in the distal bowel (Fig. 19G, arrow). Mild strictures may resolve without resection. Most strictures are single and the splenic flexure (watershed area) is the most common site.[4]

The exact etiology of NEC is unknown. Currently, most experts agree that NEC is a final common pathway for several different insults to the bowel (hypoxia, hyperosmolar feeds, stress, infection, etc.) in a susceptible host with decreased barrier function of the enteric mucosa (impaired immunity, reduced secretory function, decreased blood flow regulation and antioxidant function).[2]

- The bubbly pattern of pneumatosis is often confused with stool and is less specific than the target (Fig. 19I) or linear pattern (Fig. 19H).[4]

- The properitoneal fat line can be confused with the linear pattern.

Necrotizing enterocolitis occasionally occurs in term babies. Forty percent have predisposing risk factors such as hypoxia, hypoglycemia, polycythemia, and respiratory distress.[6] In this group, the disease usually involves the colon, occurs earlier (first 4 days), has fewer systemic symptoms, and has a higher survival rate (90%); most patients (70%) require surgery.[6] Figure 19H shows colonic involvement in a term baby with congenital heart disease.

Further Reading

1. Kosloske AM, Musemeche CA. Necrotizing enterocolitis of the neonate. *Clin Perinatol* 16(1):97–111,1989.
2. Faix RG, Adams JT. Neonatal necrotizing enterocolitis: current concepts and controversies. In: *Advances in Pediatric Infectious Diseases.* St. Louis: Mosby-Year Book; 1994:1–36.
3. Seibert JJ, Parvey LS. The telltale triangle: use of the supine cross table lateral radiograph of the abdomen in early detection of pneumoperitoneum. *Pediatr Radiol* 5:209–210, 1977.
4. Morrison SC, Jacobson JM. The radiology of necrotizing enterocolitis. *Clin Perinatol* 21(2):347–363, 1994.
5. Miller SF, Seibert JJ, Kinder DL, Wilson AR. Use of ultrasound in the detection of occult bowel perforation in neonates. *J Ultrasound Med* 12:531–535, 1993.
6. Andrews DA, Sawin RS, Ledbetter DJ, Schaller RT, Hatch EI. Necrotizing enterocolitis in term neonates. *Am J Surg* 159:507–509, 1990.
7. Edwards DK. Size of gas-filled bowel loops in infants. *AJR Am J Roentgenol* 135:331–334, 1980.

Case 20

Clinical Presentation

A 6-month-old male infant with vomiting and lethargy for 18 hours.

Radiographic Studies

Supine radiograph (Fig. 20A) of the abdomen shows distended bowel loops, no definite colonic air, and the suggestion of a mass in the right upper quadrant (RUQ). Ultrasound (US) shows a "donut" or "target" appearance in cross section with multiple concentric rings (Fig. 20B). Good blood flow in the mass is demonstrated with color flow Doppler (Fig. 20C). Air enema in a different patient confirms a convex filling defect in the colonic air column (Fig. 20D). Air-filled distal ileum and resolution of the filling defect later occur (Fig. 20E).

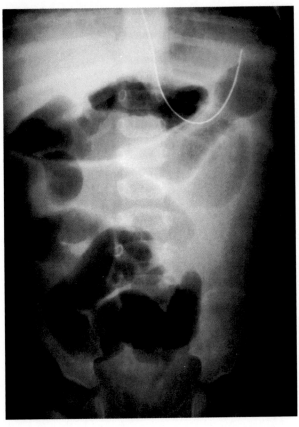

A

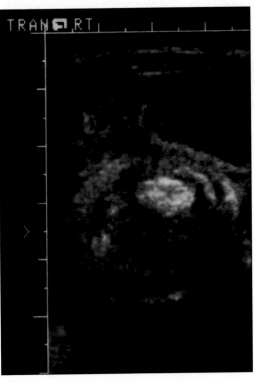

B

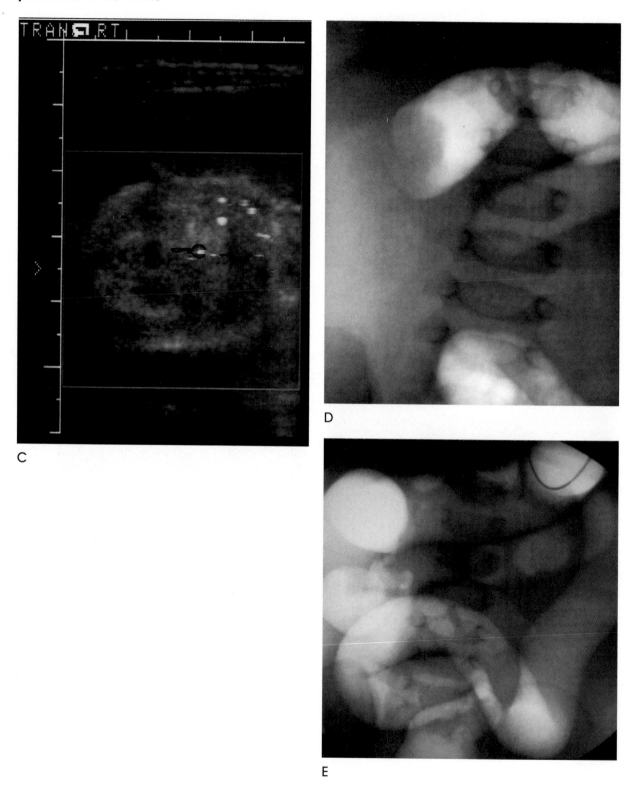

C

D

E

Diagnosis Intussusception

Discussion and Differential Diagnosis

PEARLS

• Intrauterine intussusception is a rare cause of bowel atresia.[10]

• Absolute contraindications to any enema include free air, shock, and peritonitis.[2,6]

• Lead points are more difficult to see with air. In suspicious cases, water-soluble contrast may be helpful.[5]

• Valsalva maneuver may protect against perforation and aid reduction.[8]

PITFALLS

• Air enemas with perforation can cause tension pneumoperitoneum. A 19-gauge needle should be available for rapid decompression.[5]

• Spontaneous reductions may occur after failed enema reduction.[5]

• There is a 7% recurrence rate.[3] Most cases occur in the first week of life.

• "Target" lesions on US may also be seen in feces, psoas muscle, Crohn's disease, hematoma, or volvulus.[6]

Intussusception is a common abdominal emergency in infants and children. Early diagnosis and treatment are important in preventing bowel ischemia and perforation. Although intussusception can occur at any age, most cases present in infants, aged 6 to 12 months, and the condition is more common (72%)[1] in boys. The classic triad of symptoms—intermittent colic, abdominal mass, and blood in the stool—is present in only 43%.[2] One of the most common symptoms is vomiting.[3] Less common presentations are lethargy alone,[4] restless behavior and early shock,[2] or chronic intermittent symptoms.[2]

Most intussusceptions are ileocolic (93%)[5] and are found in the transverse colon or hepatic flexure (88%).[6] Less than 10% of cases, usually the youngest[3] and oldest patients, have a lead point (polyp, Meckel's diverticulum, duplication, mesenteric adenitis).

Plain film diagnosis is definitive in only 21% of cases and equivocal in another 53%, with a diagnostic accuracy of only 40%.[7] The best plain film signs are the presence of a soft tissue mass and decreased colonic gas.[7] Erect and cross-table lateral films are useful only in rare cases with free air at presentation.[7]

Since the mid-1980s, US has been increasingly used for diagnosis, to predict reducibility, and to predict bowel necrosis. The sensitivity and specificity of US for diagnosis is excellent.[1,4,6] The US appearance is a "pseudokidney," "target," or "bulls-eye." Recently, Doppler US has been used for evaluation of blood flow in the intussusceptum (Fig. 20C, Color Plate 3). In cases with absent flow, fewer can be reduced and many are ischemic at surgery. A small amount of pelvic fluid is a common finding and should not be considered a contraindication to enema reduction.[1,6] Interloop fluid, large amounts of pelvic and abdominal fluid[2] (especially if echogenic), and paralytic ileus indicate peritonitis and predict nonreducibility.[2] Further experience may soon allow color Doppler US to be used to predict which patients should be sent directly to surgery because of a high suspicion of bowel gangrene[4] or when not to persist at attempted reduction.

Barium enema has been used for diagnosis and attempted reduction since the 1950s. Success rates range from 45 to 80%.[3,5,8] Perforation rate is less than 1 to 2.5%.[5] Since the mid-1980s, air reduction enema has been widely used. Its advantages: less mess; speed; less radiation; pressure is easier to control with a pump and pressure valve[8]; higher success rate; and perforations are less complicated. Successful reduction rates are higher than for barium enema (56 to 90%).[3,5,8,9] Although the perforation rate is higher than with liquid contrast (2.8%),[5] the rate of complication from surgical repair of perforation is lower.

Reduction rate is lower in cases of ileoileal or ileoileocolic intussusception, rectal bleeding, long duration (> 2 days), prior failed reduction, small bowel obstruction (35% reduced), and age younger than 6 months.[3,5]

- The "crescent in the doughnut sign" on ultrasound, however, is a characteristic feature of intussusception.[11] The crescent is formed by the mesentery enclosing the entering limb of the intussusceptum.

CONTROVERSY

- IV antibiotics, glucagon, and sedation are used in some centers prior to reduction.[12]

Further Reading

1. Lim K, Bae SH, Lee KH, Seo GS, Yoon GS. Assessment of reducibility of ileocolic intussusception in children: usefulness of color Doppler sonography. *Radiology* 191(3):781–785, 1994.
2. Lam AH, Firman K. Value of sonography including color Doppler in the diagnosis and management of long standing intussusception. *Pediatr Radiol* 22:112–114, 1992.
3. McDermott VG, Taylor T, Mackenzie S, Hendry GMA. Pneumatic reduction of intussusception: clinical experience and factors affecting outcome. *Clin Radiol* 49:30–34, 1994.
4. Lagalla R, Caruso G, Novara V, Derchi LE, Cardinale AE. Color Doppler ultrasonography in pediatric intussusception. *J Ultrasound Med* 13:171–174, 1994.
5. Stein M, Alton DJ, Daneman A. Pneumatic reduction of intussusception: 5-year experience. *Radiology* 183(3):681–694, 1992.
6. Verschelden P, Filiatrault D, Garel L, et al. Intussusception in children: reliability of US in diagnosis—a prospective study. *Radiology* 184:741–744, 1992.
7. Sargent MA, Babyn P, Alton DJ. Plain abdominal radiography in suspected intussusception: a reassessment. *Pediatr Radiol* 24:17–20, 1994.
8. Shiels WE II, Maves CK, Hedlund GL, Kirks DR. Air enema for diagnosis and reduction of intussusception: clinical experience and pressure correlates. *Radiology* 181:169–172, 1991.
9. Lee H-C, Yeh H-J, Leu Y-J. Intussusception: the sonographic diagnosis and its clinical value. *J Pediatr Gastroenterol Nutr* 8(3):343–347, 1989.
10. Adejuyigbe O, Odesanmi WO. Intrauterine intussusecption causing intestinal atresia. *J Pediatr Surg* 25(5):562–563, 1990.
11. del-Pozo G, Albillos JC, Tejedor D. Intussusception: US findings with pathologic correlation—the crescent-in-doughnut sign. *Radiology* 199:688–692, 1996.
12. Meyer JS. The current radiologic management of intussusception: a survey and review. *Pediatr Radiol* 22:323–325, 1992.

Case 21

Clinical Presentation

A 13-year-old boy with acute lymphocytic leukemia (ALL) presented to the emergency department with abdominal pain, vomiting, temperature of 101.4°F, neutropenia, thrombocytopenia, and shock 1 week after chemotherapy.

Radiographic Studies

Plain abdominal radiograph (Fig. 21A) shows splinting concave to the right and a generalized paucity of bowel gas. CT scan reveals a markedly thickened cecal wall, but no free fluid (Fig. 21B).

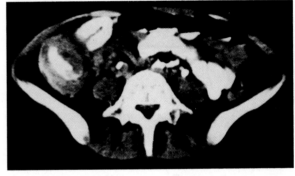

B

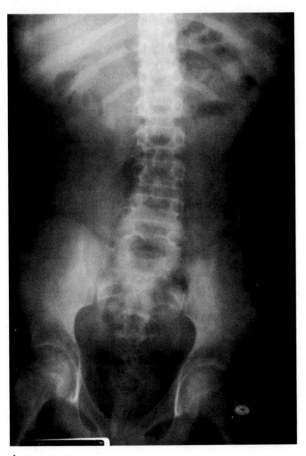

A

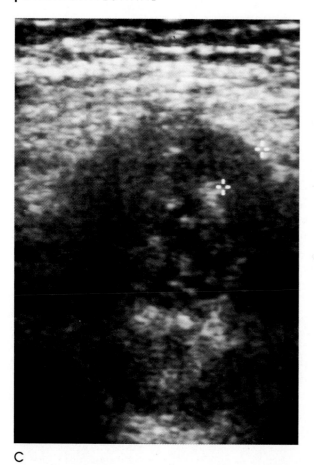

C

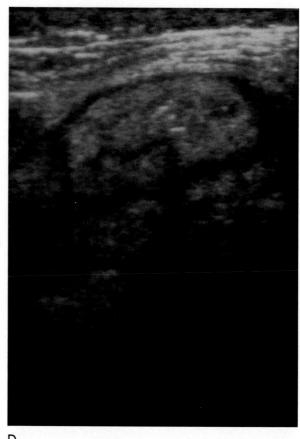

D

Diagnosis Typhlitis

Discussion and Differential Diagnosis

Typhlitis, also known as neutropenic enterocolitis, is a necrotizing colitis that was first described in 1970 as an almost uniformly fatal complication of treatment in childhood leukemia.[1] Since then, it is now known to occur in both children and adults with immune suppression of various etiologies (ALL, acute myelogenous leukemia, lymphoma, aplastic anemia, myelodysplasia, cyclic neutropenia, multiple myeloma, renal and bone marrow transplants, breast cancer, and AIDS).[2–6] Most patients have received chemotherapy, but if the underlying disease causes neutropenia, typhlitis can occur without chemotherapy.

Patients present with nonspecific signs and symptoms including abdominal pain and distention, fever, neutropenia (absolute neutrophil count usually $<0.5 \times 10^9$/ L).[7] Symptoms and physical findings are often suppressed by treatment with steroids and other drugs.

PEARLS

- Typhlitis occurs in 10 to 24% of children with leukemia. It should be suspected in any neutropenic child with abdominal symptoms.[7]

- Typhlitis has a high recurrence rate in medically treated older children and adults.[10]

The cause of typhlitis is unknown, but the number of cases diagnosed is increasing because of better diagnostic imaging and the use of more aggressive chemotherapy.[6] The pathophysiology involves many factors, including dilated cecum with a tenuous blood supply, disruption of mucosal integrity secondary to chemotherapy or leukemic infiltrate, and proliferation of bacteria because of decreased host resistance. Bowel wall necrosis, hemorrhage, perforation, sepsis, and shock may occur. Even with optimum treatment, mortality rates are greater than 50%.[6]

Other conditions such as appendicitis, intussusception, abscess, obstruction, mural hemorrhage, and pseudomembranous colitis[4,8] can have similar clinical and plain radiograph findings.

Barium enema, angiography, CT, and ultrasound have all been used to confirm the diagnosis of typhlitis. Ultrasound is now widely accepted as the preferred diagnostic modality. It provides excellent visualization of the pathology; can usually distinguish typhlitis from other entities in the differential diagnosis; is faster and less risky; and can be performed at the bedside in these often unstable patients.

The characteristic ultrasound appearance is a "target" lesion in the right lower quadrant with thickened bowel wall (Fig. 21C). There may also be marked echogenic thickening of the mucosa, sometimes with a polypoid appearance (Fig. 21D). In the other conditions in the differential diagnosis, the bowel wall thickening is hypoechoic.[8] Because typhlitis can involve only the cecum, cecum and ascending colon, cecum and distal ileum, and cecum and isolated areas of more distal colon, the US exam should attempt to determine extent of disease by following thickened bowel wall proximally and distally to normal bowel.

CT findings are similar to US appearance, with symmetric cecal wall thickening and pericecal inflammation and fluid collection if perforation has occurred.[4] Early diagnosis and determination of extent of disease are necessary so that appropriate medical treatment (bowel rest, normalization of neutrophil counts,[3,6] antibiotics, and fluid management) or surgical intervention can be instituted. Indications for surgery include perforation, persistent bleeding, sepsis that does not respond to medical management, and need for abscess drainage[9] (percutaneous drainage may be indicated).

Further Reading

1. Katz JA, Wagner ML, Gresik MV, Mahoney DH Jr, Fernbach DJ. Typhlitis: an 18-year experience and postmortem review. *Cancer* 65:1041–1047, 1990.
2. Teefey SA, Montana MA, Goldfogel GA, Shuman WP. Sonographic diagnosis of neutropenic typhlitis. *AJR Am J Roentgenol* 149:731–733, 1987.
3. Nagler A, Pavel L, Naparstek E, Muggia-Sullam M, Slavin S. Typhlitis occurring in autologous bone marrow transplantation. *Bone Marrow Transplant* 9:63–64, 1992.
4. Merine D, Nussbaum AR, Fishman EK, Sanders RC. Sonographic observations in a patient with typhlitis. *Clin Pediatr* 28(8):377–379, 1989.
5. Pestalozzi BC, Sotos GA, Choyke PL, et al. Typhlitis resulting from treatment with Taxol and doxorubicin in patients with metastatic breast cancer. *Cancer* 71(5):1797–1800, 1993.

6. Sloas MM, Flynn PM, Kaste SC, Patrick CC. Typhlitis in children with cancer: a 30-year experience. *Clin Infect Dis* 17:484–490, 1993.

7. Paulino AFG, Kenney R, Forman EN, Medeiros LJ. Typhlitis in a patient with acute lymphoblastic leukemia prior to the administration of chemotherapy. *Am J Pediatr Hematol* 16(4):384–351, 1994.

8. Alexander JE, Williamson SL, Seibert JJ, Golladay ES, Jimenez JF. The ultrasonographic diagnosis of typhlitis (neutropenic colitis). *Pediatr Radiol* 18:200–204, 1988.

9. Moir CR, Scudamore CH, Benny WB. Typhlitis: selective surgical management. *Am J Surg* 151(5):563–566, 1986.

10. Keidan RD, Fanning J, Gatenby RA, Weese JL. Recurrent typhlitis: a disease resulting from aggressive chemotherapy. *Dis Colon Rectum* 32(3):206–209, 1989.

11. Rodgers B, Seibert JJ. Unusual combination of an appendicolith in a leukemic patient with typhlitis—ultrasound diagnosis. *J Clin Ultrasound* 18:191–193, 1990.

Case 22

Clinical Presentation

A term male newborn with bilious vomiting and physical examination suggesting Down syndrome.

Radiographic Studies

Plain abdominal film shows a "double-bubble" (Fig. 22A). Upper gastrointestinal series (UGI) confirms duodenal obstruction with a rounded configuration (Fig. 22B).

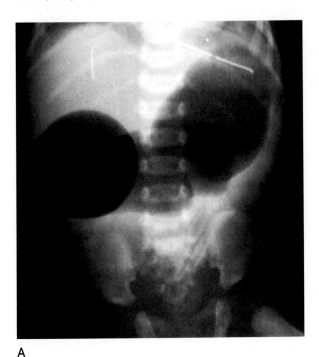

A

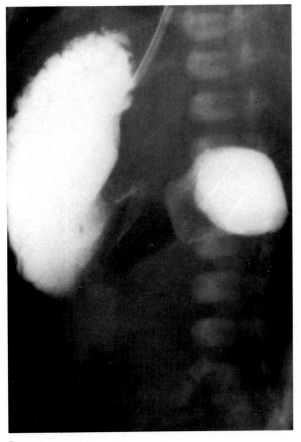

B

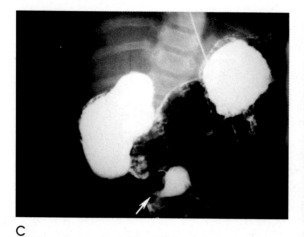

C

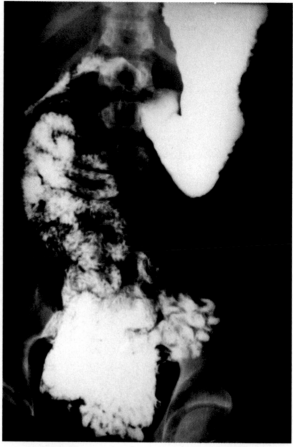

D

Diagnosis Duodenal Obstruction

Discussion and Differential Diagnosis

Many cases of duodenal obstruction are now recognized on fetal ultrasound (US) examination. Duodenal obstruction in the newborn presents as vomiting in 90% of cases. Other clinical signs include abdominal distention and dehydration. Thirty-eight percent of patients have associated anomalies such as Down syndrome, cardiac defects, other GI atresias, and CNS abnormalities.[1] Plain radiographs are diagnostic of duodenal obstruction in 58% of cases,[1] but a contrast UGI is usually performed for confirmation and to determine the cause of obstruction if obstruction is incomplete.

Causes of duodenal obstruction may be divided into two categories: intrinsic (atresia, stenosis, web) or extrinsic (malrotation, peritoneal bands, annular pancreas, duplication and anterior portal vein). Forty-five percent of patients are premature.[1]

Intrinsic forms of obstruction result from the failure of the fetal bowel to the recanalize at 12 weeks after a solid stage of development. Extrinsic causes occur as the result of duplication of the duodenum, abnormal migration of the pancreatic

Barium exam while the patient is symptomatic may detect intermittent volvulus.[7]

- Only 66% of newborns with duodenal obstruction have *bilious* vomiting.[1]

- Orogastric tube may decompress a "double-bubble."

- Situs inversus or massively enlarged liver may also cause reversal of the position of the SMA and SMV.[3]

- Appendicitis will not present in the RLQ in patients with malrotation or nonrotation.

CONTROVERSY

- Surgical treatment of nonrotation is recommended by some surgeons, but not others.

anlage resulting in concentric compression, or abnormalities of rotation (during the 10th fetal week) with resulting bands (Ladd's bands) that can obstruct. Abnormal rotation may predispose to midgut volvulus. Delay in diagnosis of volvulus leads to bowel ischemia, sepsis, perforation, and death or loss of significant small bowel.

If surgery is not performed immediately on the basis of the patient's clinical condition and radiographs, a contrast UGI can confirm obstruction. The cause of the obstruction is often difficult to determine. A rounded contour to the obstruction can be caused by stenosis, annular pancreas, peritoneal bands, or volvulus. If the ligament of Trietz is absent or not in its normal location to the left of the spine and as high as the level of the pylorus,[2] then malrotation is present. If there is also a partial "beaked" obstruction, volvulus is present (Fig. 22C).

However, if obstruction due to volvulus is complete, it usually occurs in the second or third portion of the duodenum so that the position of the ligament of Trietz cannot be determined. A twist may be evident, but the site of obstruction may be indistinguishable from other causes of obstruction. Because of this, and because about one fifth of patients have conditions resulting from a combination of causes,[1] urgent surgery is usually performed in the newborn with duodenal obstruction.

Although 90% of duodenal obstructions present in the first month of life,[2] malrotation may be identified at any age on imaging studies such as barium exams, US, CT, or MRI. Intermittent or chronic volvulus may be the cause of vomiting and abdominal pain in older children and adults. The patient in Figure 22D had intermittent symptoms. There was malrotation without volvulus at the time of the exam. For patients with chronic or intermittent symptoms, US may be the first examination performed. Reversal of the normal position of the superior mesenteric artery (SMA) and superior mesenteric vein (SMV) so that the SMV is located to the left of the SMA suggests malrotation, though this reversal may not always be present.[2] The same finding may be seen on CT or MRI.[3] In addition to SMA-SMV reversal, a dilated proximal duodenum, bowel wall edema, peritoneal fluid and location of jejunum on the right may be seen on US[4] or CT. Engorged mesenteric vessels may be noted on CT[5] in cases of volvulus.

Further Reading

1. Bailey PV, Tracy TF Jr, Connors RH, Mooney DP, Lewis JE, Weber TR. Congenital duodenal obstruction: a 32-year review. *J Pediatr Surg* 28(1):92–95, 1993.
2. Loyer E, Eggli KD. Sonographic evaluation of superior mesenteric vascular relationship in malrotation. *Pediatr Radiol* 19(3):173–175, 1989.
3. Shatzkes D, Gordon DH, Haller JO, Kantor A, De Silva R. Malrotation of the bowel: malalignment of the superior mesenteric artery-vein complex shown on CT and MR. *J Comput Assist Tomogr* 14(1):93–95, 1990.
4. Leonidas JC, Magid N, Soberman N, Glass TS. Midgut volvulus in infants: diagnosis with US. Work in progress. *Radiology* 179(2):491–493, 1991.
5. Mori H, Hayashi K, Futagawa S, Uetani M, Yanagi T, Kurosaki N. Vascular compromise in chronic volvulus with midgut malrotation. *Pediatr Radiol* 17(4):277–281, 1987.

6. Al-Salem AH, Khwaja S, Grant C, Dawodu A. Congenital intrinsic duodenal obstruction: problems in the diagnosis and management. *J Pediatr Surg* 24(12):1247–1249, 1989.
7. Berger RB, Hillemeier AC, Stahl RS, Markowitz RI. Volvulus of the ascending colon: an unusual complication of non-rotation of the midgut. *Pediatr Radiol* 12:298–300, 1982.

Case 23

Clinical Presentation

A 6-hour-old infant with choking during first feeding. Attempt to pass an orogastric tube was unsuccessful.

Radiographic Studies

Chest radiograph (Fig. 23A) shows a dilated air-filled upper esophagus. Coiled orogastric tube is faintly visualized (arrow, Fig. 23B). No upper GI tract air is seen.

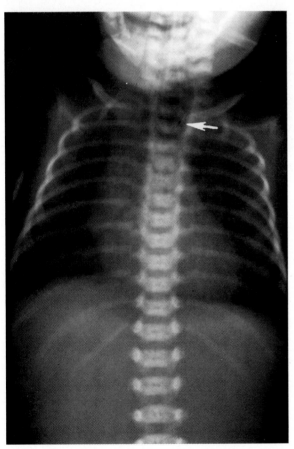

A

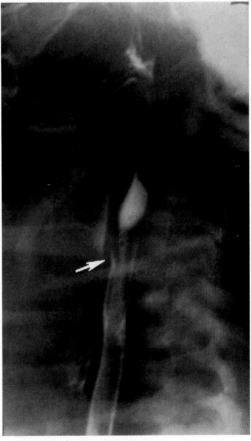

B

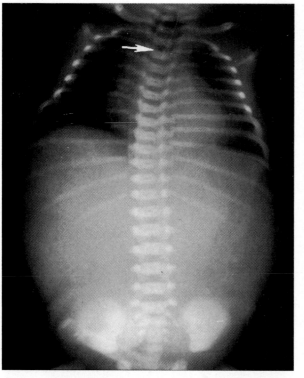

C

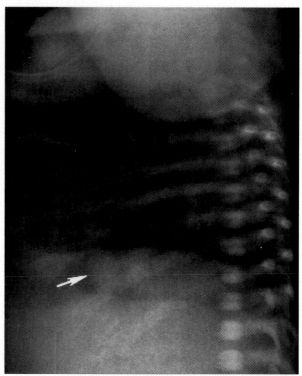

D

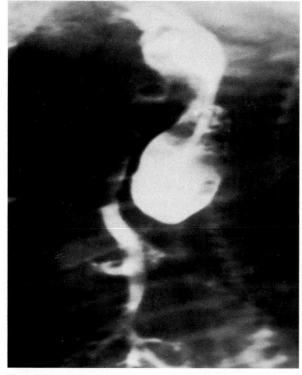

E

Diagnosis Esophageal Atresia (EA) without Tracheoesophageal Fistula (TEF)

Discussion and Differential Diagnosis

- The dilated proximal esophageal pouch in EA is seen intermittently on fetal US. Other fluid collections in the neck (cystic hygroma, teratoma, thyroglossal duct cyst) are more stable.[6]

- EA with duodenal atresia causes more dilatation of the fetal stomach and duodenum than isolated duodenal atresia and the findings are seen earlier (second trimester) than with isolated duodenal atresia (third trimester).[3,7]

- Five percent of patients with TEF have a right aortic arch. Knowing the side of the arch is important for surgical planning.

PITFALLS

- When contrast is injected for diagnosis of an H-type fistula, overdistention may cause aspiration from above that can mimic contrast in the trachea from a fistula. Video recording can prevent confusion.

Esophageal atresia and tracheoesophageal fistula result from abnormal separation of the primitive foregut into trachea and tubular esophagus. The separation occurs during weeks four or five of fetal life. These anomalies are part of the VACTERL (*v*ertebral, *a*nal, *c*ardiac, *t*racheal, *e*sophageal, *r*enal, and *l*imb) association in 30% of cases of EA with TEF. In cases with EA but no TEF, Down syndrome and other GI atresias are the most common coexisting abnormalities.[1]

Eight-two percent of cases have esophageal atresia with a fistula between the ventral surface of the distal esophagus and the distal trachea. Nine percent of cases have EA without a fistula (Fig. 23A). These two most common forms of the anomaly can be differentiated by the presence of GI tract air. Rarely, there is a fistula between the blind upper esophagus pouch and the trachea (1%) or between the proximal and distal ends of a discontinuous esophagus and the trachea (2%). In the H-type fistula, the esophagus is a continuous tube, but there is a fistula off its ventral wall into the posterior wall of the trachea (6%) (Fig. 23B, arrow).

In the most common forms, the newborn presents with excessive oral secretions, failure of a routinely placed enteric tube to pass, or regurgitation of the initial feed.[2] The atresia is usually at the level of the junction of the proximal one third and distal two thirds of the esophagus. Because the proximal pouch is intermittently dilated in utero, it may be visualized on prenatal ultrasound (US). If polyhydramnios and a small stomach are also seen, EA should be suspected. The dilated proximal pouch may also compress the fetal trachea and cause tracheomalacia.

In cases of EA without TEF and duodenal atresia, the distal esophagus, stomach, and duodenum are dilated and form a C-shaped fluid collection in the fetal abdomen and a fluid collection behind the heart on prenatal US.[3] Postnatal radiographs demonstrate an air-filled proximal esophageal pouch, a distended gasless abdomen, and a retrocardiac density (Figs. 23C, 23D, arrows).

The diagnosis of esophageal atresia can be made on plain radiographs and is usually confirmed with the visualization of a feeding tube tip or coil at the distal end of the pouch. Air may be injected for confirmation. The presence of air in the GI tract confirms a distal fistula. The injection of contrast into the pouch can cause aspiration with secondary respiratory compromise[2] (Fig. 23E).

Patients with a fistula from the upper esophagus to the trachea may present with severe respiratory distress and pulmonary infiltrates secondary to aspiration of saliva and feeds. An H-type fistula may have more subtle clinical signs and present later as coughing while the infant is feeding. Contrast must usually be used for diagnosis of H-type fistulas. Careful fluoroscopic technique includes placing the infant in the right anterior oblique (RAO) or near-prone position or using a horizontal beam while the infant swallows isotonic nonionic contrast, or careful injection of contrast through an enteric tube while it is slowly withdrawn from the esophagus with the patient in the RAO position. Repeat exams may be required to identify a small fistula.

Postoperative complications and sequelae of EA repair are common and often require multiple radiographic diagnostic procedures. They include tracheomalacia, anastamotic leaks, recurrent fistula, anastomotic stricture (frequently presenting with foreign body impaction), and gastroesophageal reflux and esophageal dysmotility.[4,5]

Further Reading

1. Cumming WA. Esophageal atresia and tracheoesophageal fistula. *Radiol Clin North Am* 13(2):277–295, 1975.
2. Hicks LM, Mansfield PB. Esophageal atresia and tracheoesophageal fistula. Review of thirteen years' experience. *J Thorac Cardiovasc Surg* 81:358–363, 1981.
3. Estroff JA, Parad RB, Share JC, Benacerraf BR. Second trimester prenatal findings in duodenal and esophageal atresia without tracheoesophageal fistula. *J Ultrasound Med* 13:375–359, 1994.
4. Spitz L, Kiely E, Brereton RJ. Esophageal atresia: five year experience with 148 cases. *J Pediatr Surg* 22(2):103–108, 1987.
5. Griscom NT, Martin TR. The trachea and esophagus after repair of esophageal atresia and distal fistula: computed tomographic observations. *Pediatr Radiol* 20:447–450, 1990.
6. Satoh S, Takashima T, Takeuchi H, Koyanagi T, Nakano H. Antenatal sonographic detection of the proximal esophageal segment: specific evidence for congenital esophageal atresia. *J Clin Ultrasound* 23(7):419–423, 1995.
7. Kessel D, de Bruyn R, Drake D. Case report: ultrasound diagnosis of duodenal atresia combined with isolated oesophageal atresia. *Br J Radiol* 66(781):86–88, 1993.
8. Rideout DT, Hayashi AH, Gillis DA, Giacomantonio JM, Lau HYC. The absence of clinically significant tracheomalacia in patients having esophageal atresia without trachoesophageal fistula. *J Pediatr Surg* 26(11):1303–1305, 1991.

Case 24

Clinical Presentation

A 4-year-old boy with bilious vomiting was brought to the emergency department. Later, a detailed history revealed a history of being "punched in the stomach" by an uncle who was baby-sitting.

Radiographic Studies

Upper gastrointestinal series (UGI) (Fig. 24A) shows obstruction of the second portion of the duodenum by a mass. Ultrasound (US) identified a 4 × 5 cm echogenic mass between the duodenum and gallbladder (Fig. 24B).

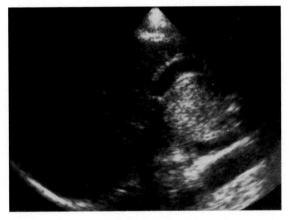

B

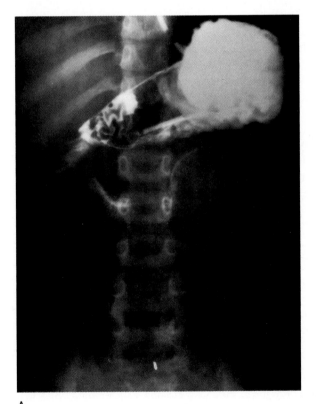

A

Diagnosis Duodenal Hematoma

Discussion and Differential Diagnosis

Blunt abdominal trauma occurs in about 0.5% of cases of child abuse. The mortality rate is 45%.[1] Injuries can include duodenal hematoma, pancreatic injury, duodenojejunal rupture, and solid organ laceration. Mortality rates are higher in children with massive hemorrhage[1] and multiple injuries.[2]

Duodenal hematoma is usually treated conservatively and resolves without sequelae in less than 10 days.[2] The classic appearance of duodenal hematoma on UGI, first described by Felson, includes duodenal obstruction, intramural mass, and a coiled spring appearance of the mucosa.[3] Irregular tapered narrowing, "picket fence" edema, and nodular filling defects may also be present.[4]

On US, a duodenal hematoma has a sonolucent rim with echogenic mucosa acutely. A clot goes through an echogenic stage and later may show fluid-fluid levels and septa as it resolves.[5] Ultrasound is useful for following resolution of the hematoma and associated solid organ and pancreatic injuries.

Some children who suffer blunt abdominal trauma as the result of child abuse, playground accidents, or motor vehicle accidents will also sustain rupture of the duodenum or jejunum. These injuries require urgent surgical treatment.[6] CT imaging using oral contrast and careful technique[7] can separate these cases from those that can be managed without surgery. Findings of thickened duodenal wall, intraperitoneal fluid, fluid in the right perirenal space and right anterior pararenal space, as well as solid viscera injury, may be seen in both duodenal hematoma and duodenal rupture.[6] However, gas and/or extravasated oral contrast in the right anterior pararenal space are indications of duodenal rupture.[6] The mechanism of injury is rapid compression of involved organs against the spine.[1]

Further Reading

1. Cooper A, Floyd T, Barlow B, et al. Major blunt abdominal trauma due to child abuse. *J Trauma* 28(10):1483–1487, 1988.
2. Winthrop AL, Wesson DE, Filler RM. Traumatic duodenal hematoma in the pediatric patient. *J Pediatr Surg* 21(9):757–760, 1986.
3. Felson B, Levin EJ. Intramural hematoma of the duodenum. *AJR Am J Roentgenol* 63:823–829, 1954.
4. Hughes JJ, Brogdon BG. Computed tomography of duodenal hematoma. *CT: J Comput Tomogr* 10(3):231–236, 1986.
5. Hayashi K, Futagawa S, Kozaki S, Hirao K, Hombo Z. Ultrasound and CT diagnosis of intramural duodenal hematoma. *Pediatr Radiol* 18:167–168, 1988.
6. Kunin JR, Korobkin M, Ellis JH, Francis IR, Kane NM, Siegel SE. Duodenal injuries caused by blunt abdominal trauma: value of CT in differentiating perforation from hematoma. *AJR Am J Roentgenol* 160:1221–1223, 1993.

PEARLS

- Delay in seeking medical help averages 13 hours after it is obvious that child is moribund. Delay may result from fear of discovery and/or lack of recognition of severity of injury.[1]

- Presenting symptoms relate to the injured organ in stable milder injuries. Hemodynamically unstable patients present with a history of "coma" of unknown cause following mild trauma such as a "bump on the head" or "fall from bed."[1]

- Bicycle handlebar accidents can cause identical abdominal injury but most such injuries caused by abuse will have associated head, soft tissue, and skeletal injuries typical of child abuse.[1]

PITFALLS

- Introduction of air during peritoneal lavage can cause small gas bubbles in the peritoneal cavity in the absence of rupture.[6]

- Intraperitoneal air in duodenal perforation may be caused by rupture of the intraperitoneal portion of the duodenum or traumatic disruption of the peritoneal membrane with escape of gas from the retroperitoneum.[6]

- An intussusception may have a similar appearance on US, but the location of a hematoma and lack of alternating echogenic and lucent bands should help to differentiate the two.[8]

7. Mirvis SE, Gens DR, Shanmuganathan K. Rupture of the bowel after blunt abdominal trauma: diagnosis with CT. *AJR Am J Roentgenol* 159:1217–1221, 1992.
8. Orel SG, Nussbaum AR, Sheth S, Yale-Loehr A, Sanders RC. Duodenal hematoma in child abuse: sonographic detection. *AJR Am J Roentgenol* 151:147–149, 1988.

Case 25

Clinical Presentation

A 3-day-old male infant with delayed passage of meconium and persistent abdominal distention. Barium enema at outside hospital at 24 hours of age was interpreted as normal.

Radiographic Studies

Plain radiographs show complete clearance of previously administered barium and multiple dilated loops of bowel with air-fluid levels and no gas in the rectum (Figs. 25A, 25B). Water-soluble contrast enema demonstrates a funnel-shaped narrowing of dilated colon at the rectosigmoid junction with a transition into smaller-than-normal-caliber rectum (rectosigmoid ratio less than 1:1) (Figs. 25C, 25D).

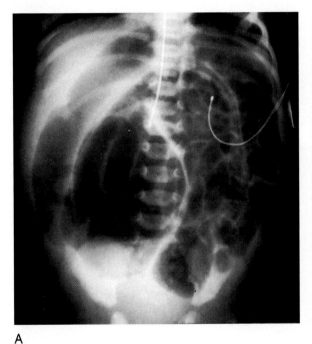

A

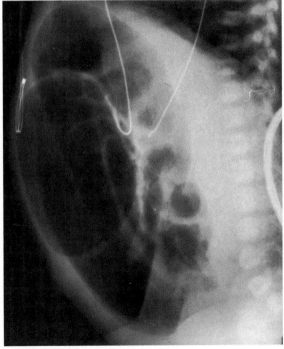

B

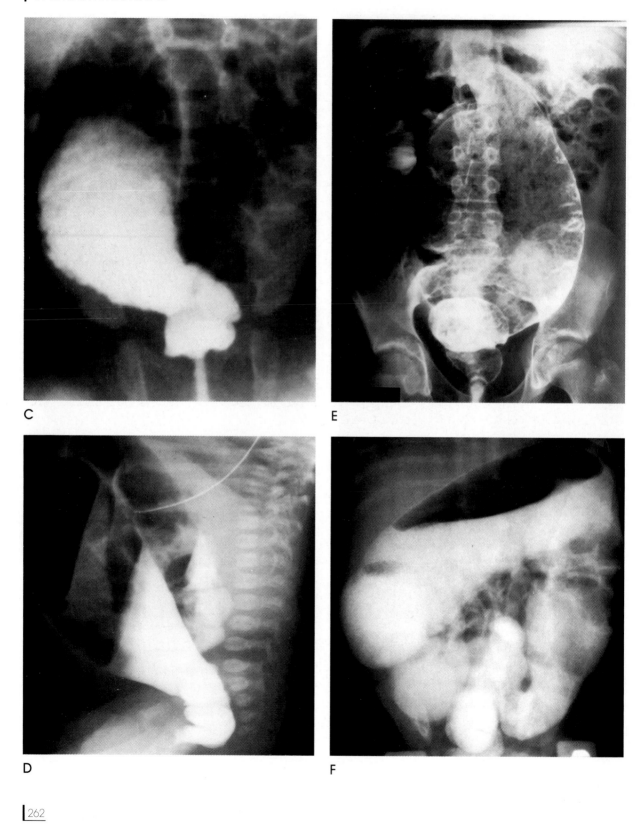

C

D

E

F

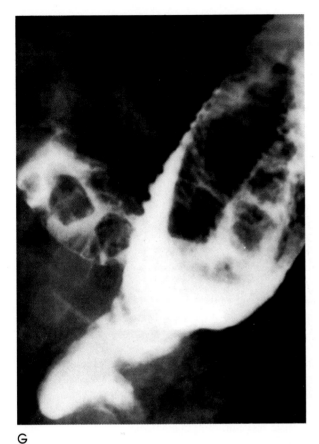

G

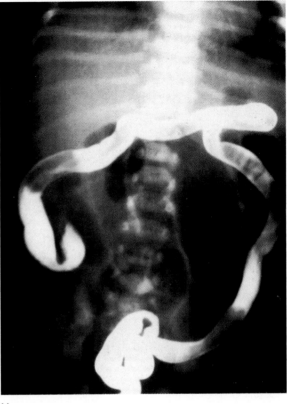

H

Diagnosis Hirschsprung's Disease

Discussion and Differential Diagnosis

Hirschsprung's disease is an important cause (1 in 5000 live births)[1] of distal bowel obstruction in the newborn and constipation in infants and children. It results from the absence of ganglion cells in the myenteric plexus of the colon. Normal colonic peristalsis does not propagate feces through the aganglionic segment. The segment remains contracted and causes functional obstruction at the level of the zone of transition from normal to aganglionic bowel. Most (67%) cases involve the rectum or rectosigmoid, 15% the left colon, 9% the proximal colon, and 9% the entire colon.[1] Three fourths of patients are diagnosed in the first year of life.[1] In the neonatal period, Hirschsprung's disease presents as failure to pass meconium in the first 48 hours (37%), abdominal distention, bilious vomiting, and, rarely, enterocolitis[1] or perforation.[2]

Older infants and children, and even adults, present with lifelong constipation and intermittent abdominal distention. Figure 25E shows a barium enema of an

(4%),[8] and neurocristopathies (neuroblastoma, pheochromocytoma, neurofibromatosis, Waardenburg's syndrome, multiple endocrine neoplasia II).[3]

- Infants with long segment or total colonic Hirschsprung's disease may present with isolated perforation of the appendix, ascending colon, or distal ileum, and this condition should be suspected in infants who present with unexplained pneumoperitoneum.[9]

- Adults may have undiagnosed Hirschsprung's disease. This is more common in females; the presentation is of long-term constipation and increasing abdominal girth.[10]

- Diagnostic contrast enemas for children with constipation should be done on an unprepped colon. Vigorous prep can obscure the zone of transition.

PITFALLS

- Patients with Hirschsprung's disease can have enterocolitis before *and* after surgical treatment. A few of these patients will have pseudomembranous colitis that can be rapidly fatal without prompt treatment. These diagnoses should be considered in any patient with Hirschsprung's disease who

11-year-old boy with constipation since birth and a narrowed, spastic rectosigmoid colon. The most common form of the disease, this obstruction at the rectosigmoid junction is four times more common in boys.

Abdominal radiographs show dilated gas- and stool-filled proximal bowel to the level of the zone of transition, usually in the sigmoid. There may be absence of rectal air (Figs. 25A, 25B) or a prone cross-table lateral film may demonstrate air in a small rectum.

In the newborn, the differential diagnosis, based on clinical findings and radiographs, includes other forms of distal small bowel and colon obstruction (meconium plug, small left colon, meconium ileus, colon atresia). The diagnosis is made by performing contrast enema on an unprepped colon. Contrast is introduced per rectum with the patient in the lateral position. Rectal and distal sigmoid caliber is usually smaller than normal. At the level of transition to normally innervated colon (the *zone of transition*), the contrast fills dilated, stool-filled bowel. If the zone of transition is in its most common location, the rectum or sigmoid, the caliber of the rectum will be smaller than the caliber of the sigmoid colon (less than 1:1). The normal rectosigmoid ratio is 1.2 to 1.4:1.[3]

The transition zone is identified in only 80% of infants with Hirschsprung's disease and a suspected transition zone can be seen in infants without Hirschsprung's disease.[4,5] In difficult cases, other helpful findings on barium exam include retained barium mixed with stool on 24- and 48-hour delayed films (Fig. 25F) and/or abnormal muscular contractions at or distal to the zone of transition on postevacuation, early delayed, or 24-hour radiographs (Fig. 25G).

Diagnosis is often confirmed by suction biopsy[4] and/or anorectal manometry[6] before surgical treatment.

Treatment consists of surgical resection of aganglionic bowel with an anal pull-through procedure (Duhamel, Soave, Swenson).[1] Two thirds of patients have normal postoperative bowel habits, and both constipation and soiling improve with time.[1] Laparoscopic pull-through procedures have recently been performed.[7]

Further Reading

1. Rescorla FJ, Morrison AM, Engles D, et al. Hirschsprung's disease. Evaluation of mortality and long-term function in 260 cases. *Arch Surg* 127(8):934–941, 1992.
2. Newman B, Nussbaum A, Kirkpatrick JA Jr. Bowel perforation in Hirschsprung's disease. *Am J Roentgenol* 148(6):1195–1197, 1987.
3. McAlister WH, Kronemer KA. Emergency gastrointestinal radiology of the newborn. *Radiol Clin North Am* 34(4):819–844, 1996.
4. Taxman TL, Yulish BS, Rothstein FC. How useful is the barium enema in the diagnosis of infantile Hirschsprung's disease? *Am J Dis Child* 140(9):881–884, 1986.
5. Rosenfield NS, Ablow RC, Markowitz RI, et al. Hirschsprung disease: accuracy of the barium enema examination. *Radiology* 150(2):393–400, 1984.
6. Lanfranchi GA, Bazzocchi G, Federici S, et al. Anorectal manometry in the diagnosis of Hirschsprung's disease—comparison with clinical and radiological criteria. *Am J Gastroenterol* 79(4):270–275, 1984.

presents with fever, abdominal distention, and diarrhea.[11]

- The colon may appear normal or almost normal in cases of total colonic involvement with Hirschsprung's disease. Usually it will appear slightly decreased in length and caliber throughout and may have the appearance of an adult colon rather than the usual redundant infant colon (Fig. 25H).

- In long-segment disease, the radiographic transition zone may lie distal to the pathologic transition zone. Delayed films may identify the true location more accurately.[12]

CONTROVERSY
- The use of 24- and/or 48-hour follow-up films following barium enema has been found to be helpful by some authors[1,12] and not helpful by others.[3,4]

7. Georgeson KE, Fuenfer MM, Hardin WD. Primary laparoscopic pull-through for Hirschsprung's disease in infants and children. *J Pediatr Surg* 30(7):1017–1021, 1995.
8. Ryan ET, Ecker JL, Christakis NA, Folkman J. Hisrschsprung's disease: associated abnormalities and demography. *J Pediatr Surg* 27(1):76–81, 1992.
9. Newman B, Nussbaum A, Kirkpatrick JA Jr, Colodny A. Appendiceal perforation, pneumoperitoneum, and Hirschsprung's disease. *J Pediatr Surg* 23(9):854–856, 1988.
10. Hung WT, Chiang TP, Tsai YW, et al. Adult Hirschsprung's disease. *J Pediatr Surg* 24(4):363–366, 1989.
11. Bagwell CE, Langham MR Jr, Mahaffey SM, et al. Pseudomembranous colitis following resection for Hirschsprung's disease. *J Pediatr Surg* 27(10):1261–1264, 1992.
12. Johnson JF, Cronk RL. The pseudotransition zone in long segment Hirschsprung's disease. *Pediatr Radiol* 10(2):87–89, 1980.

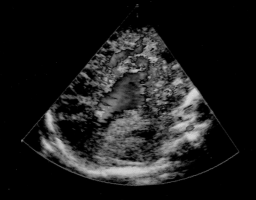

Color Plate 1.

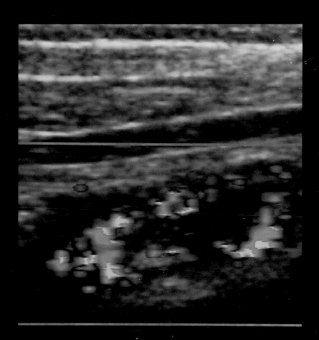

Color Plate 2.

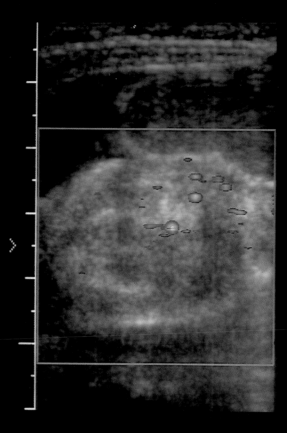

Color Plate 3.

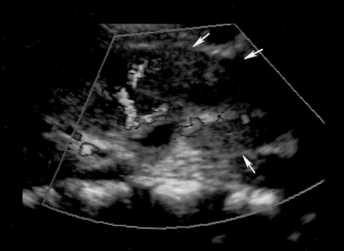

Color Plate 4.

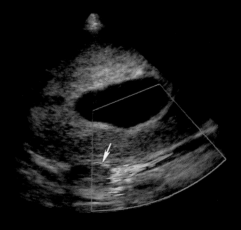

Color Plate 5.

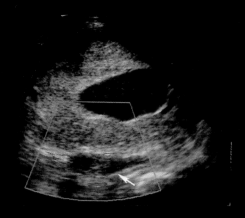

Color Plate 6.

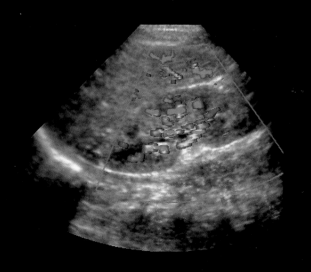

Color Plate 7.

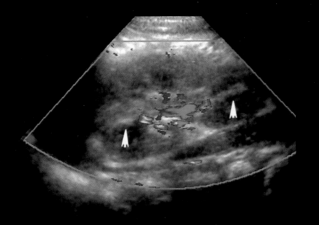

Color Plate 8.

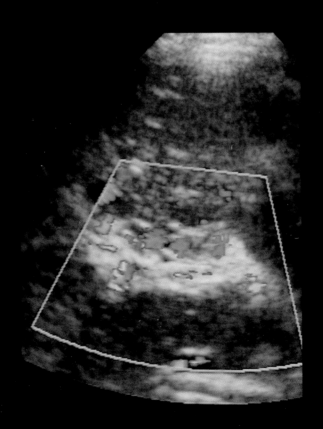

Color Plate 9.

GENITOURINARY

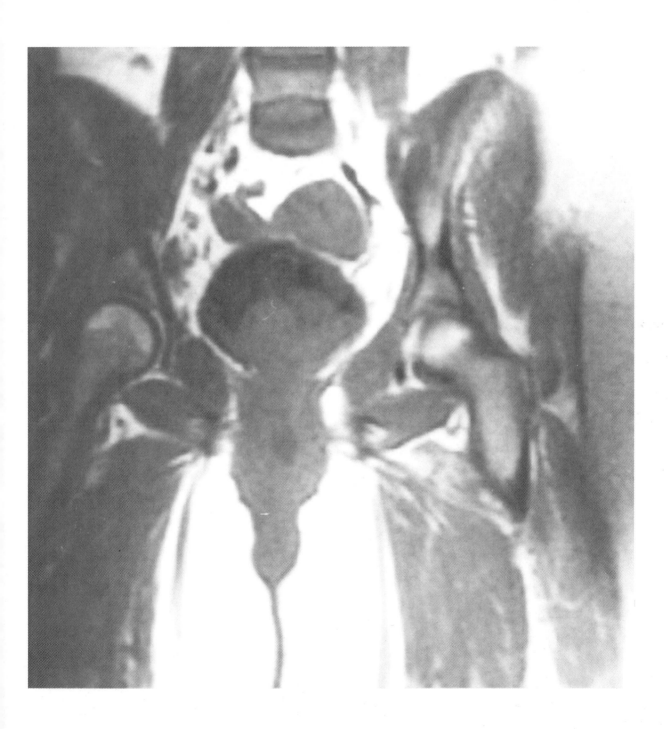

Case 1

Clinical Presentation

A 3-year-old boy with a history of urinary tract infection.

Radiographic Studies

Oblique view from a voiding cystourethrogram (Fig. 1A) shows reflux into the distal ureter (arrowhead), as well as into a periureteral outpouching (black arrows) near the ureterovesical junction. A post-void anteroposterior (AP) view of the bladder from a voiding cystourethrogram (Fig. 1B) shows residual urine in bilateral structures (arrows) with nearly empty bladder.

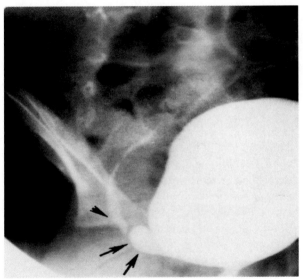 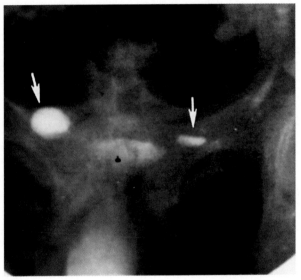

A   B

Diagnosis Bladder Diverticulum: Hutch Diverticulum with Reflux

Discussion and Differential Diagnosis

Bladder diverticula are usually best seen on oblique, lateral, or post-void images from a voiding cystourethrogram. The high pressure generated during micturition fills the bladder diverticula with contrast.[1] Post-void films usually show residual contrast in the diverticula because of delayed or incomplete diverticula emptying.[2]

Ultrasound may be useful in identifying diverticula, but they are sometimes difficult to distinguish from other cystic pelvic masses. However, color flow Doppler studies of the diverticula have been described as showing a "diverticular jet effect" because of alternating bidirectional fluid shift between the bladder and the diverticulum.[3] This jet phenomenon is probably secondary to differences in urine densities between the urine in the diverticulum and that in the bladder.[3]

A bladder diverticulum is usually secondary to protrusion of bladder mucosa through a congenital defect in the bladder muscular wall. A "Hutch" diverticulum is usually defined as a diverticulum at or near the ureterovesical junction in a patient with an otherwise normal bladder.[1] The incidence of bladder diverticula has been reported to be 1.7%, in a recent study of 5000 pediatric patients in a genitourinary database.[4] Of these patients with bladder diverticula, the incidence of reflux is reported to be as high as 93%.[5]

Bladder diverticula in children have been divided into four groups.[1,4] Primary diverticula are simply secondary to protrusion of the bladder mucosa through the bladder muscular wall. The majority of primary diverticula are Hutch diverticula at or near the ureterovesical junction.[1,2,4,6] If the Hutch diverticula are separate from the ureteral orifice, then they may be asymptomatic.[1] If, however, the ureteral orifice intersects the rim of the diverticulum or actually drains into the diverticulum, then frequently vesicoureteral reflux is present, especially as the diverticulum enlarges. When the diverticulum becomes markedly enlarged, it may actually cause obstruction of the distal ureter, or displace the bladder and cause urethral obstruction.[1] A variant of a periureteral diverticulum occurs when an ureterocele intussuscepts on itself during voiding and protrudes through the posterior bladder wall, usually at or near the ureterovesical junction.[1] Other locations of primary bladder diverticula are less common and usually insignificant unless there is urine stasis or urinary obstruction. Primary diverticula may present special problems in the newborn if diverticular size becomes so large that it causes bladder outlet obstruction or hydronephrosis.[1,5]

The second group of bladder diverticula are secondary to bladder outlet obstruction (usually secondary to posterior urethral valves, urethral strictures, or large ureteroceles),[4] or secondary to a neurogenic bladder (usually in patients with meningomyelocele/meningocele).[1,4] Bladder diverticula are uncommon in these patients; more often there is a "cellule or saccule"[1] protrusion of the bladder mucosa between hypertrophied muscle bundles rather than formation of a true bladder diverticulum.

The third group of bladder diverticula is usually iatrogenic, postsurgical in nature.[1,4] Causes include ureteral reimplantation, bladder wall weakness at the site of a previous suprapubic tube, or diverticula formation in patients who are status

diverticulum is mistaken for the bladder.[6]

- Large bladder diverticula may be difficult to differentiate from other cystic pelvic masses.[3,5]

CONTROVERSY

- Ultrasound is a rapid, inexpensive, noninvasive method of diagnosing bladder diverticula, especially if the diverticular jet effect is identified at color Doppler ultrasound.[3,5] However, most authors still advocate voiding cystourethrography as the imaging modality of choice because of the excellent visualization of bladder contour during high pressure voiding, and because of the easy visualization of associated vesicoureteral reflux.

post-repair of high anorectal malformations, with imperforate anus.[1,4]

The fourth group of bladder diverticula occurs in patients with syndromes associated with abnormal collagen structure/function or abdominal wall muscular weakness, including prune-belly syndrome, kinky-hair syndrome, Williams syndrome, Ehlers-Danlos syndrome, or cutis laxa.[2,4,6]

Bladder diverticula are usually resected if they are greater than 3 cm in length or if they are associated with urinary tract infection, reflux, or obstruction.[5] If they are associated with reflux, surgical reimplantation of the ureter is usually performed at the time of diverticulum resection.[5] If patients are asymptomatic with a small diverticulum, surgery may be avoided, but they must be followed closely because the diverticulum tends to enlarge with time and to cause urinary stasis with infection.[5]

Diverticula are usually best visualized with voiding cystourethrogram and/or ultrasound. Voiding cystourethrogram studies must include oblique and lateral views to visualize the region near the trigone, and the patient must be carefully monitored with fluoroscopy during voiding because bladder diverticula are best visualized during high pressure micturition.[1] Ultrasound identifies the bladder diverticula, and color Doppler ultrasound can identify the "diverticular jet effect" with the application of gentle abdominal palpation as previously described.[3,7]

The differential diagnosis of bladder diverticula includes ovarian cysts, seminal vesicle cysts, ascites, and intraperitoneal collections of cerebral spinal fluid secondary to ventriculoperitoneal shunt tube.[3] The entities may be difficult to differentiate at ultrasound, unless the diverticular jet effect is identified, localizing the point of communication between the diverticulum and the bladder.[3,5] However, a voiding cystourethrogram usually differentiates these entities.

Further Reading

1. Boechat MI, Lebowitz RL. Diverticula of the bladder in children. *Pediatr Radiol* 7:22–28, 1978.
2. Kelalis PP, King LR, Belman AB. *Clinical Pediatric Urology, II.* 3rd ed. Philadelphia: WB Saunders Co; 1992:612.
3. Weingardt JP, Nemcek AA Jr, Miljkovic SC. The diverticular jet effect: color Doppler differentiation of bladder diverticula from other pelvic fluid collections. *J Clin Ultrasound* 22(6):397–400, 1994.
4. Blane CE, Zerin JM, Bloom DA. Bladder diverticula in children. *Radiology* 190:695–697, 1994.
5. Vates TS, Fleisher MH, Siegel RL. Acute urinary retention in an infant: an unusual presentation of a paraureteral diverticulum. *Pediatr Radiol* 23:371–372, 1993.
6. Carty H, Brunelle F, Shaw D, Kendall B, eds. *Imaging Children.* New York: Churchill Livingstone; 1994:712.
7. Levine D, Filly RA. Using color Doppler jets to differentiate a pelvic cyst from a bladder diverticulum. *J Ultrasound Med* 13:575–577, 1994.

Case 2

Clinical Presentation

A 6-month-old female infant with a history of urinary tract infection.

Radiographic Studies

Anteroposterior (AP) view of the pelvis from a voiding cystourethrogram (Fig. 2A) shows the mass (arrows) within the right side of the bladder. Longitudinal ultrasound of the bladder (Fig. 2B) in another patient shows the mildly dilated distal ureter (arrow) and the "cobra head" (white arrowhead) in the bladder. Transverse ultrasound of the bladder (Fig. 2C) shows a cystic mass (white arrow) within the bladder lumen.

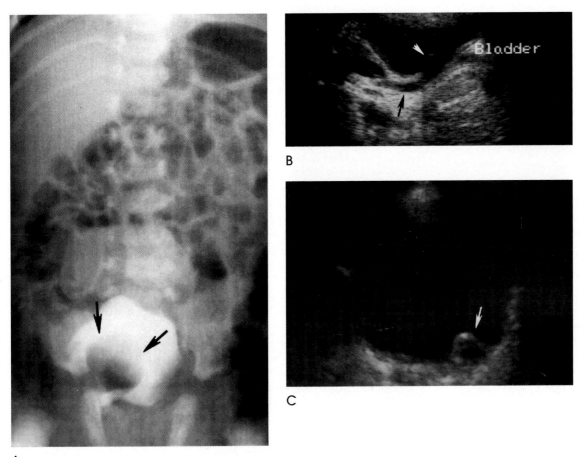

A

B

C

Diagnosis Simple Ureterocele

Discussion and Differential Diagnosis

A ureterocele is a congenital cystic dilatation of the terminal portion of the ureter.[1] Ureteroceles are classified as orthotopic (simple ureteroceles related to single upper collecting systems) or ectopic (connected to the upper pole of a duplicated collecting system and inserting in an abnormal location). The classification system is inadequate, and there is greater variability in ureter insertion than the classification system allows, but no adequate classification system has been adopted.[2]

Simple ureteroceles are of variable size and rare in the pediatric patient. There are several theories as to the cause of ureteroceles, including (1) a primary ureteromeatal obstruction, (2) incomplete muscularization of the distal ureter, and (3) excessive dilatation of the distal ureter as it is absorbed into the developing urogenital sinus and bladder neck.[2] There are varying degrees of associated renal obstruction and dysplasia, more severe if a single system ureter or ureterocele is ectopic.[3]

Pediatric patients may present with a palpable abdominal mass because of the large size of the ureterocele, with obstruction secondary to prolapse of the ureterocele into the bladder neck during voiding, with obstruction of the contralateral ureter because of the size of the ureterocele, or with distortion of the trigone and secondary reflux or infection.[2] Ureteroceles are increasingly diagnosed on obstetrical ultrasound, allowing for earlier intervention.[3] With ultrasound, they are identified as cystic masses protruding into the posterior aspect of the bladder, and can be followed into the distal ureter. The dilated proximal ureter and upper collecting system may also be identified.[3] During voiding cystourethrography, ureteroceles are identified as filling defects in the bladder, near the trigone. At excretory urography, ureteroceles are identified as a "cobra head" in the bladder base, filled from contrast from the ureter, and surrounded by a halo of radiolucent ureterocele wall.[4] The differential diagnosis includes a bladder calculus, blood clot, or air bubble within the bladder lumen; all are usually readily differentiated from an ureterocele at ultrasound.

Further Reading

1. Carty H, Brunelle F, Shaw D, Kendall B, eds. *Imaging Children.* New York: Churchill Livingstone; 1994:642–644, 646, 648.
2. Kelalis PP, King LR, Belman AB. *Clinical Pediatric Urology, II* 3rd ed. Philadelphia: WB Saunders Co; 1992:554–562.
3. Blane CE, Ritchey ML, DiPietro MA, Sumida R, Bloom DA. Single system ectopic ureters and ureteroceles associated with dysplastic kidney. *Pediatr Radiol* 1992:22:217–220.
4. Kirks DR, ed. *Practical Pediatric Imaging,* 2nd ed. Boston: Little, Brown & Co; 1991:963–966.

5. Gharagozloo AM, Lebowitz RL. Detection of a poorly functioning malpositioned kidney with single ectopic ureter in girls with urinary dribbling: imaging evaluation in five patients. *AJR Am J Roentgenol* 1995:164:957–961, 1995.

CONTROVERSY

- Treatment and management of simple ureteroceles is controversial. Some authors advocate transvesical excision of the ureterocele with ureteral reimplantation because of the high incidence of vesicoureteral reflux after endoscopic surgery.[2] However, with newer instrumentation and more controlled endoscopic incision to relieve upper tract dilatation and obstruction, many authors advocate endoscopic surgery initially. If reflux occurs, prophylactic antibiotic therapy can reduce the risk of infection while the upper tract dilatation resolves. Reflux may ultimately resolve.[2]

Case 3

Clinical Presentation

A 7-month-old male infant presents with irritability and crampy abdominal pain. A contrast enema was performed to exclude intussusception, and mass effect was identified on the distal rectum. Subsequent ultrasound demonstrated upper pole hydronephrosis and hydroureter causing rectal mass effect.

Radiographic Studies

Longitudinal ultrasound of the left kidney (Fig. 3A) shows a cystic mass at the upper pole and a relatively normal appearing lower pole moiety (arrowheads). Part of the dilated left upper pole ureter (black arrow) is seen deep to the kidney. Transverse ultrasound of the bladder (Fig. 3B) shows the dilated upper pole ureter (black arrow) posterior to the bladder and a large thin-walled cyst-like mass at the base of the bladder (white arrow). Percutaneous nephrostomy of the upper pole moiety was performed because of the patient's sepsis and clinical instability. Nephrostogram (Fig. 3C; prone image) delineates the hydronephrotic upper pole moiety and hydroureter (arrows).

Full-bladder image from a voiding cystourethrogram (VCUG) (Fig. 3D) shows reflux into the lower moiety ureter (black arrows), a partially intussuscepting mass (black arrowheads) creating an apparent paraureteral diverticulum, and the non-intussuscepted portion of the mass (white arrow) still in the bladder. Supine post-void image (Fig. 3E) shows reflux into the lower pole ureter and moiety, a nearly empty bladder, a "diverticulum" (arrow), and the nephrostomy tube draining the upper pole moiety.

Five-minute film from an excretory urogram of another patient (Fig. 3F) shows a normal left collecting system. Dilation of the right collecting system (arrows) and downward displacement is apparent. A large filling defect is identified in the bladder.

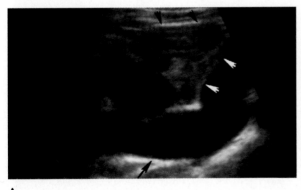

A

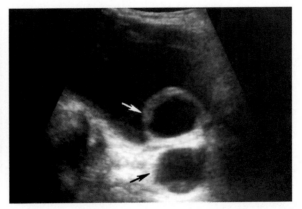

B

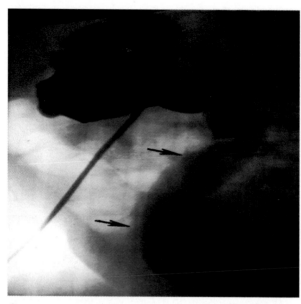

C

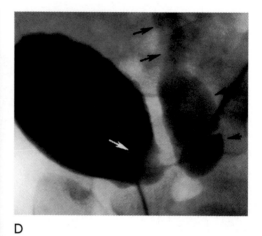

D

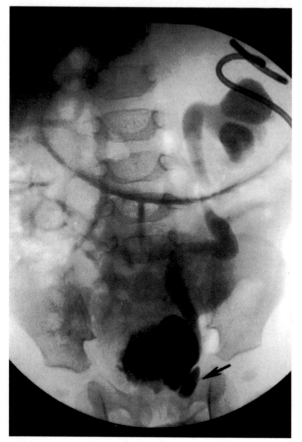

E

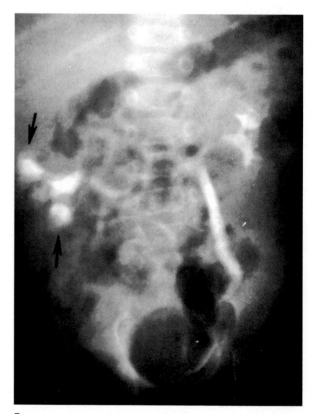

F

Diagnosis Ectopic Ureter/Ureterocele with Duplicated Collecting System

Discussion and Differential Diagnosis

Duplication is the most common anomaly of the urinary tract, seen in approximately 1 in 160 patients, and in 8% of patients with urinary tract infection.[1] The spectrum ranges from a simple bifid pelvis to complete duplication of the upper collecting system and ureter.[1] Incomplete duplication is associated with two problems: ureteropelvic junction obstruction of the lower moiety and retrograde "yo-yo" peristalsis of urine in the two ureters.[2] Complete ureteral duplication occurs in 1 in 500 patients, and is usually asymptomatic.[2] Two separate ureteral buds arise in the fetus; one ureter drains the upper moiety of the kidney and enters into the bladder more medial and caudal than usual.[2] The upper pole moiety may be hydronephrotic from obstruction, with secondary parenchymal damage or dysplasia.[2] Ectopic ureteral insertion and ureteroceles from the upper moiety are common, especially in female patients; this ectopic ureter may insert into the bladder neck, the vagina, the urethra, the uterus, or the fallopian tubes.[2] In males, this ectopic upper pole ureter/ureterocele may insert into the bladder neck, the prostatic urethra, and the male genitourinary ductal system including ejaculatory ducts or epididymis.[1,2] The lower pole ureter inserts more lateral and cephalad in the trigone than normal, has a short intravesicular mucosal tunnel, and is associated with reflux in two thirds of patients.[2]

Prenatal diagnosis may be made when upper pole and ureteral dilatation are noted, as well as dysplastic, thinned upper pole parenchyma, secondary to renal dysplasia.[3] Radiographic evaluation usually begins with screening ultrasound, to identify a dilated upper pole moiety and ureter secondary to obstruction or dysplasia, and a variably dilated lower pole moiety secondary to reflux or ureteropelvic junction obstruction.[2] Ultrasound of the bladder may show an ectopic ureterocele at the distal end of the upper moiety ureter.[3] Voiding cystourethrography usually demonstrates the ureterocele during early bladder filling and reflux into the lower moiety ureter.[3] During voiding, the upper moiety ureterocele may suddenly intussuscept on itself and evert, causing the sudden appearance of an apparent "bladder diverticulum."[4] In some cases, this everted ureterocele includes the orifice of the lower pole ureter.[4] Further evaluation of renal function with nuclear medicine studies usually confirms at least partial obstruction of the upper pole with varying degrees of renal function.[3] Excretory urography is usually unnecessary. The differential diagnosis includes multicystic dysplastic kidney, renal cyst, and adrenal hemorrhage; these entities are usually differentiated during the ultrasound, voiding cystourethrogram, and nuclear medicine studies. Adrenal hemorrhage may be difficult to clearly differentiate from an obstructed upper pole, and MRI may be helpful in showing the acute/subacute blood within the adrenal hemorrhage. Cystic neuroblastoma and nephroblastoma are more rare.[3]

Further Reading

1. Kirks DR, ed. *Practical Pediatric Imaging*, 2nd ed. Boston: Little, Brown & Co; 1991:960–963.

reserved for the neonate in whom there is marked hydronephrosis and hydroureter.[2] If the upper pole collecting system is functioning, management becomes more controversial. Many authors advocate endoscopic unroofing of the ureterocele, which usually converts an obstructed system to a refluxing system, with subsequent antibiotic prophylaxis for urinary tract infection. This approach permits subsequent reevaluation of upper pole function, and possible heminephrectomy in an older child who is a better operative risk. In some patients, if the ureterocele is unroofed early in life, renal function returns to the upper pole moiety.[2]

2. Kelalis PP, King LR, Belman AB. *Clinical Pediatric Urology, II.* 3rd ed. Philadelphia: WB Saunders Co; 1992:530–579.
3. Carty H, Brunelle F, Shaw D, Kendall B, eds. *Imaging Children.* New York: Churchill Livingstone; 1994:637–642.
4. Bellah RD, Long FR, Canning DA. Ureterocele eversion with vesicoureteral reflux in duplex kidneys: findings at voiding cystourethrography. *Am J Roentgenol* 165:409–413, 1995.
5. Fernbach SK, Zawin JK, Lebowitz RL. Complete duplication of the ureter with ureteropelvic junction obstruction of the lower pole of the kidney: imaging findings. *AJR Am J Roentgenol* 164:701–704, 1995.

Case 4

Clinical Presentation

A 2-year-old boy presents with fever, irritability, and flank pain. Urinalysis and culture indicate urinary tract infection.

Radiographic Studies

Longitudinal ultrasound of the pelvis (Fig. 4A) shows a dilated distal ureter (arrows) deep in the pelvis, which apparently does not communicate with the bladder. Figure 4B, from a voiding cystourethrogram taken during micturition, shows a radiopaque catheter in the male urethra with its tip in the bladder base, and a dilated ureter (arrows) inserting into the prostatic urethra (arrowhead) and filling with refluxed contrast. Figure 4C is an oblique view of the pelvis showing the extremely dilated contrast-filled bladder anteriorly, and reflux into the tortuous dilated left ureter (black arrow) and hydronephrotic left upper collecting system (white arrow).

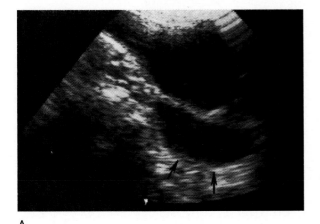

A

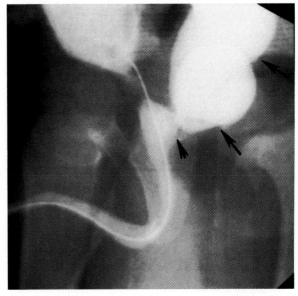

B

- Ectopic ureters and ureteroceles associated with a single, nonduplicated upper collecting system have a much higher incidence of complications than those associated with duplicated collecting systems. An investigation for associated anomalies and other organ system abnormalities is necessary.[4]

- Bladder outlet obstruction may be the presenting symptom secondary to the ureterocele size, ectopic insertion, or prolapse into the urethra.[4]

- In many patients with an ectopic ureter or ureterocele in a single system, nephrectomy may be necessary because of associated dysplasia of the upper collecting system.[4]

- When performing voiding cystourethrography, it is very important to use dilute contrast in small amounts during the initial portion of the exam and film in lateral, oblique, and AP positions to delineate a ureterocele with the ectopic ureter.[2] In males, it is very important to visualize the entire urethra during the voiding phase.

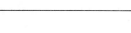

- If only one kidney is identified at screening ultrasound, then a diligent investigation for a

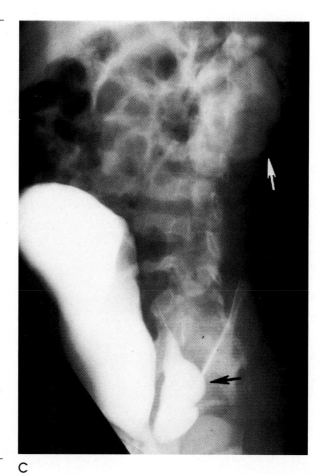

C

Diagnosis Ectopic Ureter/Ureterocele with Nonduplicated Collecting System

Discussion and Differential Diagnosis

Ectopic ureters are defined as ureters that do not insert in the posterior lateral angle of the trigone and have many presentations.[1] They occur more commonly in females than in males and are usually associated with duplicated collecting systems in approximately 80% of the cases. However, in 10% to 20% of cases, an ectopic ureter arises from a solitary nonduplicated renal pelvis.[1,2] Ectopic ureters from nonduplicated collecting systems are much more common in male patients and have various insertions, including the posterior urethra, ejaculatory ducts, seminal vesicles, vas deferens, or even the rectum.[1–3] In female patients, ectopic ureters from nonduplicated systems may insert into the urethra, vagina uterus, rectum, vestibule, or labia.[1–3] In many cases, the upper collecting system is hypoplastic or dysplastic, or markedly abnormal as a result of obstruction and chronic infection.[1,4]

Ectopic ureters and ureteroceles from single systems usually present in males with

malpositioned, poorly functioning
dysplastic kidney is necessary.[5]

CONTROVERSY
- Some authors maintain that the
  degree of renal dysplasia is
  determined by the degree of in
  utero obstruction.[4] Other
  authors maintain that the renal
  dysplasia is secondary to
  abnormal insertion of the
  ureteric bud into the
  metanephros during fetal life.[6]
  Other authors believe that the
  greater the distance the ureter
  is inserted from its normal
  location, the greater the
  dysplasia of the upper
  collecting system.

symptoms relating to obstruction, or occasionally, a pararectal mass is identified during rectal examination.[2] In female patients, symptoms are usually more often secondary to incontinence with constant dampness.[1,2] In newborn patients or on prenatal ultrasound, ectopic ureters can present as a multiseptated cystic abdominal mass, secondary to massive dilatation and tortuosity of the ectopic ureter. In addition, the screening ultrasound may identify the dilated ureter deep into the pelvis, not connected to the bladder. The upper collecting system and renal parenchyma are frequently hyperechoic, with loss of the corticomedullary junction, and variable-sized cysts indicative of renal dysplasia.[2,4] If only one kidney is identified at screening ultrasound or excretory urography, then an extensive workup should be performed to detect a malpositioned kidney.[5] Nuclear medicine imaging is often necessary to localize the malpositioned/ectopic kidney, followed by directed CT scan to evaluate the kidney.[5] In all patients, voiding cystourethrography should be performed to delineate a ureterocele and/or reflux into the ectopic ureter. In females with continuous urine dribbling or dampness who are toilet trained and have otherwise normal voiding habits, cystoscopy, vaginoscopy, or vaginography may be necessary to identify and cannulate an ectopic ureteral orifice.[1,2,4,5] The differential diagnosis of a cystic intraabdominal mass includes a multiseptated ectopic ureter, lymphangioma, cystic Wilms' tumor, and teratoma; these can usually be delineated from each other by the imaging studies as described above.[1]

Further Reading

1. Nussbaum AR, Dorst JP, Jeffs RD, Gearhart JP, Sanders RC. Ectopic ureter and ureterocele: their varied sonographic manifestations. *Radiology* 159:227–235, 1986.
2. Kirks DR, ed. *Practical Pediatric Imaging*, 2nd ed. Boston: Little, Brown & Co; 1991:960–963.
3. Carty H, Brunelle F, Shaw D, Kendall B, eds. *Imaging Children*. New York: Churchill Livingstone; 1994:642–646.
4. Blane CE, Ritchey ML, DiPietro MA, Sumida R, Bloom DA. Single system ectopic ureters and ureteroceles associated with dysplastic kidney. *Pediatr Radiol* 22:217–220, 1992.
5. Gharagozloo AM, Lebowitz RL. Detection of a poorly functioning malpositioned kidney with single ectopic ureter in girls with urinary dribbling: imaging evaluation in five patients. *Am J Roentgenol* 164:957–961, 1995.
6. Eklöf O, Mäkinen. Ectopic ureterocele: a radiological appraisal of 66 consecutive cases. *Pediatr Radiol* 2:111–120, 1974.

Case 5

Clinical Presentation

A 7-year-old boy who presents with hematuria and flank pain after minimal trauma has a palpable mass in the left flank at physical examination. Neonates may present simply with abdominal distention and a palpable mass. Patients of any age may present with urinary tract infection.

Radiographic Studies

Longitudinal scan of the left kidney (Fig. 5A) shows dilatation of multiple calyces, communicating centrally. A more medial longitudinal scan of the left kidney (Fig. 5B) shows marked dilatation of the left renal pelvis. A transverse image of the left kidney (Fig. 5C) shows dilated calyces lateral to the markedly dilated large left renal pelvis. Posterior image from a furosemide (Lasix) renogram at 2 minutes (Fig. 5D) shows a photopenic central collecting system on the left (arrow). A later posterior image (Fig. 5E), 20 minutes after the administration of furosemide (Lasix), shows the dilated left upper collecting system (black arrows) filled with radioisotope. The right collecting system radioisotope has almost completely cleared. Figure 5F is a time activity curve from the renogram, showing increasing counts of radioisotope in the left kidney after the administration of furosemide (Lasix), with no evidence of washout.

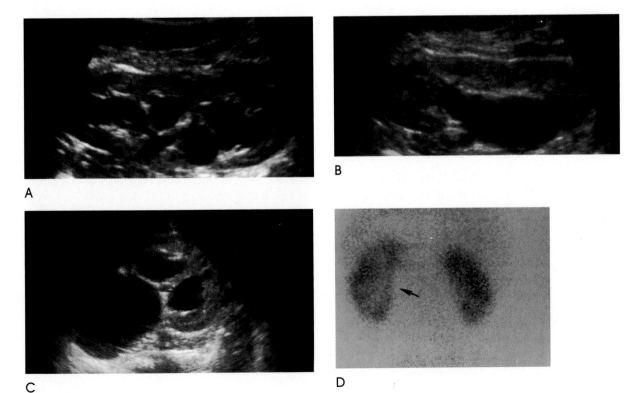

A

B

C

D

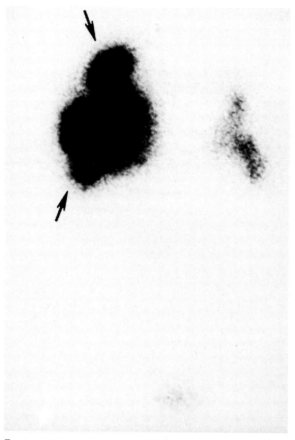

E

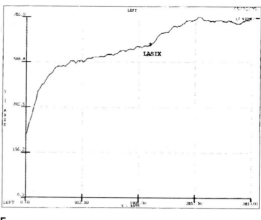

F

PEARLS

- In rare cases, the cause of UPJO may be renal stone with subsequent stricture formation, atypical valve at the ureteropelvic junction, or intraluminal polyps or masses.[3]

Diagnosis Ureteropelvic Junction Obstruction (UPJO)

Discussion and Differential Diagnosis

Ureteropelvic junction obstruction is the most common congenital obstruction of the urinary tract; its incidence is cited at between 1 in 800 and 1 in 1500.[1] Sixty-five percent of patients are male; 5% of obstructions are bilateral.[1] Ureteropelvic junction obstructions are often found in the lower pole moiety in patients with complete renal duplication and should be considered when there is dilatation of the lower pole moiety.[2] Associated anomalies include contralateral multicystic dysplastic kidney, VATER (vertebral, anal, tracheal, esophageal, and renal) anomalies, congenital heart disease, and ipsilateral reflux in 10% of patients.[1] Intrinsic anomalies of

- Duplex Doppler is an excellent modality for post-op evaluation of UPJO repair.[5,7]

- Duplex Doppler sonography of multicystic dysplastic kidney usually yields resistive indices that are extremely elevated (0.98 or greater).[7]

PITFALLS

- With long-standing dilatation secondary to obstruction and secondary cortical loss, duplex Doppler ultrasound may be normal secondary to compensated vascular resistance.[5]

- In patients with acute renal infection, the resistive index may be equivocal or normal.[7]

- When the Whitaker test is necessary, it is important to evaluate the patient in multiple positions, including those positions that accentuate the patient's symptoms. Intermittent ureteral obstruction from ureteral kinking, ureteral tortuosity, malpositioned kidneys, or previous surgery may occur.[8]

the ureteropelvic junction are the most common cause, and include ureteric stenosis and adynamic ureteric segment secondary to muscle discontinuity.[3] Extrinsic compression of the ureteropelvic junction is less common and is usually secondary to ureteral kinking, fibrous bands, or vascular compression.[1,3]

Ureteropelvic junction obstructions are frequently diagnosed prenatally. Renal pelvis diameter of 5 mm or less in the second or third trimester is normal; renal pelvic diameter of 5 to 10 mm may resolve spontaneously during pregnancy or at birth, and renal pelvis dilatation greater than 10 to 12 mm is definitely abnormal and requires evaluation after birth.[3] The investigation includes an initial ultrasound to confirm the abnormality; this should be performed after 2 days of life, to allow for neonatal dehydration to resolve.[1] Ultrasound of the renal pelvis and calyces shows dilatation of the central renal pelvis communicating with dilated calyces at the lateral margins of the kidney. The ureter is not dilated. Parenchymal thinning may be seen secondary to severe distention, long-standing obstruction, and resultant atrophy.[4] Voiding cystourethrography should be performed to differentiate dilatation secondary to UPJO from dilatation secondary to vesicoureteral reflux.[1] Functional evaluation is performed with diuretic nuclear renography to evaluate the degree of obstruction[1]; in the newborn, it is best to wait approximately 3 to 4 weeks after birth, for complete renal function to develop. If the time for drainage of half of the radioisotope from the upper collecting system is greater than 20 minutes after the administration of furosemide (Lasix), then the patient has obstruction and surgery is usually indicated. This time can be artificially elongated if the patient has extremely poor renal function on the affected side. If the time for drainage of half of the radioisotope from the collecting system is between 15 and 20 minutes, then the patient may have intermittent or partial obstruction.[1] The Whitaker test is reserved for patients in whom the furosemide renogram is inconclusive. The test involves simultaneous pressure monitoring of the collecting system and bladder during controlled percutaneous antegrade infusion of the upper collecting system. Nuclear medicine renography with Tc-99m-DTPA or MAG3 usually shows a photon-deficient area centrally, with progressive slow accumulation of radioisotope in the collecting system. Delayed images at 4 to 6 hours may be helpful in identifying the level of obstruction.[4] Excretory urography is usually not indicated in the evaluation of UPJO.

Duplex Doppler ultrasound of the kidney is helpful in discerning UPJO from nonobstructive renal pelvis dilatation.[5] In patients with obstruction, the increased renal vascular resistance causes a secondary decrease in renal diastolic flow and therefore the resistive indices are elevated. In patients with unilateral UPJO, the resistive indices in the arcuate arteries of the obstructed kidney are greater than 0.70, and there is an absolute difference in the resistive indices between the kidneys, with the obstructed kidney's resistive index at least 0.08 higher than that of the nonobstructed kidney.[5] Applying these two criteria yields a sensitivity of 100% and a specificity of 94% in differentiating unilateral UPJO from nonobstructed dilated upper collecting systems.[5] Postdiuretic evaluation of the resistive indices in UPJO shows further elevation of the resistive index in the obstructed kidneys after the administration of diuretics.[6] Other authors have confirmed these findings in pediatric patients and have documented that after repair of the UPJO, the resistive index decreases to a more normal range in the repaired UPJO, and that there may be an associated slight increase in the resistive index in the contralateral kidney.[7]

The differential diagnosis of UPJO includes ureterovesicular junction obstruction (UVJO), multicystic dysplastic kidney, and dilated nonobstructed collecting system. Ureterovesical junction obstruction shows similar findings, but a dilated ureter is identified behind the bladder at ultrasound.[3] Duplex Doppler ultrasound is not helpful in these patients, probably because the dilated ureter acts as a compliant reservoir for urine and therefore renal vascular resistance does not increase.[5] On ultrasound, the sonolucent cystic structures of multicystic dysplastic kidneys do not communicate with one another or with a large central medial renal pelvis.[3] Patients with reflux may show dilated upper collecting systems, but voiding cystourethrography delineates these patients. Dilated nonobstructed collecting systems are differentiated from UPJO by nuclear diuretic renography and/or duplex Doppler ultrasound.

Further Reading

1. Kelalis PP, King LR, Belman AB. *Clinical Pediatric Urology, II.* 3rd ed. Philadelphia: WB Saunders Co; 1992:693–722.
2. Fernbach SK, Zawin JK, Lebowitz RL. Complete duplication of the ureter with ureteropelvic junction obstruction of the lower pole of the kidney. *Am J Roentgenol* 164:701–704, 1995.
3. Carty H, Brunelle F, Shaw D, Kendall B, eds. *Imaging Children.* New York: Churchill Livingstone; 1994:609–617.
4. Kirks DR, ed. *Practical Pediatric Imaging,* 2nd ed. Boston: Little, Brown & Co; 1991:1038–1043.
5. Kessler RM, Quevedo H, Kankau CA. Obstructive vs. nonobstructive dilatation of the renal collecting system in children: distinction with duplex sonography. *Am J Roentgenol* 160:353–357, 1993.
6. Ordorica RC, Lindfors KK, Palmer JM. Diuretic Doppler sonography following successful repair of renal obstruction in children. *J Urol* 150:774–777, 1993.
7. Riccabona M, Ring E, Fueger G, et al. Doppler sonography in congenital ureteropelvic junction obstruction and multicystic dysplastic kidneys. *Pediatr Radiol* 23:502–505, 1993.
8. Ellis JH, Campo RP, Marx MV. Positional variation in the Whitaker test. *Radiology* 197:253–255, 1995.
9. Tublin ME, Dodd GD, Verdile VP. Acute renal colic: diagnosis with duplex Doppler US. *Radiology* 193:697–701, 1994.

10. Platt JF, Rubin JM, Ellis JH. Acute renal obstruction: evaluation with intrarenal duplex Doppler and conventional US. *Radiology* 186:685–688, 1993.
11. Platt JF. Looking for renal obstruction: the view from renal Doppler US. *Radiology* 193:610–612, 1994.
12. Lee HJ, Kim SH, Jeong YK, Yeun KM. Doppler sonographic resistive index in obstructed kidneys. *J Ultrasound Med* 15:613–618, 1996.

Case 6

Clinical Presentation

A male newborn presents with a prenatal diagnosis of left ureteral dilatation. Older patients may present with hematuria, flank pain or mass, urinary tract infection, and enuresis.

Radiographic Studies

Longitudinal ultrasound of the left flank at 3 days of age (Fig. 6A) shows the tortuous ectatic dilated ureter, with abrupt transition to normal caliber at the distal end (arrow). Longitudinal ultrasound of the bladder (Fig. 6B) shows no ureteral dilatation posterior to the bladder. Figure 6C is a prone view during right nephrostogram that shows dilatation of the collecting system and a tortuous dilated ureter to the level of the bladder.

Figure 6D is a posterior image from a nuclear medicine diuretic renogram taken 30 minutes after administration of furosemide; it shows persistent concentration of radioisotope in the right collecting system and ureter in another patient.

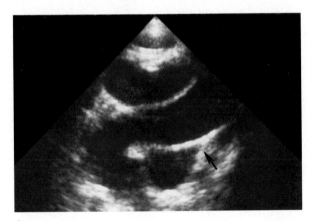

A

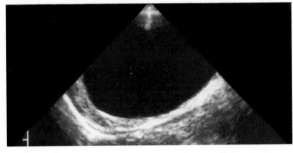

B

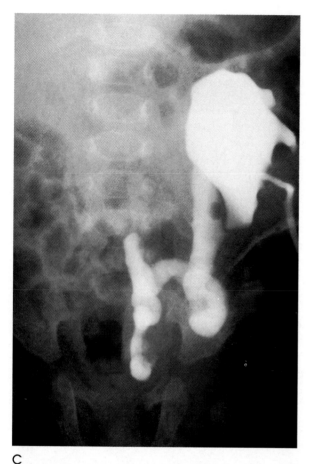

C

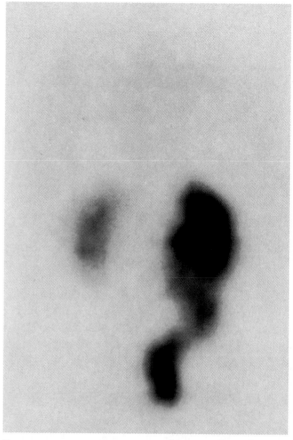

D

Diagnosis Megaureter

Discussion and Differential Diagnosis

Megaureter or megaloureter is a general term used to describe ureteral dilatation greater than 5 to 7 mm in diameter, with variable degrees of dilatation of the collecting system.[1] The term is not defined as a distinct entity and, in fact, incorporates ureteral dilatation with multiple causes and diverse pathology.[1] Multiple systems have been proposed in an attempt to classify abnormalities of the ureterovesical junction; none are absolutely comprehensive. The most common cause of distal ureteral obstruction is primary megaureter,[2] defined as varying degrees of proximal ureteral dilation above a normal or narrowed distal ureteral segment.[1,3] The distal ureteral lumen is patent; the ureteral location at the trigone is normal, and there may or may not be vesicoureteral reflux. However, with primary megaureter, there is absence of the normal peristaltic wave through the distal ureteral segment; this is believed to be secondary to a predominance of distal ureteral circular muscle fibers, a paucity of distal ureteral longitudinal muscle fibers, and an excess of collagen infiltration in the terminal

- After a voiding cystourethrogram, delayed drainage of refluxed contrast from a dilated ureter above a normal or narrowed ureterovesical junction may be initial evidence of primary megaureter with or without obstruction.[1]

- Congenital megacystis/ megaureter syndrome is a different entity, usually detected in utero or just after birth, in which the ureters, urinary bladder, and upper collecting systems are grossly dilated, secondary to massive reflux during voiding. Initially, bladder contractility is normal, but ultimately there is massive bladder dilatation and dysfunction with large residual urine volumes. Patients so afflicted usually succumb to renal failure.[1,2]

- Megacystis-microcolon-hypoperistalsis syndrome describes another entity, with massive dilatation of the urinary tract, vesicoureteral reflux, functional intestinal obstruction, short dilated hypoactive small bowel, and microcolon. These patients probably have a degenerative smooth muscle disorder.[1]

PITFALLS

- Retrocaval ureter may cause ureteral dilatation and has a typical appearance involving only the proximal one third of the ureter.[1] There are varying degrees of histological abnormalities in the terminal ureteral segment, and these may account for the varying clinical presentations of megaureter.[1] Some megaureters develop peristaltic waves, and the obstruction resolves spontaneously. This may be secondary to growth of distal ureteral longitudinal muscle, creating a more normal ratio between circular and longitudinal muscle fibers.[1]

The diagnosis of megaureter may be made prenatally when a tubular anechoic structure is identified behind the bladder and at the renal pelvis, with varying degrees of renal pelvis dilatation and varying degrees of renal dysplasia.[2,4] Postnatal ultrasound usually confirms the dilated ureter with peristaltic waves identified proximally. Ultrasound can assess the degree of hydronephrosis and the presence of a ureterocele. Contrast voiding cystourethrography is necessary to exclude bladder outlet obstruction or neurogenic bladder, and to evaluate for reflux.[1] Nuclear medicine diuretic renography can assess renal function as well as evaluate for obstruction.[1] If the radioisotopic clearance half-time after diuretic administration is less than 15 minutes, no obstruction is present. If it is between 15 and 20 minutes, the examination is indeterminate. If it is greater than 20 minutes, and there is adequate renal function, obstruction is present.[1] If the nuclear medicine diuretic renogram is equivocal, the Whitaker test/pressure-perfusion study, which evaluates urine flow during maximal diuresis and measures the pressure gradient between the collecting system and the bladder, can be performed.[1]

If these examinations define primary megaureter with no evidence of obstruction, and no secondary cause of megaureter, then surgery is not indicated. However, regular follow-up including diuretic renography is necessary because these patients may later develop obstruction. Antibiotic prophylaxis may be indicated for several years, until stability of the lesion is determined.[1] If obstruction is identified at the ureterovesical junction from the primary megaureter, resection of the abnormal terminal ureter and reimplantation are indicated, before development of obstructive renal damage. If there is significant renal dysplasia—and, in particular, if the ipsilateral kidney shows less than 20% of the total renal function, even after upper collecting system diversion—then nephrectomy may be indicated.[1,4]

Another common cause of distal ureteral dilatation is severe vesicoureteral reflux.[2] Other causes include postoperative ureteral reimplantation, stricture, calculus, post-inflammatory or infectious change including granulomatous infection,[3] and retroperitoneal fibrosis.[2] Congenital causes of distal ureteric dilatation include obstruction secondary to ureterocele, extrinsic ureteric compression at the ureterovesical junction, usually secondary to a persistent left umbilical artery or prominent right ovarian vein, congenital ureteric diverticula, which may occur anywhere along the ureter and cause obstruction or infection, and rare congenital ureteric strictures.[2] Congenital bladder dysfunction (secondary to meningomyelocele) or acquired bladder dysfunction (from spinal cord injury) may cause a neurogenic bladder and associated dilatation of the distal ureters.[1]

Further Reading

1. Kelalis PP, King LR, Belman AB. *Clinical Pediatric Urology, II.* 3rd ed. Philadelphia: WB Saunders Co; 1992:781–812, 834.

right ureter; it may be mistaken for ureteropelvic junction obstruction at ultrasound.[1]

- If primary megaureter is associated with a severely dysplastic kidney that is not visualized at ultrasound, then the differential for the tortuous dilated ureter becomes more extensive and includes the differential for cystic abdominal masses such as mesenteric cysts, ovarian cysts, and duplication cysts.[4]

CONTROVERSY

- The major controversy with primary megaureter involves difference of opinion in terms of classification systems, and whether to include both obstructed and nonobstructed systems in the term *primary megaureter.*

- In some patients, the diuretic renogram and Whitaker test are both equivocal; the management of these patients and, specifically, whether distal ureteral resection and reimplantation are indicated is controversial. Most authors agree that surgical intervention is necessary before renal damage occurs.[1]

2. Carty H, Brunelle F, Shaw D, Kendall B, eds. *Imaging Children.* New York: Churchill Livingstone; 1994:617–628.
3. Kirks DR, ed. *Practical Pediatric Imaging,* 2nd ed. Boston: Little, Brown & Co; 1991:1043.
4. Alcantara AL, Amundson GM, Chang CH. Megaureter associated with severe renal dysplasia. *J Clin Ultrasound* 21;274–277, 1993.

Case 7

Clinical Presentation

This patient is a neonate who presented with obstructive symptoms.

Radiographic Studies

Voiding cystourethrogram (Fig. 7A) shows a dilated and elongated prostatic urethra (arrow). Transabdominal ultrasound (Fig. 7B) shows the dilated prostatic urethra (arrows). Anteroposterior (AP) image of another patient (Fig. 7C) shows a trabeculated bladder with a thickened bladder wall, and multiple diverticula or cellules of varying sizes. This patient had a large postvoid residual urine volume. Transverse ultrasound of the bladder (Fig. 7D) shows dilated distal ureters, with bladder wall thickening. Ultrasound of the upper urinary tracts showed hydronephrosis.

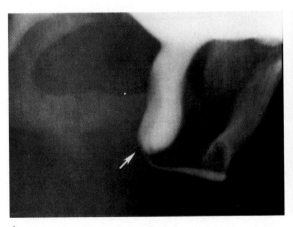

A

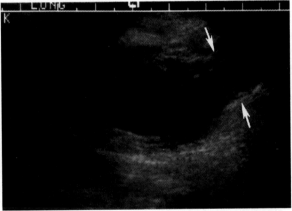

B

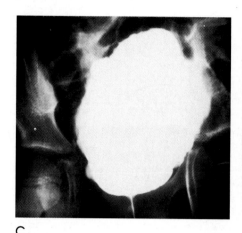

C

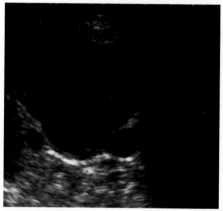

D

Diagnosis Posterior Urethral Valves

Discussion and Differential Diagnosis

The clinical presentation of posterior urethral valves falls into two groups: (1) those with obstructive symptoms, commonly neonates, and (2) those with infectious symptoms, more commonly older children.[1] Other presentations include: (1) prenatal ultrasound diagnosis in patients with hydronephrosis, dilated bladder, and dilated posterior urethra, (2) neonates with a urine leak with ascites and urinoma,[1–3] and (3) older children with failure to thrive and chronic renal failure.

Posterior urethral valves are the most common cause of urinary tract obstruction and end-stage renal disease in males. The incidence varies between 1 in 5000 and 1 in 8000.[4] Posterior urethral valves are divided into three types: type I valves account for almost all cases and are mucosal folds extending anteroinferiorly from the verumontanum and fusing lower in the urethra.[1]

Type I valves are derived from the plicae colliculi.[1] Type II posterior urethral valves are mucosal folds that extend anterosuperiorly from the verumontanum toward the bladder neck; these valves are quite rare.[1] Type III valves are a disc-like membrane unrelated to the verumontanum and located more distally in the urethra.[1]

Posterior urethral valves cause urine outflow obstruction with secondary bladder wall hypertrophy and trabeculation. There are frequently alterations in the ureterovesical junction, sometimes associated with Hutch diverticula. Massive hydronephrosis is common, either secondary to ureterovesical incompetence with vesicoureteral reflux, or secondary to obstruction. In either case, renal dysplasia is common with chronic renal failure and end-stage renal disease. Even after ablation of the valves, hydronephrosis may persist secondary to a hypertrophied noncompliant bladder.[1] If reflux persists after valve ablation, the patient may have renal dysplasia.[5] An urinoma may be associated with the hydronephrosis, particularly in the neonate, because of the high-grade outflow obstruction and/or reflux.[2,3]

The diagnosis of posterior urethral valves is usually made with a voiding cystourethrogram, which delineates the urethral obstruction and assesses for vesicoure-

PEARLS

- Transient hydronephrosis of the newborn may be a normal variant seen on prenatal ultrasound and may resolve spontaneously.[1,6]

- There are many normal variants to the appearance of the male urethra, and nonobstructed urethral ectasia or kinking should not be confused with posterior urethral valves.[1]

- Transperineal ultrasound delineating the linear echogenic structure representing the valves within the urethra helps differentiate patients with posterior urethral valves from patients with urethral strictures.[4]

- In patients with posterior urethral valves, 50% have

vesicoureteral reflux at presentation; of these, 50% have bilateral reflux.

- A male newborn who presents with isolated ascites most likely has posterior urethral valves.[7]

PITFALLS

- Urethral strictures can be confused with posterior urethral valves, but strictures are usually irregular in outline and in a different location. Urethral strictures are inflammatory, congenital, traumatic, or iatrogenic in origin.[1]

- Urethral polyps and hypertrophy of the verumontanum are rare but may cause a filling defect in the proximal urethra, deviating the urine stream around the defect, and thus may resemble posterior urethral valves.[1]

- A patient is less likely to have a good response to valve ablation if the bladder is small, with a thickened wall; this bladder configuration is thought to be secondary to intravesical urine extravasation into the bladder wall, reducing compliance and inducing bladder wall hypertrophy.[8]

CONTROVERSY

- The treatment and management of patients with

teral reflux. Renal ultrasound may demonstrate hydronephrosis and hydroureter from obstruction or reflux, and may identify an associated urinoma. Ultrasound of the posterior urethra may demonstrate a dilated urethra, with a linear echogenic structure within it, representing the posterior urethral valve membrane.[4] Nuclear medicine studies may be useful in assessing renal function and the degree of residual obstruction after valve ablation.

The differential diagnosis includes bilateral ureteropelvic junction obstruction or bilateral ureterovesical obstruction; these patients usually have a normal bladder. Prune-belly syndrome is indistinguishable from posterior urethral valves in utero, but at birth, the absence of abdominal musculature confirms the diagnosis of prune-belly syndrome. The urethra in prune-belly syndrome may be dilated (because of prostatic hypoplasia) but is not elongated. Megacystis/megaureter syndrome usually occurs in females and is frequently associated with dilated bowel from hypoperistalsis.[1] Multicystic kidney disease, polycystic kidney disease, and ovarian cyst may have a similar presentation on ultrasound, but these patients all have normal bladders.[1]

Further Reading

1. Macpherson RI, Leithiser RE, Gordon L, Turner WR. Posterior urethral valves: an update and review. *Radiographics* 6(5):753–791, 1986.
2. Morgan CL Jr, Grossman H. Posterior urethral valves as a cause of neonatal uriniferous perirenal pseudocyst (urinoma). *Pediatr Radiol* 7:29–32, 1978.
3. Fernbach SK, Feinstein KA, Zaontz MR. Urinoma formation in posterior urethral valves: relationship to later renal function. *Pediatr Radiol* 20:543–545, 1990.
4. Cohen HL, Susman M, Haller JO, Glassberg KI, Shapiro MA, Zinn DL. Posterior urethral valve: transperineal US for imaging and diagnosis in male infants. *Radiology* 192:261–264, 1994.
5. Johnston JH. Vesicoureteric reflux with urethral valves. *Br J Urol* 51:100–104, 1979.
6. Kelalis PP, King LR, Belman AB. *Clinical Pediatric Urology, II.* 3rd ed. Philadelphia: WB Saunders Co; 1992:835–848.
7. Scott TW. Urinary ascites secondary to posterior urethral valves. *J Urol* 116:87–91, 1976.
8. Lebowitz R. Society of Pediatric Radiology, Toronto, 1979.

posterior urethral valves is complicated and controversial.[1,5] In older children, primary valve ablation through a transurethral approach is usually the treatment of choice. In patients with severe bladder hypertrophy, bladder outflow obstruction and/or reflux may persist. If reflux persists, prophylactic antibiotic therapy is necessary; if reflux occurs in a nonfunctioning renal unit, nephroureterectomy is the treatment.[5] Sometimes a combined approach with urinary diversion, either through vesicostomy or ureterostomy, may be necessary. Ultimately, these patients may need renal transplantation.[1]

- In the infant, the management is more controversial. The urethra may be too small to accommodate the urethroscope/cystoscope. If a scope that is too large is forced into the urethra, complications such as urethral strictures, diverticula, or incontinence are common. In these small patients, temporary urinary diversion with vesicostomy may be necessary until the urethra grows larger and the patient is more stable. However, a "dry" urethra may make the urethral obstruction worse.[2,5]

Case 8

Clinical Presentation

A 4-year-old boy with new onset of fever, abdominal pain, a palpable midline hypogastric mass, and urinary frequency. Urinalysis and culture documented the presence of urinary tract infection.

Radiographic Studies

Longitudinal (Fig. 8A) and transverse (Fig. 8B) ultrasound scans of the hypogastric region show a 2-cm cystic mass (arrows and caliper markers), with mixed internal echogenicity representing internal debris. Thick echogenic walls are identified with surrounding low echogenicity that represents edema. The mass is compressing and displacing the adjacent dome of the bladder (white arrows) and is located between the anterior abdominal wall and the bladder.

   Figure 8C is an oblique image from a voiding cystourethrogram of patient with prune-belly syndrome, showing an outpouching (arrows) located at the dome of the bladder.

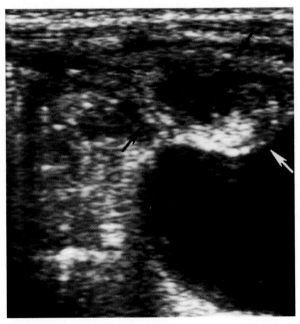

A

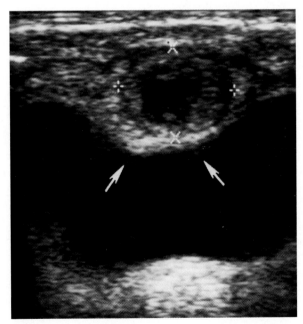

B

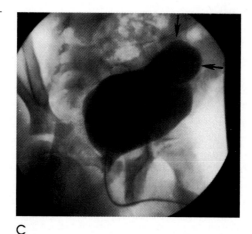

C

Diagnosis   Urachal Cyst Anomalies

Discussion and Differential Diagnosis

The urachus is the fibrous remnant of the allantoic stalk connecting the bladder and umbilicus.[1] In the fetus, the urachal channel progressively narrows after 4 to 5 months' gestation,[2] and by birth, it is usually fibrosed and obliterated. In the older patient, the urachal remnant sometimes may be seen by ultrasound as an approximately 3-mm relatively echolucent mass in the superficial abdominal wall between the rectus muscles.[1] This fibrous remnant of the urachus may contain remnants of one or both umbilical arteries, which occasionally form tiny punctate calcifications.[1] Patency of the urachus is reported in autopsy series, with an incidence varying between 1 in 1000 and 1 in 5000, depending on the pediatric autopsy series.[1,3]

Urachal anomalies are classified into four subgroups.[1,4] A completely patent urachus is secondary to failure of obliteration of the urachal channel in the fetus and frequently presents in the newborn.[1,4] The urachus may be widely patent, with free flow of urine from the umbilicus, often seen in patients with prune-belly syndrome, posterior urethral valves, or ventral abdominal wall defects such as omphalocele.[5,6] In some patients, the fistula may be tiny, with only intermittent and sparse urine drainage.[2] Ultrasound often demonstrates a fluid-containing channel between the dome of the bladder and the umbilicus, and voiding cystourethrography shows contrast filling the patent channel and draining from the umbilicus.[5]

The second subgroup of urachal anomalies is made up of patients with an urachal sinus—a blind-ending sinus tract that opens into the umbilicus.[1,2,4] Symptoms may occur at any age and are usually secondary to infected discharge from the sinus.[2] The diagnosis is usually made by direct injection of contrast into the sinus orifice at the umbilicus.[4,5]

The third subgroup of urachal anomalies includes patients with urachal diverticula.[1,2,4] An urachal diverticulum opens into the bladder.[5] At ultrasound, an urachal diverticulum is identified as a cystic structure connecting with the superior aspect

cysts are frequently thick-walled and contain internal echogenic debris from infection.

CONTROVERSY

● Infected urachal cysts may be treated with drainage and antibiotic therapy. However, there is an approximately 30% recurrence rate of infected urachal cysts in patients who are treated only with drainage and antibiotic therapy.[2,4] Therefore, most authors advocate complete resection of the urachal tract from umbilicus to bladder, including resection of a cuff of the dome of the bladder.[2] In addition, complete resection is advocated because there is a small risk of the late development of urachal carcinoma in patients with a persistent patent urachal anomaly.[6]

● In adults, urachal anomalies are frequently acquired secondary to bladder outlet obstruction. In the pediatric patient, urachal anomalies are more often an isolated congenital anomaly and less often related to bladder outlet obstruction.[3]

of the distended bladder.[5] It may also be identified at voiding cystourethrography as an irregular-shaped diverticulum at the dome of the bladder.[5] Urachal diverticula may be incidental findings at ultrasound or voiding cystourethrography. If these diverticula enlarge, they may present as symptoms secondary to stone formation within the diverticulum, or stasis with urinary tract infection.[2]

The fourth subgroup of urachal anomalies,[1,2,4] urachal cysts, is probably the most interesting. The cysts form within the isolated urachal channel, and the lumen enlarges over time secondary to desquamated or degenerative tissue.[2] Urachal cysts/urachal anomalies may be identified in utero as cystic masses within the umbilical cord, sometimes connected with the fetal bladder.[7] These masses show no flow within them, but color flow interrogation shows splaying of both umbilical arteries around the lateral walls of this cyst.[7] After birth, the cysts are usually asymptomatic until infected[3]; skin and bladder serve as portals for infection.[4] If direct communication with the bladder occurs, infection is common.[2] Complications include rupture of the infected cysts into the preperitoneal tissues and rupture into the intraperitoneal tissues with secondary peritonitis.[2] A rare complication includes inflammation of adjacent bowel loops with secondary enteric fistulas.[2] The diagnosis of infected urachal cysts can be made at ultrasound as shown in Figures 8A, B, or the diagnosis can be made with CT.[4] CT findings of pyourachus include a conical-shaped mass with the apex at the umbilicus extending with its base toward the bladder, deep to the rectus abdominis muscles. The mass begins abruptly at the umbilicus, and the adjacent tissue surrounding the umbilicus shows inflammatory changes.[4] CT and voiding cystourethrography may both confirm the communication with the bladder.

A rare fifth group of urachal anomalies includes the uncommon tumors of the urachus[4] usually seen as a solid mass at ultrasound. Frequently, further evaluation with CT or MRI is required to delineate the extent of the disease.[1,4] Reported solid tumors of the urachus include adenoma, fibroma, yolk sac tumor, and adenocarcinoma.[6]

The differential diagnosis of urachal cyst includes ovarian cyst and mesenteric cyst.[1,2] Differentiation can usually be made with ultrasound and voiding cystourethrograms (VCUG) based on location and configuration of the anomaly. Rarer entities in the differential diagnosis include non-Hodgkin's lymphoma,[4] but these abdominal masses (nodes) are usually solid and spherical rather than cystic and conical. Desmoplastic round cell tumor is a well-defined tumor[4] (usually solid at ultrasound) that may be found in the midline.

Further Reading

1. Carty H, Brunelle F, Shaw D, Kendall B, eds. *Imaging Children.* New York: Churchill Livingstone; 1994:714–775.
2. Kelalis PP, King LR, Belman AB. *Clinical Pediatric Urology, II* 3rd ed. Philadelphia: WB Saunders Co; 1992:613–616.
3. Fuchkar Z, Mozetich V, Dimec D. Sonographic diagnosis of an inflamed urachal cyst. *J Clin Ultrasound* 21:52–54, 1993.

4. Herman TE, Shackleford GD. Pyourachus: CT manifestations. *J Comput Assist Tomogr* 19(3):440–443, 1995.

5. Kirks DR, ed. *Practical Pediatric Imaging.* 2nd ed. Boston: Little, Brown & Co; 1991:969.

6. Suita S, Nagasaki A. Urachal remnants. *Semin Pediatr Surg* 5(2):107–115, 1996.

7. Sepulveda W, Bower S, Dhillon H, et al. Prenatal diagnosis of congenital patent urachus and allantoic cyst: the value of color flow imaging. *J Ultrasound Med* 14:47–51, 1995.

Case 9

Clinical Presentation

A female newborn presents with complex congenital anomalies, including sacral agenesis, anorectal malformation with imperforate anus, and a palpable midline abdominal/pelvic mass.

Radiographic Studies

Transverse ultrasound of the pelvis (Fig. 9A) shows a large, incompletely septated, primarily cystic pelvic mass (white arrows). The mass contains a large volume of inhomogeneous echogenic debris. A small cystic structure is displaced anteriorly, against the abdominal wall, and represents a nearly empty compressed bladder (arrowheads).

Figure 9B is an anteroposterior radiograph taken after percutaneous puncture of this cystic abdominal mass, partial drainage of the contents, and injection of radiopaque contrast. The contrast demonstrates a very distended, nearly completely septated mass. Percutaneous drainage was performed in this patient to decompress the cystic mass and relieve the upper urinary tract obstruction, prior to correcting the anorectal malformation/imperforate anus.

Transverse ultrasound after percutaneous drainage (Fig. 9C) shows the nearly completely septated mass, greatly reduced in size, with fluid/debris levels in both portions of the mass.

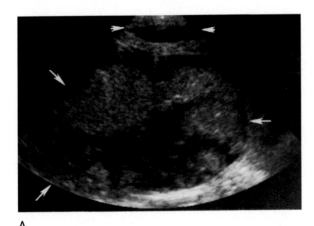

A

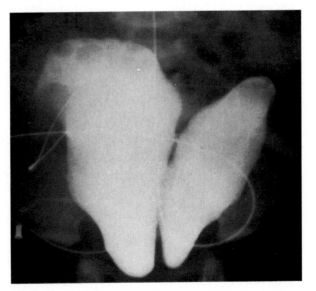

B

- If there is simple isolated vaginal outlet obstruction, the fluid identified in the vagina at ultrasound is usually homogeneous.[3] If there are associated complex anomalies causing hydrocolpos/hydrometrocolpos, then usually the fluid identified at ultrasound is inhomogeneous, with clumps of echogenic debris scattered throughout the fluid.[3] Figure 9A shows such findings.

- Kaufman-McKusick syndrome is an autosomal recessive triad including hydrometrocolpos, polydactyly, and cardiac malformations.[3]

- At the time of diagnosis, it is important to evaluate the upper urinary tract for obstruction. Hydronephrosis and hydroureter may be present due to compression of the distal ureters and subsequent obstruction by the large pelvic mass.[3]

- MRI may be helpful in evaluating these patients if the ultrasound diagnosis is uncertain.

- In patients with associated congenital anomalies, the vagina and uterus may be septated/duplicated.[1,3]

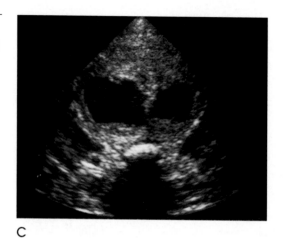

C

Diagnosis   Hydrocolpos/Hydrometrocolpos

Discussion and Differential Diagnosis

Hydrocolpos is defined as "dilatation of the vagina proximal to a congenital obstruction."[1] Hydrometrocolpos is present if there is dilatation of the uterus as well as the vagina.[1] In its simplest form, the obstruction is secondary to an imperforate hymen, and simple lysis of the hymen provides resolution of the problem.[2,3] In more complex forms, vaginal atresia or stenosis is the cause of the obstruction. These patients have other complicated congenital anomalies, including anorectal malformations, cloacal abnormalities with a common urogenital sinus, duplicated/septated uterus or vagina, rectovaginal fistula, and renal anomalies with hydronephrosis.[2,3] These conditions are obviously more complicated, and correction of hydrocolpos or hydrometrocolpos must be coordinated with correction of the other complex anomalies.

The typical patient is a female newborn with a palpable pelvic/abdominal mass. Diagnosis may be delayed, and the patient may present at puberty, when there is an increased accumulation of menstrual blood and secretions causing uterine and vaginal distention.[3] In these patients, hydrocolpos/hydrometrocolpos was present at birth but unnoticed.[3]

The differential diagnosis includes ovarian cysts, mesenteric cysts, anterior meningoceles, and sacrococcygeal teratomas.[3] In patients with ovarian cysts and mesenteric cysts, the uterus and vagina are usually identified by ultrasound but may be difficult to visualize because of severe compression or displacement. Ultrasound of patients with anterior meningocele and sacrococcygeal teratomas usually shows that the masses are related to the sacrum or distal neural canal. In patients whose diagnosis is uncertain, or if further delineation of adjacent structures is necessary, an MRI of the pelvis may prove helpful.

Further Reading

1. Reed MH, Griscom NT. Hydrometrocolpos in infancy. *Am J Roentgenol Rad Ther Nucl Med* 118(1):1–58, 1973.
2. Kirks DR, ed. *Practical Pediatric Imaging.* 2nd ed. Boston: Little, Brown & Co; 1991:975–978.
3. Mirk P, Pintus C, Speca S. Ultrasound diagnosis of hydrocolpos: prenatal findings and post natal follow-up. *J Clin Ultrasound* 22(1):55–58, 1994.
4. Graivier L. Hydrocolpos. *J Pediatr Surg* 4(5):563–568, 1969.

PITFALLS

- If the bladder is completely empty, or markedly compressed against the anterior abdominal wall, it may not be identified on ultrasound. In these patients, the dilated vagina/uterus may be confused with a dilated bladder.[3]

- Correct diagnosis is important before any therapy. If hydrocolpos/ hydrometrocolpos is confused with a pelvic mass, unnecessary laparotomy, which has a reported perioperative mortality of up to 35%,[4] or unnecessary hysterectomy may be performed.[3]

Case 10

Clinical Presentation

A female newborn with bulging flanks and feeding difficulty.

Radiographic Studies

Supine view of the abdomen (Fig. 10A) shows a large soft tissue mass in the pelvis, extending into the left side of the abdomen, with displacement of the bowel gas pattern into the right upper quadrant. Longitudinal ultrasound (Fig. 10B) shows a large cystic mass extending from the pelvis into the upper abdomen. Transverse ultrasound (Fig. 10C) shows the large anterior cystic mass and two normal kidneys posteriorly. Longitudinal ultrasound of the mass (Fig. 10D) shows internal septations (arrowhead) and echogenic debris (arrows) within the mass.

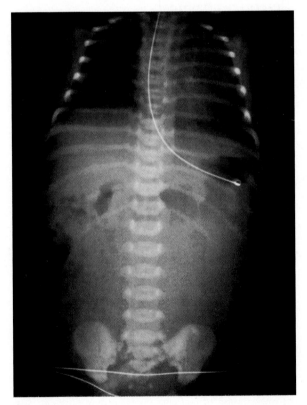

A

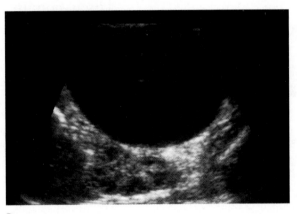

B

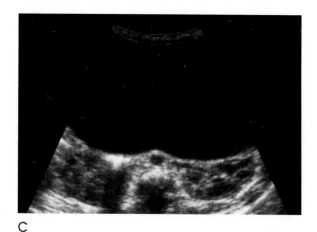

C

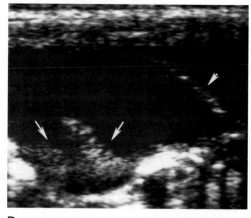

D

Diagnosis Ovarian Cyst

Discussion and Differential Diagnosis

In the neonate, small follicular and lutein cysts are common and are generally asymptomatic.[1] At ultrasound, the cysts are identified as thin-walled cystic masses, usually up to approximately 3 cm in diameter with good posterior wall-through transmission.[1] These generally resolve spontaneously in the days to weeks following birth.[1]

Occasionally, in the fetus, the ovarian cyst may become very large, which is thought to be secondary to in utero maternal chorionic gonadotropin stimulation,[1] and at birth, the newborn presents with an abdominal/pelvic mass.[2] These large cysts may be identified prenatally, with a variable ultrasound appearance, depending on torsion, and/or hemorrhage into the cyst.[3] There is an increased incidence of large ovarian cysts in infants of diabetic mothers and in infants whose prenatal history includes maternal toxemia or maternal isoimmunization.[1] Serial prenatal ultrasound scans show a changing appearance to the fetal ovarian cyst.[3]

Shortly after birth, the diagnosis of a large ovarian cyst is usually made with ultrasound, which identifies a unilocular or septated cyst, with or without internal echoes.[1] The differential diagnosis of large ovarian cystic masses includes hydronephrosis, enteric duplication cysts, hydrocolpos, and urachal cysts.[1] In assessing the mass, hydronephrosis is usually excluded by identifying two normal kidneys. An enteric duplication cyst frequently has a thin hyperechoic rim of smooth muscle just beneath the cyst capsule,[1] which helps to distinguish it from an ovarian cyst. Urachal cysts and hydrocolpos are both usually midline. If two normal ovaries are identified, a large ovarian cyst is unlikely.[1] Ultrasound cannot definitively separate benign from malignant masses, but in the neonate, ovarian malignancies are extremely rare.[1] In the older child, the presentation of ovarian cyst is entirely different, and the differential diagnosis includes a hemorrhagic/torsed ovary, an ectopic pregnancy, pelvic inflammatory disease, or appendicitis.[1]

PEARLS

- Unilocular anechoic cysts are benign, regardless of the patient's age or size.[4]

- Most cysts smaller than 5 cm resolve spontaneously.[1]

- The presence of septations, echogenic debris, or fluid levels within ovarian cysts usually indicate previous torsion and hemorrhage into the cyst.[3]

- Ovarian malignancies are extremely rare in the neonate.[1]

PITFALLS

- The use of the resistive index (RI) and pulsatility index (PI) with Doppler ultrasound may prove helpful in evaluating some masses,[5] but the PI and RI cannot be reliably used to differentiate benign from malignant lesions.[6] The lack of demonstrable color flow does not exclude malignancy.[6,7]

CONTROVERSY

- The management of ovarian cysts in the neonate is controversial. Some authors indicate that cysts larger than 6 cm or with complex ultrasound characteristics need surgery.[2] Others state that neither the size nor the character of the cyst predict clinical outcome,[8] and ovarian cysts even larger than 5 to 6 cm in diameter can be safely managed with serial ultrasound examinations, because most cysts decrease in size or resolve.[8] The decision for surgery should be based on the symptoms (feeding difficulties, respiratory difficulties, or GI obstruction), diagnostic evaluation suggestive of a nonovarian source of the mass, evidence of neoplasm, complications of the mass such as extensive hemorrhage, or failure of resolution or decrease in size.[8]

Further Reading

1. Carty H, Brunelle F, Shaw D, Kendall B, eds. *Imaging Children.* New York: Churchill Livingstone; 1994:769–772.
2. Kirks DR, ed. *Practical Pediatric Imaging.* 2nd ed. Boston: Little, Brown & Co; 1991:1028–1030.
3. Shozu M, Akasofu K, Yamashiro G, Omura K. Changing ultrasonographic appearance of a fetal ovarian cyst twisted in utero. *J Ultrasound Med* 12:415–417, 1993.
4. Atri M, Nazarian S, Bret P, et al. Endovaginal sonographic appearance of benign ovarian masses. *Radiographics* 14:747–760, 1994.
5. Levine D, Feldstein V, Babcock C, Filly R. Sonography of ovarian masses: poor sensitivity of resistive index for identifying malignant lesions. *Am J Roentgenol* 162:1355–1359, 1994.
6. Brown D, Frates MC, Laing FC, et al. Ovarian masses: Can benign and malignant lesions be differentiated with color and pulsed Doppler US? *Radiology* 190:333–336, 1994.
7. Salem S, White LM, Lai J. Doppler sonography of adnexal masses: the predictive value of the pulsatility index in benign and malignant disease. *Am J Roentgenol* 163:1147–1150, 1994.
8. Warner BW, Kuhn JC, Barr LL. Conservative management of large ovarian cysts in children: the value of serial pelvic ultrasonography. *Surgery* 112:749–755, 1992.

Case 11

Clinical Presentation

A newborn male patient with complex gastrointestinal/genitourinary anomalies including imperforate anus, vesicocolic fistula, dilated neurogenic bladder with grade 4 bilateral reflux, urinary stasis, and hypospadia.

Radiographic Studies

Longitudinal ultrasound of the pelvis (Fig. 11A) performed shortly after birth shows a dilated irregularly contoured bladder, with debris (arrows) within the bladder lumen, which may be secondary to the vesicocolic fistula, or urinary stasis. Transverse ultrasound of the bladder at 15 months of age (Fig. 11B) shows a dilated neurogenic bladder with an 8-mm echogenic density (caliper markers) lodged at the bladder base. The density casts a posterior acoustical shadow.

An anteroposterior (AP) view of the abdomen in another patient (Fig. 11C) shows a large calcified bladder mass. Ultrasound of the bladder in this patient (Fig. 11D) shows a large echogenic bladder mass (arrow), with posterior acoustical shadowing.

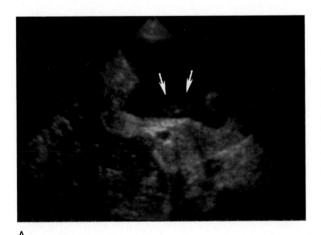

A

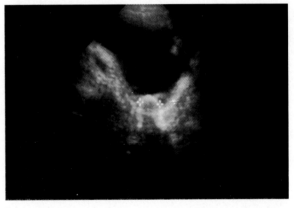

B

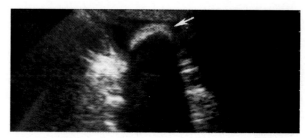

D

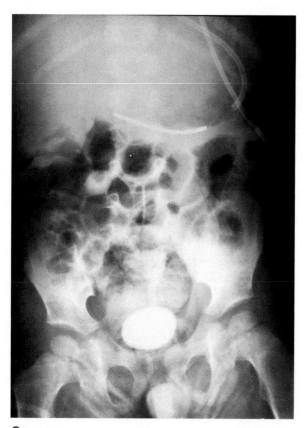

C

Diagnosis   Urolithiasis: Bladder Stone

Discussion and Differential Diagnosis

Bladder stones are uncommon in children in the Western hemisphere and are usually related to anatomical or functional anomalies of the urinary tract. The stones arise locally in patients with urinary stasis, congenital GU anomalies, or neurogenic bladder, or from a foreign body nidus. Bladder stones have also been identified in patients who have had bladder augmentation or ileal surgery.[1,2] Occasionally, stones arise in the upper urinary tract and migrate to the bladder; they rarely cause obstruction but may serve as a focus for infection.[3]

Ultrasound is the examination of choice; it usually shows a mobile, echogenic mass within the bladder lumen, with posterior acoustical shadowing. The differential diagnosis includes rhabdomyosarcoma, which is usually a polypoid irregularly contoured mass within the bladder lumen and adherent to the bladder wall, without acoustical shadowing. Blood clots may also form within the bladder wall, without acoustical shadowing.

PEARLS

• Bladder stones are significant health problems in developing countries, particularly in Asia. Many are presumed to be secondary to a diet high in oxalate and deficient in phosphate. They are also presumed to be secondary to infection, infestation, and dehydration.

• Any patient with urinary stasis is highly susceptible to developing bladder stones.

Further Reading

1. Carty H, Brunelle F, Shaw D, Kendall B, eds. *Imaging Children.* New York: Churchill Livingstone; 1994:703.
2. Currarino G. The genitourinary tract. In: Silverman FN, ed. *Caffey's Pediatric X-ray Diagnosis.* 8th ed. Chicago: Yearbook Medical Publishers; 1985:1361.
3. Rumack CM, Wilson SR, Charboneau GW. *Diagnostic Ultrasound, I & II.* St. Louis: Mosby Yearbook; 1991:249, 1226.
4. Kelalis PP, King LR, Belman AB. *Clinical Pediatric Urology, II.* 3rd ed. Philadelphia: WB Saunders Co; 1992:1343.

PITFALLS

- In patients with an augmented bladder, the bladder contours are irregular, and a pseudomass may be seen at ultrasound, secondary to bowel folds, mucus, or intussuscepted bowel wall.[4] Trapped air within the folds may cause "dirty" acoustical shadowing and may be confused with bladder stones.

Case 12

Clinical Presentation

A 9-year-old girl presents with acute onset of left flank pain and hematuria.

Radiographic Studies

Longitudinal ultrasound of the left kidney (Fig. 12A) shows hydronephrosis. Longitudinal ultrasound through a distended bladder (Fig. 12B) shows left distal ureteral dilatation with an echogenic density (arrow) casting a posterior shadow at the ureterovesicular junction.

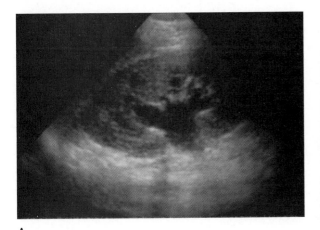

A

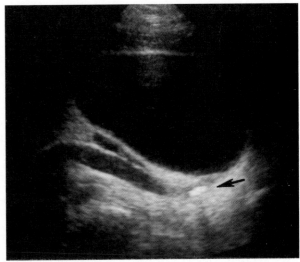

B

315

Diagnosis Urolithiasis: Ureteral Stone

Discussion and Differential Diagnosis

Urolithiasis, usually defined as calculus formation within the collecting system of the kidney and distal urinary tract,[1] is less frequent in children than in adults.[2] Calcium stones are the most common and are usually radiodense. Magnesium ammonium phosphate stones (struvite stones) are usually associated with urinary tract infection and are less likely to be radiopaque than are calcium stones. Uric acid and cystine stones are less common and are of variable radiodensity.[3]

The calculi are usually formed in the kidney and pass into the distal urinary tract.[1] Etiology of urolithiasis includes:

1. Urinary stasis, which may be secondary to an anatomic anomaly, urinary tract infection, or foreign body[3]

2. Metabolic disorders causing hypercalciuria, including renal tubular acidosis, hyperparathyroidism, and medullary sponge kidney[4]

3. Idiopathic[2]

The differential diagnosis in pediatric patients is limited, and includes appendicolith and calcified ovarian mass.[2] Both are usually distinguishable by imaging procedures.

Further Reading

1. Kirks DR, ed. *Practical Pediatric Imaging.* 2nd ed. Boston: Little, Brown & Co; 1991:942.

2. Carty H, Brunelle F, Shaw D, Kendall B, eds. *Imaging Children.* New York: Churchill Livingstone; 1994:698–706.

3. Currarino G. The genitourinary tract. In: Silverman FN, ed. *Caffey's Pediatric X-ray Diagnosis.* 8th ed. Chicago: Yearbook Medical Publishers; 1985:1702–1706.

4. Shultz PK, Strife JL, Strife CF, McDaniel JD. Hyperechoic renal medullary pyramids. *Radiology* 181:163–167, 1991.

Case 13

Clinical Presentation

A 3-week-old low-birth weight premature neonate receiving long-term furosemide therapy.

Radiographic Studies

Figure 13 is a longitudinal ultrasound scan of the kidney (caliper markers) with hyperechoic medullary pyramids (arrows).

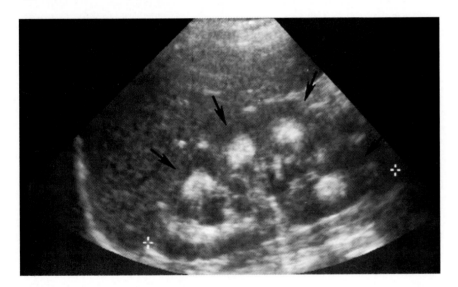

Diagnosis Nephrocalcinosis

PEARLS

• Incidence of nephrocalcinosis in very low birthweight neonates is significantly higher in white infants and in those with a positive family history of renal stones/nephrocalcinosis.[6]

• The incidence of nephrocalcinosis in premature infants is increased because of their decreased glomerular filtration rate and abnormal urine acidification; nephrocalcinosis may occur even without diuretics. Dissolved urinary calcium oxalate levels may be so high in premature patients that the calcium oxalate crystals precipitate in their own solid phase.[7]

• Nephrocalcinosis and nephrolithiasis have been reported in asphyxiated full-term newborns secondary to fat necrosis and subsequent hypercalcemia. In these patients, the hypercalcemia may be so severe that the infants develop seizures or even die.[8]

PITFALLS

• Hyperechoic renal pyramids resembling medullary nephrocalcinosis are an unusual presentation of autosomal recessive polycystic kidney disease.[9] The

Discussion and Differential Diagnosis

Nephrocalcinosis is defined as the deposition of calcium compounds within the renal parenchyma,[1] usually in tubules, the tubular epithelium, and interstitial tissues.[2] Ninety percent of nephrocalcinosis occurs in the medullary pyramids.[1] Less often, nephrocalcinosis occurs in the renal cortex, seen either as diffuse linear cortical calcifications (secondary to cortical ischemia or necrosis)[1] or focal nephrocalcinosis in a portion of the kidney (secondary to chronic inflammatory disease, tumor, or vascular lesion).[1] Renal calcifications may be seen as granular or stippled densities on routine X ray,[2] but ultrasound is more sensitive and is the preferred modality for screening for nephrocalcinosis.[1] Normally, in the pediatric patient, the medullary pyramids are hypoechoic compared to the renal cortex.[3] In patients with nephrocalcinosis, the renal pyramids are hyperechoic, with reversal of the normal corticomedullary echogenicity relationship.[2,3] Acoustical shadowing is usually not identified.[3] CT is occasionally used to identify nephrocalcinosis.[4]

There are multiple causes of nephrocalcinosis, and the majority are associated with hypercalcemia.[3] The most common include long-term furosemide therapy in neonates with bronchopulmonary dysplasia, congenital heart disease, or asphyxia. Other causes include Bartter syndrome, type I renal tubular acidosis,[3] hyperthyroidism, Williams syndrome, prolonged immobilization, steroid therapy, and hypophosphatasia.[2,3]

Hyperechoic renal medullary pyramids do not always indicate nephrocalcinosis. The differential diagnosis of hyperechoic renal medullary pyramids includes transient renal insufficiency, with tubular blockade and subsequent protein precipitation, oliguria secondary to chemotherapy or precipitated Tamm-Horsfall proteins,[5] sickle cell hemoglobinopathies with vascular congestion and early papillary necrosis,[3,5] early renal vein thrombosis,[3,5] and infection with cytomegalovirus or *Candida*.[5] It may be impossible to differentiate hyperechoic medullary pyramids in patients with nephrocalcinosis from the other causes of hyperechoic renal medullary pyramids.

Further Reading

1. Carty H, Brunelle F, Shaw D, Kendall B, eds. *Imaging Children*. New York: Churchill Livingstone; 1994:704–706.
2. Kirks DR, ed. *Practical Pediatric Imaging*. 2nd ed. Boston: Little, Brown & Co; 1991:942–944.
3. Shultz PK, Strife JL, Strife CF, McDaniel JD. Hyperechoic renal medullary pyramids in infants and children *Radiology* 163–167, 1991.
4. Lucaya J, Enriquez G, Nieto J, et al. Renal calcifications in patients with autosomal recessive polycystic kidney disease: prevalence and cause. *Am J Roentgenol* 160:359–362, 1993.
5. Hernanz-Schulman M. Hyperechoic renal medullary pyramids in infants and children. *Radiology* 181:9–11, 1991.

ultrasound appearance may be indistinguishable from that of other causes of nephrocalcinosis. In these patients, liver ultrasound may show echogenic periportal regions or slightly dilated biliary ducts, providing clues that the diagnosis may be autosomal recessive polycystic kidney disease.[9]

- Nephrocalcinosis is common in older children with autosomal recessive polycystic kidney disease, secondary to renal failure and urine acidification defects. These older patients typically present with other manifestations of autosomal recessive polycystic kidney disease and have hepatic fibrosis.[4]

CONTROVERSY

- In some patients, no simple explanation or clearly defined cause for nephrocalcinosis can be identified,[5] despite a systematic approach including patient history, measurement of serum and urine calcium concentrations, and renal function evaluation to search for a specific diagnosis for this condition.[3]

6. Karkowicz MG, Katz ME, Adelman RD, et al. Nephrocalcinosis in very low birth weight neonates: family history of kidney stones and ethnicity as independent risk factors. *J Pediatr* 122:635–638, 1993.
7. Campfield T, Braden G, Flynn-Valone P, et al. Urinary oxalate excretion in premature infants: effect on human milk versus formula feeding. *Pediatrics* 94:674–678, 1994.
8. Gu LL, Daneman A, Binet A, et al. Nephrocalcinosis and nephrolithiasis due to subcutaneous fat necrosis with hypercalcemia in two full-term asphyxiated neonates: sonographic findings. *Pediatr Radiol* 25:142–144, 1995.
9. Herman TE, Siegel MJ. Pyramidal hyperechogenicity in autosomal recessive polycystic kidney disease resembling medullary nephrocalcinosis. *Pediatr Radiol* 21:270–271, 1991.

Case 14

Clinical Presentation

A 3-year-old girl with dysuria, urgency, and frequency.

Radiographic Studies

Transverse ultrasound (Fig. 14A) shows uniform bladder wall thickening (caliper markers) with echogenic debris within the bladder. Longitudinal ultrasound (Fig. 14B) shows the bladder wall thickening.

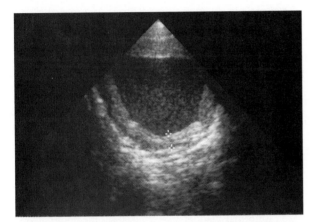

A

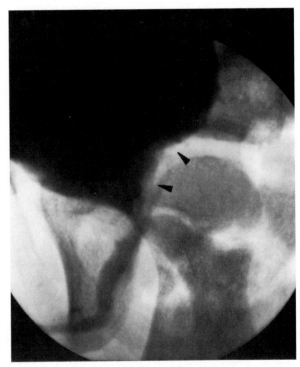

C

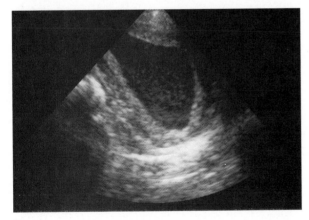

B

Diagnosis Cystitis

Discussion and Differential Diagnosis

Cystitis, or inflammation of the bladder wall, has multiple causes, but is most frequently secondary to bacterial infection in the bladder.[2] Infants and children present with unexplained fever, irritability, vomiting, diarrhea, or failure to thrive.[1] Older children who have been toilet trained present with urgency, frequency, dysuria, and secondary-onset enuresis. Fever and systemic symptoms are less common in older children.[1] Cystitis may occur as an isolated entity or be associated with pyelonephritis.[2] Hemorrhagic cystitis may result from *E. coli* infection.[1,3] Other causes include viral infection, drugs (Cytoxan), immune deficiency, and eosinophilic cystitis.[1–3] Cystitis is also associated with voiding dysfunction in patients with abnormally large bladders, who rarely completely empty the bladder.[1]

Ultrasound is the imaging modality of choice for cystitis; bladder wall thickening greater than 3 to 4 mm is usually identified with a distended bladder.[1,2] Inflammatory edema may be so prominent that it may protrude into the bladder lumen,[3] or cause focal bladder wall thickening,[4] simulating an invasive neoplasm. Patients with hemorrhagic cystitis may present with echogenic debris within the bladder lumen, representing blood clots.[2] In all patients with a culture-documented urinary tract infection, further evaluation with a contrast cystogram is recommended to detect congenital anomalies, reflux, ureteroceles, or other bladder pathology.[1] Nuclear cystography may be used for follow-up evaluation of reflux, or screening of asymptomatic siblings,[1] but contrast cystography is initially recommended because of its superior delineation of the urethra and bladder mucosa.[1] Cystography is performed when the patient is no longer symptomatic and when the urine is sterile.[1]

The differential diagnosis of abnormal bladder wall thickening includes cystitis, tumor, neurofibromatosis, chronic granulomatous disease, bladder outlet obstruction, and chemotherapy cystitis.[3] Imaging studies cannot clearly delineate the causes, and if the presentation is atypical, cystoscopy and biopsy are necessary for an accurate diagnosis, particularly in cases in which the bladder wall thickening/metaplasia mimics a bladder mass/polyp or causes bladder outlet obstruction.[4]

Further Reading

1. Kelalis PP, King LR, Belman AB. *Clinical Pediatric Urology, II.* 3rd ed. Philadelphia: WB Saunders Co; 1992:291–320.
2. Kirks DR, ed. *Practical Pediatric Imaging.* 2nd ed. Boston: Little, Brown & Co; 1991:924–930.
3. Carty H, Brunelle F, Shaw D, Kendall B, eds. *Imaging Children.* New York: Churchill Livingstone; 1994:710–711.
4. Hoeffel JC, Drews K, Gassner I, Arnaudin A. Pseudotumoral cystitis. *Pediatr Radiol* 23:510–514, 1993.
5. Fernbach SK, Feinstein KA. Abnormalities of the bladder in children: imaging findings. *AJR Am J Roentgenol* 162:1143–1150, 1994.
6. Ditchfield MR, De Campo JF, Cook DJ, et al. Vesicoureteral reflux: an accurate predictor of acute pyelonephritis in childhood urinary tract infection? *Radiology* 190:413–415, 1994.

Case 15

Clinical Presentation

A 3-year-old girl with a history of dysuria, frequency, and irritability. Urine culture and sensitivity show evidence of a urinary tract infection.

Radiographic Studies

A posterior image from a radionuclide cystogram (Fig. 15A) shows isotope in the left ureter and collecting system. An anteroposterior (AP) image of the pelvis from a voiding cystourethrogram (VCUG) in a 4-year-old male patient (Fig. 15B) shows contrast in a dilated tortuous left ureter (arrows) and subtle contrast in a mildly dilated right ureter (arrowheads). Contrast in the left collecting system (Fig. 15C) with hydronephrosis and calyceal clubbing is identified, as well as subtle contrast in the right collecting system (arrows).

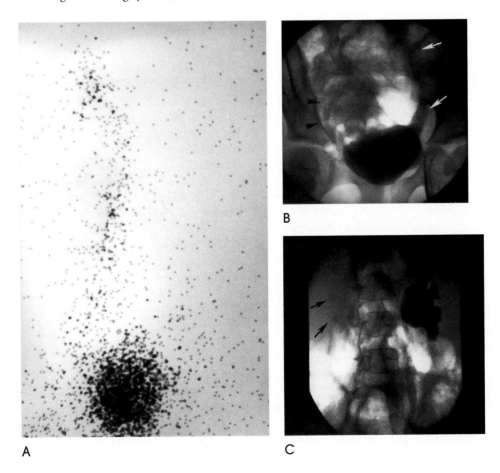

A

B

C

Diagnosis Vesicoureteral Reflux

PEARLS

- There is an inverse correlation between the severity of reflux and the likelihood of resolution.[2]

- There is an increased incidence of reflux in patients with posterior urethral valves, multicystic dysplastic kidneys, ectopic ureters, prune-belly syndrome, and ureteropelvic junction obstruction.[3]

- Renal scars do not occur if reflux occurs in the absence of infection,[5] unless there is an element of bladder outlet obstruction. It is the obstruction that causes the renal damage.[6]

- Once renal parenchymal infection has occurred, ultimate renal scarring is independent of the presence or absence of vesicoureteral reflux.[5] Renal scarring depends on the virulence of the bacteria, the host defense mechanisms, and bacterial adherence to uroepithelial cells.[6]

PITFALLS

- Acute pyelonephritis in the absence of vesicoureteral reflux is common.[6]

- Acute pyelonephritis is the more accurate predictor for the development of renal scars than the presence or absence of vesicoureteral reflux.[7]

Discussion and Differential Diagnosis

Vesicoureteral reflux is the most common anomaly of the urinary tract in children. It is seen in approximately 35% of patients with urinary tract infection.[1] Reflux is usually an isolated anomaly, but it is important to evaluate for other urinary tract pathology, including obstruction and duplication. Vesicoureteral reflux is seen in up to 45% of asymptomatic siblings of patients with reflux and urinary tract infection.[2] Reflux usually resolves spontaneously in one third of cases each year of life.[1]

Vesicoureteral reflux is secondary to incompetence of the valve at the vesicoureteral junction; this is usually secondary to a short distal ureteric submucosal tunnel through the posterior bladder wall, leading to an incompetent orifice.[3] This abnormal configuration of the ureteral orifice causes abnormal function at the ureterovesical junction. There is an increased risk of reflux if there is an associated paraureteral diverticulum.[2,3]

Vesicoureteral reflux can be imaged with either a nuclear cystogram or a voiding cystourethrogram. Both studies involve urethral catheterization, with retrograde filling of the bladder. Imaging is usually delayed until antibiotic therapy has been complete and the urine is sterile, in order to decrease bladder irritability and secondary underfilling of the bladder, thereby avoiding false-negative examinations.[1] In addition, high pressure reflux to the kidney with infected urine has been reported to increase damage to the kidney.[8] With nuclear medicine cystography, radioisotope mixed with saline is instilled into the bladder. This study allows for constant monitoring of the bladder during the examination and low radiation dose. It is ideal for girls but lacks anatomic detail. Subtle bladder wall or urethral abnormalities may not be detected.[1] Voiding cystourethrography is done by infusing radiographic contrast into the bladder, intermittent monitoring of bladder filling for reflux, and detailed evaluation of the urethra during voiding. This technique allows visualization of detailed bladder wall and urethral anatomy, and is ideal for male patients, who have a higher incidence of urethral abnormalities than do female patients. The technique is also useful for female patients with a history or physical examination suggestive of urethral pathology, such as dribbling, or abnormalities of the external genitalia.[1] Some authors recommend that for routine reflux, the initial study should be a standard voiding cystourethrogram, and follow-up examinations should be performed with nuclear medicine cystography, in order to minimize radiation exposure.[8]

The severity of vesicoureteral reflux is graded according to the International Reflux Classification Standard,[2] and reflux is graded as follows[4]:

Grade I: Ureter only

Grade II: Ureter, pelvis, and calyceal; no dilatation, normal calyceal fornices.

Grade III: Mild or moderate dilatation and/or tortuosity of the ureter and mild or moderate dilatation of the renal pelvis; no, or slight, blunting of the fornices.

CONTROVERSY

- It has been assumed that vesicoureteral reflux is the primary risk factor for the development of renal scars in patients with urinary tract infections. Therefore, screening for reflux was assumed to assess for the risk of scarring. Patients with grade II or greater reflux are routinely treated with suppressive antibiotic therapy to prevent recurrent urinary tract infections and scarring. Patients with grade I reflux or no reflux are routinely not treated with suppressive antibiotics. However, new data suggest that renal parenchymal infection occurs commonly in patients who do not have reflux; any patient with renal parenchymal infection is at risk for developing scars. Nuclear medicine renal cortical scanning is an accurate tool for identifying acute pyelonephritis and renal scars. Several researchers believe that the presence of renal parenchymal involvement in patients with urinary tract infection, documented on renal cortical nuclear medicine scanning, is a more important indicator for patients at risk of developing renal scars,[1,5,6] and may be a more important indicator for antibiotic prophylaxis, particularly in a younger patient, than the presence or absence of vesicoureteral reflux.[1,7]

Grade IV: Moderate dilatation and/or tortuosity of the ureter and moderate dilatation of the ureter and moderate dilatation of the renal pelvis and calyces; complete obliteration of the sharp angle of the fornices but maintenance of the papillary impressions in the majority of calyces.

Grade V: Gross dilatation and tortuosity of the ureter; gross dilatation of the renal pelvis and calyces; the papillary impressions are no longer visible in the majority of the calyces.

Surgery for correction of vesicoureteral reflux is usually reserved for patients with ureteral diverticula, ureteral obstruction with reflux, ureters with a "golf hole" orifice with no submucosal tunneling, or persistent urinary tract infections despite antibiotic therapy.[2]

Further Reading

1. Andrich MP, Majd M. Diagnostic imaging in the evaluation of the first urinary tract infection in infants and young children. *Pediatrics* 90(3):436–441, 1992.
2. Kelalis PP, King LR, Belman AB. *Clinical Pediatric Urology, I.* 3rd ed. Philadelphia: WB Saunders Co; 1992: 441–500.
3. Carty H, Brunelle F, Shaw D, Kendall B, eds. *Imaging Children, I.* New York: Churchill Livingstone; 1994:648–670.
4. Lebowitz RL, Olbing H, Parkkulainen KV, et al. International system of radiographic grading of vesicoureteric reflux. *Pediatr Radiol* 15:105–109, 1985.
5. Rushton HG, Majd M, Jantausch B, et al. Renal scarring following reflux and nonreflux pyelonephritis in children: evaluation with ^{99m}Technetium-dimercaptosuccinic acid scintigraphy. *J Urol* 147:1327–1332, 1992.
6. Majd M, Rushton HG. Renal cortical scintigraphy in the diagnosis of acute pyelonephritis. *Semin Nucl Med* 22(2):98–111, 1992.
7. Ditchfield MR, De Campo JF, Cook DJ, et al. Vesicoureteral reflux: an accurate predictor of acute pyelonephritis in childhood urinary tract infection? *Radiology* 190:413–415, 1994.
8. Kirks, DR, ed. *Practical Pediatric Imaging.* 2nd ed. Boston: Little, Brown and Co.; 1991:984–990.

Case 16

Clinical Presentation

An 8-year-old boy presents with fever, flank pain, and intermittent hematuria. Clinical data include leukocytosis, pyuria, bacteriuria, and a positive urine culture.

Radiographic Studies

Longitudinal ultrasound scan of the kidney (Fig. 16A) shows blurring of the corticomedullary junction secondary to diffuse renal edema, poorly defined hypoechoic wedge-shaped lucencies (arrows) within the renal parenchyma, and mild dilatation of the central renal pelvis (arrowhead). Longitudinal ultrasound scan of the kidney (Fig. 16B) shows a poorly defined focal hypoechoic area (caliper markers) within the lower pole renal parenchyma.

CT scan (Fig. 16C) shows wedge-shaped streaky zones of low attenuation (arrowheads) after contrast administration in another patient. Mild renal enlargement is noted, with dilatation of the renal pelves bilaterally.

Posterior image from a DMSA (dimercaptosuccinic acid) renal cortical scan (Fig. 16D) shows several zones of decreased cortical uptake (arrows), without volume loss, in the upper and lower poles of the right kidney of the 8-year-old patient.

Longitudinal color Doppler ultrasound image of the lower pole of the kidney (Fig. 16E, Color Plate 4) shows multiple focal areas of decreased flow (arrows) at the mid and lower portions of the kidney.

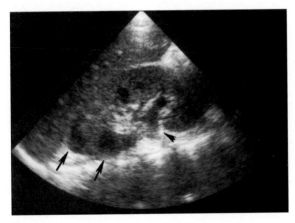

A

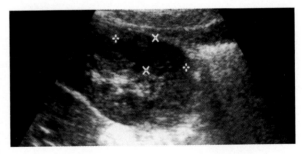

B

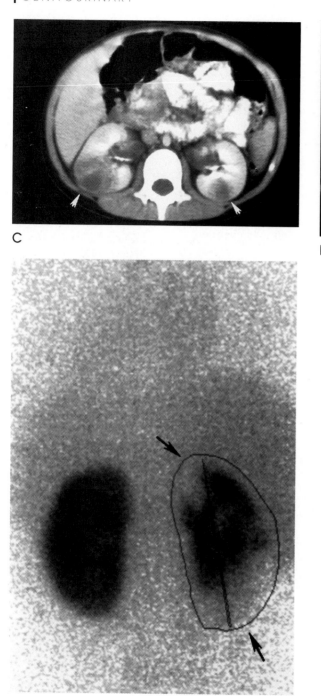

C

D

E

Diagnosis Acute Pyelonephritis

Discussion and Differential Diagnosis

Acute pyelonephritis is defined as a bacterial infection of the kidney with acute inflammation, involving the renal pelvis and parenchyma, usually along one or more medullary rays.[1,2] The pathology is usually secondary to ascending infection from the bladder, with inflammatory cells in the tubules and interstitial tissues.[2] The mechanism of infection also may be hematogenous, usually found in patients who are IV drug abusers or immunosuppressed, or in patients with an extra-renal infection source, such as skin, teeth, or heart valves. Hematogenous infection may be very difficult to distinguish from ascending infection.[2]

Acute pyelonephritis is the most important clinical issue in a patient with a febrile urinary tract infection. Recent studies have shown clinical and laboratory data to be inadequate in diagnosing acute pyelonephritis.[3] Acute pyelonephritis is a cause of major morbidity in children with urinary tract infection because it may lead to irreversible renal scarring, with secondary growth retardation, hypertension, and chronic renal failure.[4] Early diagnosis and treatment are of critical importance in preventing the development of renal scars.[3] Vesicoureteral reflux is identified in approximately 30 to 50% of patients with acute pyelonephritis. However, acute pyelonephritis in the absence of reflux is also common.[4]

The pathogenesis is controversial and depends on bacterial virulence, the adherence of bacteria to uroepithelial cells, host defense mechanism,[4] bladder outlet obstruction, and possibly the presence of reflux. Parenchymal infection is a prerequisite for acquired renal scarring, and scarring occurs only at sites corresponding to areas of previous acute pyelonephritis.[5]

Multiple studies have demonstrated that radionuclide renal cortical scanning is an excellent modality for imaging renal parenchymal involvement (acute pyelonephritis) during acute urinary tract infection.[3–6] The sensitivity of renal cortical scanning is 90%, and the specificity is 99%.[1,3] The radioisotope glucoheptonate may be a superior screening radiopharmaceutical for detecting acute pyelonephritis and also for imaging renal function.[6] Approximately 20% of glucoheptonate is bound to tubules, allowing imaging of renal cortex; the remainder is excreted into the urine, providing dynamic excretory data to assess functional abnormalities of the collecting system.[4] In patients with urinary tract infections, almost all abnormalities are detected by combined radionuclide imaging with glucoheptonate and voiding cystourethrography.[6]

The radioisotope DMSA is an extremely sensitive, reliable renal cortical imaging agent. Uptake with DMSA occurs only in the renal cortex and depends on renal blood flow and tubular cell function. With acute pyelonephritis, there are varying degrees of decreased cortical uptake secondary to renal ischemia and tubular cell dysfunction. With acute pyelonephritis, there is decreased cortical uptake, but no volume loss. Imaging with DMSA does not show the collecting system.[4] Gallium 67 and indium 111 are not used for renal cortical imaging, because of their excessive radiation dose.

- Prophylactic antibiotic therapy may be more important in patients with renal cortical scanning evidence of acute pyelonephritis during acute urinary tract infection.[4,5]

CT is not routinely performed in children, because of the relatively higher radiation dose and the necessity for intravenous contrast. Sensitivity of CT is approximately equal to that of renal cortical scanning, greater than 90%.[1] CT is routinely used in adults; it shows wedge-shaped streaky zones of low attenuation with variable, but decreased enhancement compared to normal renal parenchymal tissue after administration of contrast. There may be absent or delayed enhancement and focal swelling or renal enlargement.[2,3]

Ultrasound has a lower sensitivity for the detection of, and underestimates the extent of, acute pyelonephritis.[4] However, power Doppler sonography may be useful in children.[1] Recent studies with power Doppler sonography show a sensitivity of 75%, with a specificity of 100% in children with pyelonephritis. Power Doppler images show perfusion defects similar to those seen at renal cortical scanning. Power Doppler may prove very useful and can be performed in patients without sedation. Motion artifact remains a significant problem, especially when attempting to identify a small focus of infection. Diffuse cortical involvement from pyelonephritis may not be seen at power Doppler sonography.[1]

The differential diagnosis with renal cortical scanning is primarily between acute pyelonephritis (decreased cortical uptake) and renal scarring (renal parenchymal loss), identified as parenchymal thinning, flattening, and wedge-shaped cortical defects.[4,5]

Further Reading

1. Winters WD. Power Doppler sonographic evaluation of acute pyelonephritis in children. *J Ultrasound Med* 15:91–96, 1996.
2. Talner LB, Davidson AJ, Lebowitz RL, et al. Acute pyelonephritis: Can we agree on terminology? *Radiology* 192:297–305, 1994.
3. Andrich MP, Majd M. Diagnostic imaging in the evaluation of the first urinary tract infection in infants and young children. *Pediatrics* 90(3):436–441, 1992.
4. Majd M, Rushton HG. Renal cortical scintigraphy in the diagnosis of acute pyelonephritis. *Semin Nucl Med* 22(2):98–111, 1992.
5. Rushton HG, Majd M, Jantausch B, et al. Renal scarring following reflux and nonreflux pyelonephritis in children: evaluation with [99m]Technetium-dimercapto-succinic acid scintigraphy. *J Urol* 147:1327–1332, 1992.
6. Sreenarasimhaiah V, Alon US. Uroradiologic evaluation of children with urinary tract infection: Are both ultrasonography and renal cortical scintigraphy necessary? *J Pediatr* 127:373–377, 1995.

Case 17

Clinical Presentation

A 13-year-old patient with spinal dysraphism, bladder augmentation, and a history of multiple previous urinary tract infections presents with decreasing renal function.

Radiographic Studies

Longitudinal ultrasound of the right kidney (Fig. 17A) shows a focal area of parenchymal loss (arrows) at the right upper pole. Prone longitudinal ultrasound scan of the left kidney (Fig. 17B) shows extensive parenchymal thinning (white arrows) along the anterolateral cortex (caliper markers). A right posterior oblique image from a DMSA renal cortical scan (Fig. 17C) shows a focal wedge-shaped defect (arrow) at the upper pole of the right kidney and a smaller left kidney. A left posterior oblique image from a DMSA renal cortical scan (Fig. 17D) shows the extensive defect (arrows) along the anterolateral portion of the smaller left kidney.

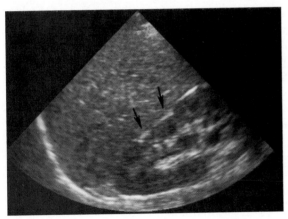

A

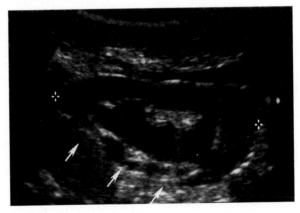

B

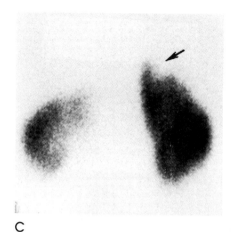

C

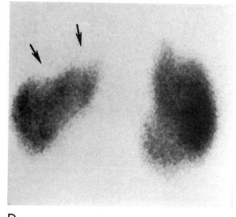

D

PEARLS

- Recent studies indicate that acquired renal scars occur commonly after urinary tract infections, even in the absence of vesicoureteral reflux.[4]

- Other studies have demonstrated that patients with moderate to severe reflux are at increased risk for the development of renal scars.[1]

- Bladder pathology is a major risk factor in the development of renal scars, regardless of reflux, especially if there is functional or anatomic bladder outlet obstruction.[2]

CONTROVERSY

- The current goal of therapy is to prevent the development of renal scars or to prevent their progression. Low-dose prophylactic antibiotic therapy is the current treatment

Diagnosis Cortical Scars

Discussion and Differential Diagnosis

Renal scars are focal areas of parenchymal loss, usually resulting from previous bacterial infection. The scar begins as localized fibrosis in the medulla, eventually involves the entire renal thickness, and causes the outer renal margin to be retracted inward and the renal papilla to be pulled outward. Renal scars occur more often at the upper or lower pole of the kidneys. Some authors consider renal scars to be a direct result of intrarenal reflux with infected urine and maintain that scars rarely occur without reflux. Some authors have even postulated a direct correlation between the grade of reflux and the degree of scarring.[1] Other authors maintain that the incidence of renal parenchymal infection depends on bacterial virulence, bacterial adherence to uroepithelial cell walls causing ascending infection, and host defense mechanisms, regardless of the presence or absence of vesicoureteral reflux.[2] Almost all authors agree that renal scarring occurs with urinary tract infection when the patient has bladder outlet pathology, particularly obstruction, regardless of the presence or absence of vesicoureteral reflux.[2] Reflux without urinary tract infection and without bladder obstruction does not cause renal scarring.[2]

Regardless of etiology, the sequelae of renal scarring are extensive and must be avoided. Renal scars may lead to growth retardation, hypertension, or chronic renal failure.[6] The goal of therapy is to identify patients at risk for renal scarring, and prevent development and progression of the scars. The sensitivity of nuclear medicine renal cortical scanning is approximately 90%, with a specificity of 99%, for detecting renal scars.[6] The scans demonstrate an irregular contour with focal parenchymal thinning, parenchymal loss, or wedge-shaped parenchymal defects.[3] The radiopharmaceuticals DMSA and glucoheptonate have both been used as imaging agents.[2,4,5] The differential diagnosis includes fetal lobulation, but the parenchyma is not usually thinned with this entity.[1] Previous renal vein thrombosis with secondary renal scar may be difficult to differentiate, but if there is a history of renal vein thrombosis, the affected kidney is usually significantly smaller.[1]

regimen and is usually based on the presence of reflux. Severe reflux or recurrent infection despite antibiotics may necessitate ureteral reimplantation. However, recent studies demonstrate that renal scarring occurs in patients with a history of acute urinary tract infections, even without reflux. Some authors suggest that prophylactic antibiotic therapy should be based on renal cortical scan evidence of parenchymal involvement at the time of urinary tract infection.[6]

• Another controversy is that some authors advocate renal ultrasound to screen for the presence of renal cortical scars because it is available, involves no radiation, and allows the visualization of other organs in the abdomen. However, multiple studies have shown that renal ultrasound has low sensitivity in detecting renal cortical scars, and it underestimates both the number and extent of scars.[4,5] More recent studies indicate that nuclear medicine renal cortical scanning is much more reliable and is probably more useful clinically.[5]

Further Reading

1. Kirks DR, ed. *Practical Pediatric Imaging: Diagnostic Radiology of Infants and Children.* 2nd ed. Boston: Little, Brown & Co; 1991:984–994.
2. Rushton HG, Majd M, Jantausch B, et al. Renal scarring following reflux and nonreflux pyelonephritis in children: evaluation with ^{99m}Technetium-dimercapto-succinic acid scintigraphy. *J Urol* 147:1327–1332, 1992.
3. Carty H, Brunelle F, Shaw D, Kendall B. *Imaging Children, I.* New York: Churchill Livingstone; 1994:648–669.
4. Majd M, Rushton HG. Renal cortical scintigraphy in the diagnosis of acute pyelonephritis. *Semin Nucl Med* 22(2):98–111, 1992.
5. Sreenarasimhaiah V, Alon US. Uroradiologic evaluation of children with urinary tract infection: are both ultrasonography and renal cortical scintigraphy necessary? *J Pediatr* 127:373–377, 1995.
6. Andrich MP, Majd M. Diagnostic imaging in the evaluation of the first urinary tract infection in infants and young children. *Pediatrics* 90(3):436–441, 1992.

Case 18

Clinical Presentation

A 10-year-old girl with hematuria and right flank pain.

Radiographic Studies

Longitudinal scan of the right kidney (Fig. 18A) shows multiple variable-sized renal cysts (arrows), involving the cortex and the medulla, separated by areas of normal parenchyma. No hydronephrosis, hydroureter, or renal calculi are identified. Longitudinal scan of the right kidney at age 15 years (Fig. 18B) shows interval renal growth, with proportional interval growth of the renal cysts (arrows). There are still large areas of normal renal parenchyma between the cysts. CT scan of the kidneys at age 15 years (Fig. 18C) shows multiple nonfunctioning (low attenuation) renal cysts, adjacent to areas of normally enhancing (high attenuation) renal cortex. Cysts with hemorrhage may be of higher attenuation than the other cysts.

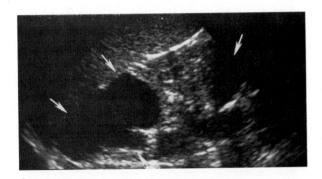

A

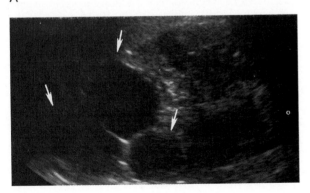

B

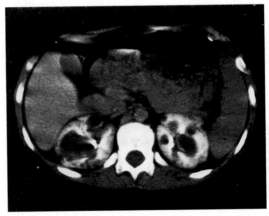

C

Diagnosis Autosomal Dominant Polycystic Kidney Disease (ADPKD)

Discussion and Differential Diagnosis

Autosomal dominant polycystic kidney disease (adult—Potter III) usually presents in the third or fourth decade of life as hypertension, hematuria, or slowly progressive renal failure.[1] These patients have enlarged kidneys, and from 13 to 74% have associated hepatobiliary cysts (intrahepatic cysts and peribiliary cysts).[2] In pancreas, thyroid, ovaries, and testes,[3] a variable incidence of cysts has also been reported. Approximately 10 to 40% of patients have intracranial aneurysms.[1,4]

ADPKD may present in early childhood with a flank mass, hematuria, or flank pain. Patients may also present in the neonatal period with multiple small renal cysts that may be difficult to differentiate from autosomal recessive polycystic kidney disease (ARPKD).[5]

Patients with ADPKD usually do not have portal fibrosis or bile duct proliferation. However, rare cases of hepatic fibrosis have been reported in ADPKD with associated portal hypertension.[6] This may be secondary to an independent allele that may modify the phenotype of ADPKD.[6] Portal hypertension and congenital hepatic fibrosis may be the initial presentation of ADPKD, and screening for the above in families with ADPKD may be warranted.[6]

In patients with suspected ADPKD, ultrasound is usually the initial imaging modality. Findings at ultrasound include asymmetric bilateral renal enlargement, with multiple renal cysts of varying sizes, involving the cortex and the medulla.[3,5] The calyces and renal pelves are frequently grossly distorted.[3,5] The cysts of patients with ADPKD are usually larger than those of patients with ARPKD. Further imaging with CT shows nonfunctioning cysts of varying sizes with distortion of the collecting systems and calyces.[3] CT of the liver shows both discrete intrahepatic cysts and peribiliary cysts, which represent cystic dilatation of the extramural peribiliary glands.[2] With progression of the disease, the renal cysts enlarge, the normal renal parenchyma is compressed and destroyed, the collecting system is distorted, and renal failure develops.[3] The differential diagnosis includes tuberous sclerosis and Turner's syndrome; these patients also have sonolucent renal cysts.[1,5,7]

Further Reading

1. Kelalis PP, King LR, Belman AB. *Clinical Pediatric Urology, II.* 3rd ed. Philadelphia: WB Saunders Co; 1992:1143–1147.
2. Itai Y, Ebihara R, Eguchi N, et al. Hepatobiliary cysts in patients with autosomal dominant polycystic kidney disease: prevalence and CT findings. *Am J Roentgenol* 164:339–342, 1995.
3. Kirks DR, ed. *Practical Pediatric Imaging.* 2nd ed. Boston: Little, Brown & Co; 1991:948–954.
4. Ruggieri PM, Poulos N, Masaryk TJ, et al. Occult intracranial aneurysms in polycystic kidney disease: screening with MR angiography. *Radiology* 191:33–39, 1994.

5. Carty H, Brunelle F, Shaw D, Kendall B, eds. *Imaging Children*. New York: Churchill Livingstone; 1994:2:597–600.

6. Lipschitz B, Berdon WE, Defelice AR, Levy J. Association of congenital hepatic fibrosis with autosomal dominant polycystic kidney disease. *Pediatr Radiol* 23:131–133, 1993.

7. Herman TE, Siegel MJ. Renal cysts associated with Turner's syndrome. *Pediatr Radiol* 24:139–140, 1994.

8. Kogutt MS, Robichaux WH, Boineau FG, Drake GK, Simonton SC. Asymmetric renal size in autosomal recessive polycystic kidney disease: a unique presentation. *AJR Am J Roentgenol* 160:835–836, 1993.

9. Blickman JG, Bramson RT, Herrin JT. Autosomal recessive polycystic kidney disease: long-term sonographic findings in patients surviving the neonatal period. *AJR Am J Roentgenol* 164:1247–1250, 1995.

10. Black WC. Intracranial aneurysm in adult polycystic kidney disease: Is screening with MR angiography indicated? Editorial. *Radiology* 191:18–20, 1994.

Case 19

Clinical Presentation

A newborn with an enlarged abdomen and respiratory problems.

Radiographic Studies

An anteroposterior (AP) view of the chest and upper abdomen (Fig. 19A) shows a bell-shaped thorax secondary to mild pulmonary hypoplasia, a moderate-sized right pneumothorax, and bilateral abdominal/flank masses, with central displacement of the bowel gas. Coronal ultrasound of the abdomen (Fig. 19B) shows bilateral markedly enlarged echogenic kidneys, with loss of corticomedullary differentiation, without dilatation of the collecting systems or ureters.

Longitudinal renal ultrasound in another patient (Fig. 19C) shows marked distortion of the renal architecture, loss of corticomedullary differentiation, and nephromegaly.

A noncontrast abdomen CT (Fig. 19D) in a different patient shows nephromegaly, with punctate renal parenchymal densities (arrows), most likely tiny renal calcifications. The enhanced CT scan (Fig. 19E) shows the typical radial streaking of contrast in the dilated collecting tubules, without dilatation of the renal pelves. In older patients, the nephromegaly may be so massive that it completely fills the abdomen.

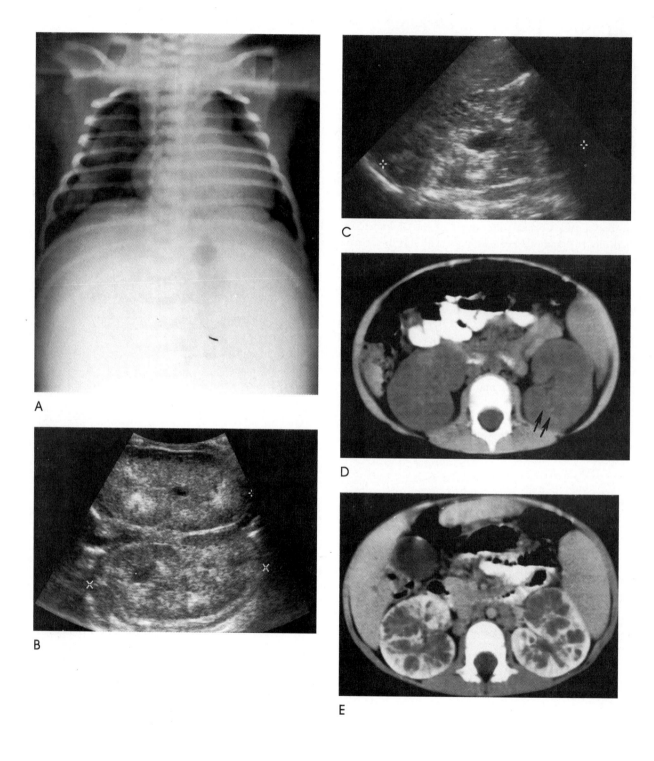

A

B

C

D

E

Diagnosis Autosomal Recessive Polycystic Kidney Disease (ARPKD)

Discussion and Differential Diagnosis

Patients with ARPKD may present in utero with changes seen on ultrasound during the third trimester of pregnancy, including oligohydramnios and bilateral large echogenic kidneys. Ultrasound findings of the kidneys earlier in pregnancy may be normal; it is postulated that the renal enlargement and increased echogenicity occur when renal function begins and the tubules dilate.[1]

The more typical patient presents as a newborn with an enlarged abdomen secondary to bilateral flank masses, and associated respiratory problems including pulmonary hypoplasia, pneumothoraces, and respiratory insufficiency, which may lead to death.[2]

A less common presentation occurs after the first year of life and during early childhood. Patients present with mild renal tubular ectasia, variable periportal hepatic fibrosis, and biliary duct ectasia.[3,4] They may have hepatosplenomegaly and portal hypertension. The liver is uniformly involved in all patients.[2]

Ultrasound of ARPKD shows nephromegaly, with kidneys usually greater than 8 cm in length, and hyperechogenicity, secondary to the dilated ectatic tubules and the multiple tiny cysts.[1] There may be a surrounding rim of relatively normal or echolucent renal cortex,[1] but there is uniform loss of the corticomedullary differentiation throughout the kidneys. CT scan shows massively enlarged kidneys, with radial streaking of contrast in the dilated tubules.[2] Noncontrast CT scan may show tiny renal calcifications, postulated secondary to urinary stagnation with precipitation of calcium or changes in excretion or solubility of urinary calcium salts.[3] The differential diagnosis of bilateral renal enlargement includes bilateral hydronephrosis, which is usually easily excluded at ultrasound. The uniform echogenicity of ARPKD excludes bilateral multicystic dysplastic kidneys and bilateral mesoblastic nephromas. Bilateral renal vein thrombosis is excluded because of the hyperechoic medulla in the early stages of renal vein thrombosis, compared to the uniform increased echogenicity of ARPKD.[2]

The prognosis for ARPKD is usually poor in patients who present with serious respiratory distress in the neonatal period. However, in patients who survive the neonatal period, the long-term follow-up of ARPKD shows gradual decrease or stabilization in renal size, decrease in renal echogenicity, and a progressive evolution of the appearance of the kidneys toward that seen with autosomal dominant polycystic kidney disease, with more isolated cysts identified.[6] In older children, therefore, it may be difficult to differentiate the sonographic findings of long-term autosomal recessive polycystic kidney disease from early changes of autosomal dominant polycystic kidney disease.[6] However, ARPKD patients usually present with symptoms of hypertension, chronic renal failure, and/or symptoms related to the liver disease including portal hypertension, hepatic fibrosis, and hepatosplenomegaly.[6]

PEARLS

- There is overlap between ARPKD and ADPKD; radiographic differentiation between the two may be difficult in older children, and renal biopsy may be necessary for diagnosis.[5]

- When the patient presents in childhood with several renal cysts, the differential diagnosis must include the childhood presentation of autosomal dominant polycystic kidney disease, tuberous sclerosis, and Turner's syndrome.[7]

- Patients who present in childhood usually have fewer symptoms in reference to renal failure, but more symptoms in reference to liver involvement, including portal hypertension, varices, and hepatic fibrosis.[2]

PITFALLS

- Transient nephromegaly can occur in the neonate, secondary to intratubular renal obstruction of unknown cause, or sometimes secondary to intravenous contrast. This diagnosis may be mistaken for ARPKD and follow-up examinations and/or renal biopsy are important.[2]

Further Reading

1. Carty H, Brunelle F, Shaw D, Kendall B, eds. *Imaging Children.* New York: Churchill Livingstone; 1994:597–600.
2. Kelalis PP, King LR, Belman AB. *Clinical Pediatric Urology, II.* 3rd ed. Philadelphia: WB Saunders Co; 1992:1135–1143.
3. Lucaya J, Enriquez G, Nieto J, et al. Renal calcifications in patients with autosomal recessive polycystic kidney disease: prevalence and cause. *Am J Roentgenol* 160:359–362, 1993.
4. Kirks DR, ed. *Practical Pediatric Imaging.* 2nd ed. Boston: Little, Brown & Co; 1991:948–954.
5. Kogutt MS, Robichaux WH, Boineau FG, Drake GK, Simonton SC. Asymmetric renal size in autosomal recessive polycystic kidney disease: a unique presentation. *Am J Roentgenol* 160:835–836, 1993.
6. Blickman JG, Bramson RT, Herrin JT. Autosomal recessive polycystic kidney disease: long-term sonographic findings in patients surviving the neonatal period. *Am J Roentgenol* 164:1247–1250, 1995.
7. Herman TE, Siegel MJ. Renal cysts associated with Turner's syndrome. *Pediatr Radiol* 24:139–140, 1994.
8. Lipschitz B, Berdon WE, Defelice AR, Levy J, Association of congenital hepatic fibrosis with autosomal dominant polycystic kidney disease. *Pediatr Radiol* 23:131–133, 1993.

CONTROVERSY

- Recent literature reports have indicated even more overlap between the clinical and imaging manifestations of ARPKD and ADPKD, including two cases of asymmetric renal size in ARPKD (rather than the uniform massive nephromegaly that is usually seen).[5] In addition, other reports have indicated the presence of hepatic fibrosis in both ARPKD and ADPKD.[8] Other authors have described that the long-term sonographic findings in patients with ARPKD evolve into a pattern similar to that seen in patients with ADPKD.[6]

Case 20

Clinical Presentation

Masses noted on prenatal ultrasound examination.

Radiographic Studies

Longitudinal ultrasound scan of the left kidney (Fig. 20A, caliper markers) shows multiple cysts of varying sizes, which do not communicate at real-time ultrasound. There is absence of a large medial or central cyst. Echogenic parenchyma, lacking the normal renal architecture, is wedged between the cystic masses. No ureter, and particularly no ureteral dilatation, is visualized. Transverse ultrasound scan of the kidney (Fig. 20B) shows similar findings.

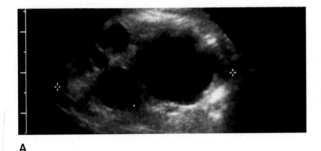

A

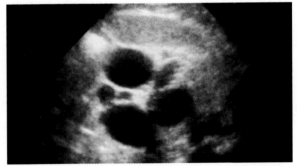

B

Diagnosis Multicystic Dysplastic Kidney

Discussion and Differential Diagnosis

Multicystic dysplastic kidney is the most common or second most common abdominal mass in the neonate.[1,2] The cause is usually thought to be secondary to complete ureteral obstruction early in fetal life (at 8 to 10 weeks' gestational age), presumed secondary to failure of the ureteric bud to unite with or properly divide and stimulate the metanephric blastema.[3] Histologically, the cysts represent dilated calyces or parts of the pelvocalyceal system, interspersed with clusters of rudimentary dysplastic renal parenchyma.[1]

The primary differential is between multicystic dysplastic kidney and hydronephrosis. Multicystic dysplastic kidney, as described above, usually consists of multiple noncommunicating cysts of varying sizes, adjacent to abnormal echogenic renal parenchyma. With nuclear medicine imaging, multicystic dysplastic kidney usually shows no function at 4 hours.

At sonography, hydronephrosis typically consists of a dilated central renal pelvis with radiating, communicating, relatively uniformly dilated calyces. With nuclear medicine imaging, hydronephrosis usually is identified by crescents of functioning renal tissue, with eventual presence of radioisotope in the central renal pelvis.

Further Reading

1. Kirks DR, ed. *Practical Pediatric Imaging.* 2nd ed. Boston: Little, Brown & Co; 1991:954–957.
2. Carty H, Brunelle F, Shaw D, Kendall B, eds. *Imaging Children.* New York: Churchill Livingstone; 1994:601–603.
3. Kelalis PP, King LR, Belman AB. *Clinical Pediatric Urology, II.* 3rd ed. Philadelphia: WB Saunders Co; 1992:1154–1166.
4. Strife JL, Souza AS, Kirks DR, Strife CF, Gelfand MJ, Wacksman J. Multicystic dysplastic kidney in children: US follow-up. *Radiology* 186:785–788, 1993.

PEARLS

- The contralateral kidney is abnormal in up to 30% of cases; the abnormality is usually a ureteropelvic junction obstruction or vesicoureteral reflux.[2] Other anomalies include ureterovesicular junction obstruction and bladder outlet obstruction.[3]

- Involution of the multicystic dysplastic kidney may occur before or after birth. Hemorrhage may occur into the cyst of a multicystic dysplastic kidney, creating echogenic cysts or fluid-fluid levels within this cyst.[2]

- Multicystic dysplastic kidney may present as a calcified cystic renal mass in older children and adults.[1]

- In follow-up ultrasound scans, two thirds of multicystic dysplastic kidneys showed decrease in size. There is a small risk of hypertension developing, so blood pressure examinations should be a routine part of the clinical follow-up.[4]

PITFALLS

- Five to 20% of multicystic dysplastic kidneys may have well-differentiated renal tissue present, and 24- to 48-hour delayed nuclear medicine scans sometimes show radioisotope activity in the cysts secondary to residual function in the renal parenchyma.[1]

- In approximately 5 to 10% of cases, a "hydronephrotic" type of multicystic dysplastic kidney is identified. At ultrasound, a dilated renal pelvis or central cyst is seen, and it may be difficult to differentiate multicystic dysplastic kidneys from hydronephrosis in these cases.[1]

CONTROVERSY

- Management is usually conservative, with serial ultrasound examinations documenting involution of the multicystic dysplastic kidney. Some authors have reported rare malignant degeneration,[2,4] but most authorities still advocate conservative management.[1,3,4]

Case 21

Clinical Presentation

A term newborn with a nontender right upper quadrant mass detected at routine physical examination in the nursery.

Radiographic Studies

Longitudinal ultrasound (Fig. 21A) shows a right upper quadrant mass of mixed echogenicity, indistinguishable from the kidney. A multicystic component is identified superiorly, and at Doppler ultrasound, the mass was hypervascular. CT scan of the abdomen (Fig. 21B) shows a large complex retroperitoneal mass, with cystic or necrotic tissue superolaterally and solid tissue inferomedially. The mass replaces the right kidney. There is faint contrast accumulation at the periphery of the mass (arrowheads).

Coronal T1-weighted MR scan of the abdomen in a different patient (Fig. 21C) shows a large heterogeneous solid right renal mass, indistinguishable from normal parenchyma. Post-gadolinium coronal T1-weighted MR image (Fig. 21D) shows enhancement of this solid right renal mass with multiple nonenhancing cysts within the lesion. Contrast within a displaced renal collecting system is noted (arrows).

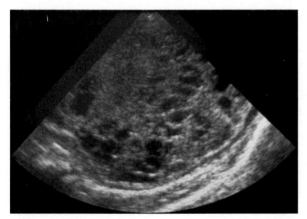

A

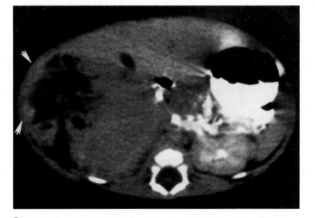

B

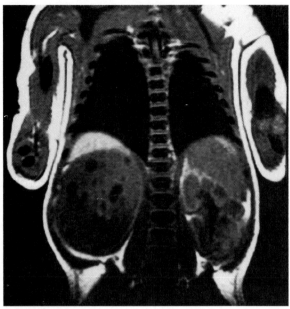

C

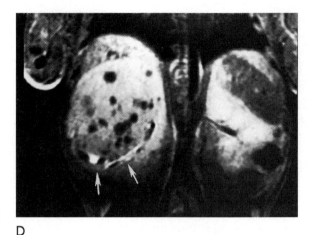

D

Diagnosis Mesoblastic Nephroma

Discussion and Differential Diagnosis

Mesoblastic nephroma, also know as fetal renal hamartoma, is the most common solid renal tumor in the newborn; a mean age at diagnosis is approximately 3 months. The mass is usually solid, unilateral, and of variable size.[1] Mesoblastic nephroma may be identified as a solid renal mass at prenatal ultrasound, and is sometimes associated with polyhydramnios[2] and prematurity.[3]

Mesoblastic nephroma is usually benign, but a clinicopathologic spectrum exists.[3] It is an unique lesion, distinct clinically and pathologically from Wilms tumor.[4] The tumor consists of interlacing spindle cells in a collagen background.[3] The cut surface has a whorled appearance, resembling a uterine fibroid.[5] The margins of the tumor blend imperceptibly with the normal renal parenchyma.[5] Imaging studies usually define a relatively solid renal mass, which rarely calcifies and cannot be distinguished from Wilms tumor radiographically.[3] At ultrasound, the mass is usually of mixed echogenicity and may have some cystic component.[6] CT shows a nonspecific renal mass of variable attenuation[3] that does not invade the pedicle and does not extend into the renal pelvis.[5] MRI may be useful in assessing the involvement of adjacent venous structures.[3]

Differential diagnosis includes hydronephrosis and multicystic dysplastic kidney, both of which are easily distinguished from mesoblastic nephroma at renal ultrasound.[1] Segmental renal vein thrombosis may be difficult to distinguish from mesoblastic nephroma. The differential diagnosis also includes renal cyst and multilocular cysts, but these are usually distinguished at ultrasound or CT.[7]

is rare in the neonate and is the most common solid renal mass of childhood.[7]

CONTROVERSY

- Atypical mesoblastic nephroma has been described. It is characterized as densely cellular, with abundant mitotic activity and occasional necrosis.[8] This form of mesoblastic nephroma has variable behavior, and rare local recurrence as well as pulmonary metastases have been described.[3] Some authors advocate adjuvant chemotherapy or radiation therapy if the tumor has malignant-appearing histology or behavior.[3] Others caution against the overzealous use of chemotherapy or radiation therapy.[5,7]

Further Reading

1. White KS, Grossman H. Wilms and associated renal tumors of childhood. *Pediatr Radiol* 21:81–88, 1991.
2. Kelalis PP, Mesrobian H-GJ. Tumors of the upper urinary tract. In: Kelalis PP, King LR, Belman AB, eds. *Clinical Pediatric Urology, II.* 3rd ed. Philadelphia: WB Saunders; 1992:1414.
3. Rieumont MJ, Whitman GJ. Mesoblastic nephroma. *Am J Roentgenol* 162:76, 1994.
4. Bolande RP. Congenital mesoblastic nephroma of infancy. *Perspect Pediatr Pathol* 1:227, 1973.
5. Bisset, Strife, Kirks DR. Multilocular cystic nephroma. In: Kirks DR, ed. *Practical Pediatric Imaging.* 2nd ed. Boston: Little, Brown & Co; 1991:1004–1008.
6. Ferraro EM, Klein SA, Fakhry J, Weingarten MJ, Rose JS. Hypercalcemia in association with mesoblastic nephroma: report of a case and review of the literature. *Pediatr Radiol* 16:516–517, 1986.
7. Hartman DS, Lesar MSL, Madewell JE, Lichtenstein JE, Davis CJ Jr. Mesoblastic nephroma: radiologic-pathologic correlation of 20 cases. *Am J Roentgenol* 136:69–74, 1981.
8. Goldberg J, Liu P, Smith C. Congenital mesoblastic nephroma presenting the hemoperitoneum and shock. *Pediatr Radiol* 24:54–55, 1994.

Case 22

Clinical Presentation

A 2-year-old boy with abdominal mass discovered by mother when bathing child.

Radiographic Studies

Longitudinal ultrasound (Fig. 22A) shows a large primarily echogenic mass at the upper pole of the kidney, with central cystic necrosis or hemorrhage. Distorted, echolucent calyces are draped over the inferior pole of the renal mass (arrows). Longitudinal color Doppler ultrasound (Fig. 22B, Color Plate 5) shows tumor extension (arrow), from the renal vein into the inferior vena cava, with blood flow surrounding the tumor thrombus. Longitudinal color Doppler scan (Fig. 22C, Color Plate 6) shows the tumor thrombus in the inferior vena cava, with flow around the thrombus. Contrast-enhanced CT (Fig. 22D) shows a well-defined mass of renal origin, with residual functioning renal parenchyma (arrows), displaced medially and draped over the mass. Central low density within the mass represents necrosis/hemorrhage. The wedge density (arrowhead) in the contralateral kidney indicates bilateral tumor.

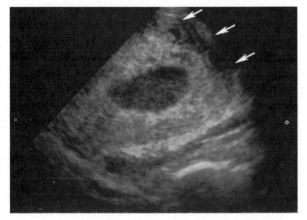

A

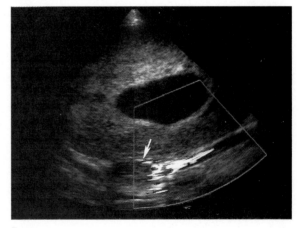

B

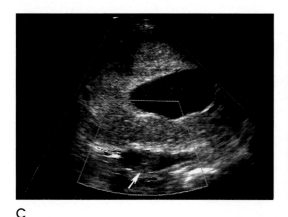

C

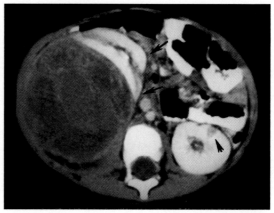

D

Diagnosis Wilms Tumor (Nephroblastoma)

Discussion and Differential Diagnosis

Wilms tumor is the most common pediatric malignant renal tumor and represents 8% of all childhood malignancies. Seven percent are bilateral; associated anomalies include aniridia, hemihypertrophy, cryptorchidism, and hypospadias.[1]

Ultrasound is the screening modality of choice, and Doppler sonography is very useful in demonstrating tumor extension into the renal vein and inferior vena cava. CT defines the organ of origin and may identify calcifications in 15% of patients.[2]

Wilms tumor must be distinguished from neuroblastoma, an extrarenal tumor, which is usually more ill-defined, involves adjacent lymph nodes, encases vascular structures, and may extend across the midline.[2] Nephroblastomatosis complex is a precursor of Wilms, includes rests of nephrogenic tissue or renal blastoma, and resembles Wilms microscopically but lacks mitoses.[2] Mesoblastic nephroma, a non-tender neonatal renal mass, is distinguished by earlier clinical presentation but is indistinguishable from Wilms by ultrasound and CT.[2] Multilocular cystic nephroma, a cystic neoplasm, is difficult to distinguish from a well-differentiated cystic Wilms except at pathology.[2] Renal cell carcinoma is a nonspecific solid renal mass indistinguishable by ultrasound from Wilms tumor, but usually occurs in older patients.[2]

Further Reading

1. Green DM, D'Angio GJ, Beckwith JB, et al. Wilms tumor. *Cancer* 46:46–63, 1996.
2. Kirks DR, ed. *Practical Pediatric Imaging,* 2nd ed. Boston: Little, Brown & Co; 1991:994–1004.
3. White KS, Grossman H. Wilms and associated renal tumors of childhood. *Pediatr Radiol* 21:81–88, 1991.

PEARLS

- Wilms tumor is probably congenital in origin (arising from primitive and embryonal renal tissue), and data from familial cases supports that this may be a genetic disease.[3]

- Tumor thrombus extending into the left renal vein may obstruct the left gonadal vein, and cause a varicocele, an uncommon problem in young children, and rarely the initial presentation of Wilms tumor.[4]

- Tumor thrombus may extend into the renal vein, the inferior vena cava, and the right atrium, occasionally causing inferior vena caval obstruction, and pulmonary tumor emboli. It is critical to assess the inferior vena cava and right atrium at the time of initial evaluation of the Wilms tumor; if right atrial involvement is identified, cardiopulmonary bypass may be necessary at the time of tumor resection.[4]

PITFALLS

• A renal mass with a CNS lesion (metastasis or a coexisting primary brain tumor) is exceedingly rare and is characteristic of rhabdoid tumor of the kidney and not Wilms tumor.[5] A peripheral crescent of fluid attenuation on CT is characteristic of rhabdoid tumor.[6]

• A renal mass with bone metastasis is characteristic of clear cell sarcoma of the kidney and not Wilms tumor.[7]

CONTROVERSY

• There are three existing controversies in the imaging of Wilms tumor:

1. Is CT scan of the chest needed for staging?

2. Is CT scan of the abdomen necessary for initial evaluation?

3. Are both radiographic skeletal surveys and nuclear medicine scans required to evaluate bone metastases in clear cell sarcoma? Most pediatric radiologists believe that CT scan of the chest and abdomen is important for the evaluation of Wilms tumor and that nuclear imaging is all that is necessary for the evaluation of bone metastases in clear cell sarcoma.[8]

4. Navoy JF, Royal SA, Vaid YN, Mroczek-Musulman EC. Wilms tumor: unusual manifestations. *Pediatr Radiol* 25 Suppl 1:S76–86, 1995.
5. Chung CJ, Lorenzo R, Rayder S, et al. Rhabdoid tumors of the kidney in children: CT findings. *Am J Roentgenol* 164(3):697–700, 1995.
6. Argons GA, Kingsman KD, Wagner BJ, Sotelo-Avila C. Rhabdoid tumor of the kidney in children: a comparative study of 21 cases. *Am J Roentgenol* 168:447–451, 1997.
7. Carcassonne M, Raybaud C, Lebreuil G. Clear cell sarcoma of the kidney in children: a dinstict entity. *J Pediatr Surg* 16(4 Suppl 1):645–648, 1981.
8. Cohen MD. Commentary: imaging and staging of Wilms tumors: problems and controversies. *Pediatr Radiol* 26(5):307–311, 1996.

Case 23

Clinical Presentation

A 3-year-old boy with hematuria and dysuria.

Radiographic Studies

A transverse ultrasound of the bladder (Fig. 23A) shows an intraluminal mass of mixed echogenicity arising from the bladder base in 3-year-old boy with hematuria and dysuria. A composite of two images from a voiding cystourethrogram (VCUG) (Fig. 23B) shows prolapse of the mass into the prostatic urethra (arrow) during voiding. The irregular trabeculated bladder wall is secondary to bladder outlet obstruction. Transverse pelvic ultrasound in a 5-year-old boy (Fig. 23C) shows a large inhomogeneous mass (caliper markers) arising from the prostate, displacing the bladder anteriorly.

Sagittal proton density MR scan in a 3-year-old girl (Fig 23D) shows tumor mass arising from the vagina, infiltrating the bladder base (arrowhead), protruding through the introitus (arrows), and displacing the rectum posteriorly. Coronal T1-weighted MR image (Fig. 23E) shows similar findings. T1-weighted sagittal MRI of the vaginal tumor (Fig. 23F) shows tumor mass (arrows) protruding through the introitus and infiltrating the bladder base.

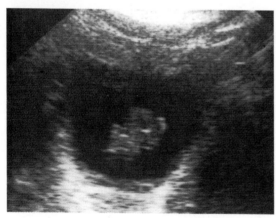

A

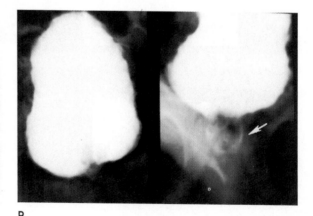

B

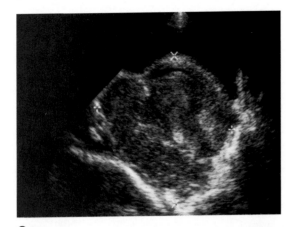

C

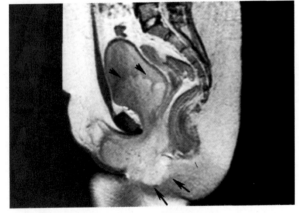

D

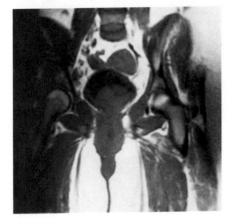

E

F

Diagnosis Rhabdomyosarcoma

Discussion and Differential Diagnosis

Presentation varies according to the site. In the lower urinary tract, patients usually present with hematuria, palpable abdominal mass, or obstructive symptoms such as acute urinary retention[1] resulting from tumor mass prolapsing into the urethra, causing urethral obstruction, or invading the trigone, causing hydroureter and hydronephrosis.[2] Vaginal masses may present as urinary symptoms resulting from invasion of the bladder, or may present as bloody vaginal discharge or as polypoid grape-like masses protruding through the introitus.[1] Testicular tumors may present as a scrotal mass. Paratesticular tumor may present as a mass in the testicular appendage, tunica, or adjacent lymph nodes.[2]

Rhabdomyosarcoma is the most common pediatric soft tissue sarcoma, and the primary tumor can occur in virtually any site in the body except for the brain.[3] It accounts for 10% of all childhood solid tumors, with an equal incidence in males and females, and peaks in children aged between 2 and 6 years.[3] The most frequent location is either the pelvis/GU tract, or the head and the neck.[2,3] Histologically, there are three types. Embryonal rhabdomyosarcoma is the most common and includes botryoid rhabdomyosarcoma, which usually invades hollow visceral organs such as the bladder.[2] Alveolar and pleomorphic/undifferentiated histologic types are less common, and usually involve the limbs or large muscle groups.[2,3] Metastatic disease is common, most frequently to the lung, but it also may involve regional lymph nodes, bone, brain, or liver.[2,3] Rhabdomyosarcoma invades adjacent organs in the pelvis, and it may be difficult to differentiate tumor arising from the bladder base, the vagina, or the prostate.[4] In all patients with bladder wall masses, cystoscopy and biopsy are necessary to establish the diagnosis of rhabdomyosarcoma before initiation of any therapeutic measures for malignancy.[2,4]

The differential diagnosis of pelvic rhabdomyosarcoma includes neurofibroma, hemangioma, or other primary neoplasms, including the rare pheochromocytoma.[2–5] Infiltration and inflammation of the bladder wall from eosinophilic cystitis may cause asymmetric bladder wall thickening (pseudotumor cystitis), trigone and ureteral wall invasion with obstruction, and bladder outlet obstruction; all are impossible to differentiate from rhabdomyosarcoma.[6]

Ultrasound is usually the initial imaging modality; it frequently defines an intravesical mass of mixed echogenicity.[1,7] However, contrast-enhanced CT and MRI are superior at defining the extension into adjacent soft tissues, nodes, bone, and large bowel.[4,7] CT is excellent for defining pulmonary metastases.[2] MRI defines invasion into adjacent soft tissues; the tumor is high signal on T2-weighted images and variable signal on T1-weighted images.[2] If the bladder is involved, a voiding cystourethrogram is helpful in defining tumor prolapse into the urethra with bladder outlet obstruction.[3] Nuclear medicine bone imaging is usually performed to assess bone metastases.[2]

PEARLS

- Hydronephrosis is a relatively common presentation of rhabdomyosarcoma, secondary to bladder wall thickening, bladder outlet obstruction, or direct trigone or ureteral invasion.[1,3,4]

- Ultrasound, CT, and MRI may not be able to delineate the organ of origin of large pelvic rhabdomyosarcomas.[3]

PITFALLS

- The intravesical portion of the rhabdomyosarcoma may not be visualized with CT because it is obscured by the dilute contrast in the bladder, especially when the tumor mass begins to decrease in size following therapy. Ultrasound is necessary to assess the intravesical portion of the tumor mass.[4]

- Frozen section at cystoscopy may be inaccurate. Therapy should begin only after histology of the permanent section confirms the diagnosis of rhabdomyosarcoma.[4]

- Intravesical rhabdomyosarcoma is easily confused with intravesical blood clot at ultrasound.[3]

- Eosinophilic cystitis may mimic rhabdomyosarcoma on all imaging studies.[6]

Further Reading

1. Kelalis PP, King LR, Belman AB. *Clinical Pediatric Urology, II.* 3rd ed. Philadelphia: WB Saunders; 1992:1100–1101,1445–1450.
2. Carty H, Brunelle F, Shah D, Kendall B, eds. *Imaging Children.* New York: Churchill-Livingstone; 1994:679–682,841,1325–1327.
3. Kirks DR. *Practical Pediatric Imaging: Diagnostic Radiology of Infants and Children.* Boston: Little, Brown & Co; 1991:1032–1035.
4. Fernbach SK, Feinstein KA. Abnormalities of the bladder in children: imaging findings. *Am J Roentgenol* 162:1143–1150, 1994.
5. Crecelius SA, Bellah R. Pheochromocytoma of the bladder in an adolescent: sonographic and MR imaging findings. *Am J Roentgenol* 165:101–103, 1995.
6. Hoeffel JC, Drews K, Gassner I, Arnaudin A. Pseudotumoral cystitis. *Pediatr Radiol* 23:510–514, 1993.
7. Geoffray A, Couanet D, Montagne JP, Leclère J, Flamant F. Ultrasonography and computed tomography for diagnosis and follow-up of pelvic rhabdomyosarcomas in children. *Pediatr Radiol* 17:132–136, 1987.

Case 24

Clinical Presentation

A 3-year-old male patient presents with weight loss, irritability, and a large abdominal mass on physical exam.

Radiographic Studies

Longitudinal ultrasound (Fig. 24A) shows a 10-cm right upper quadrant echogenic mass (arrows) displacing the kidney (caliper markers) inferiorly. Transverse ultrasound (Fig. 24B) shows the large primarily echogenic mass (caliper markers), in the expected location of the adrenal. Nonenhanced CT scan of the abdomen (Fig. 24C) shows the large right adrenal mass containing multiple stippled calcifications. The mass extends into the right lobe of the liver, and there is associated massive adenopathy encasing the inferior vena cava and celiac axis, and extending into the splenic hilum. Contrast-enhanced CT (Fig. 24D) shows the nonenhancing mass invading the right lobe of the liver, with associated massive adenopathy encasing the celiac axis (arrowheads), compressing the inferior vena cava (arrow), and displacing the aorta anteriorly.

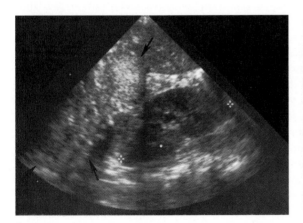

A

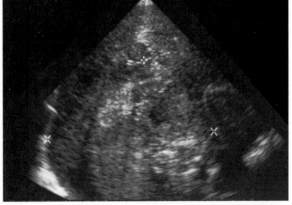

B

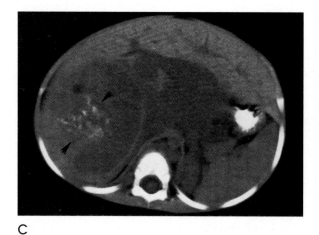

C

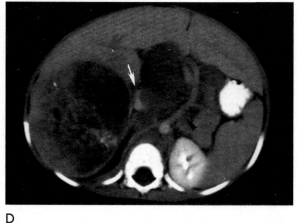

D

Diagnosis Neuroblastoma

Discussion and Differential Diagnosis

Neuroblastoma arises from the neural crest cells of the adrenal medulla and the sympathetic chain ganglia.[1] Neuroblastoma is the most common extracranial solid malignancy in children.[2] Two thirds of neuroblastomas arise in the abdomen, and of those, two thirds are adrenal in origin.[2] Neuroblastoma usually presents as a large, often ill-defined, abdominal mass filling the central abdominal cavity and frequently crossing the midline. The tumor mass usually displaces the kidney inferiorly, and may displace or invade adjacent abdominal organs. Massive adenopathy is frequently identified, with encasement of the aorta and inferior vena cava. The tumor may also arise in the thorax, in the abdomen in the organ of Zuckerkandl, or anywhere along the sympathetic chain.[3] Ninety-five percent of tumors have elevated urinary metabolites of catecholamine production.[3]

Initially, imaging is usually performed with ultrasound, as a screening examination. The mass is frequently of mixed echogenicity, with associated adenopathy. Further delineation is accomplished with CT scanning, which usually better defines the organ of origin and the relationship of the tumor mass to adjacent abdominal structures. At CT scan, approximately 80% of neuroblastomas have calcification[3]; on routine radiographs of the abdomen, greater than 50% are calcified.[4] Neuroblastoma is frequently disseminated at presentation and may involve skin, lymph, liver, bone marrow, or cortical bone. Metastatic involvement may be identified with CT scan, with MRI scan, or with nuclear medicine imaging.[4]

The differential diagnosis includes Wilms tumor (renal origin; approximately 15% with calcifications[4]), rhabdomyosarcoma, teratoma, lymphoma.[1] Neuroblastoma has been described as the only abdominal mass that displaces the aorta anteriorly from the spine.[1] Ganglioneuroma is the mature benign variant of neuroblastoma, which may produce local invasion. Ganglioneuroblastoma is the intermediate form of the tumor, between the benign ganglioneuroma and the malignant neuroblastoma.[1]

PEARLS

- Neuroblastoma may be multifocal, with a synchronous or metachronous presentation. It is important to always look for multifocal primary lesions, especially if there is a positive family history of neuroblastoma.[5]

- With the increasing frequency of prenatal ultrasound, neuroblastoma is sometimes detected prenatally. In these cases, surgical resection is usually curative, with a favorable prognosis.[6]

- Neuroblastoma may occasionally produce ascites because of peritoneal seeding; this is an unusual manifestation, and is more often seen with Wilms tumor, clear cell sarcoma, germ cell tumors, or ovarian lesions.[7]

Further Reading

1. Carty H, Brunelle F, Shah D, Kendall B, eds. *Imaging Children.* New York: Churchill-Livingstone; 1994:682–691.
2. Bousvaros A, Kirks DR, Grossman H. Imaging of neuroblastoma: an overview. *Pediatr Radiol* 16:89–106, 1986.
3. Kelalis PP, King LR, Belman AB. *Clinical Pediatric Urology, II.* 3rd ed. Philadelphia: WB Saunders 1992:1383–1389.
4. Kirks DR. *Practical Pediatric Imaging: Diagnostic Radiology of Infants and Children.* Boston: Little, Brown & Co; 1991:1010–1023.
5. Cohen MD, Auringer ST, Grosfeld JL, et al. Multifocal primary neuroblastoma. *Pediatr Radiol* 23:463–466, 1993.
6. Ho PTC, Estroff JA, Kozakewich H, et al. Prenatal detection of neuroblastoma: 10 year experience from the Dana-Farber Cancer Institute and Children's Hospital. *Pediatrics* 92:358–364, 1993.
7. Fernbach SK. Ascites produced by peritoneal seeding of neuroblastoma. *Pediatr Radiol* 23:569, 1993.
8. Dessner DA, DiPietro MA, Shulkin BL. MIBG detection of neuroblastoma: correlation with CT, US and surgical findings. *Pediatr Radiol* 23:276–280, 1993.
9. Abramson SJ, Berdon WE, Ruzal-Shapiro C, et al. Cervical neuroblastoma in eleven infants—tumor with favorable prognosis: clinical and radiologic (US, CT, MRI) findings. *Pediatr Radiol* 23:253–357, 1993.

PITFALLS

• Meta-iodobenzyl guanidine (MIBG) is a very useful nuclear imaging agent for detection of local or distant metastases. However, it is significantly less sensitive for the detection of hepatic disease, because there is normal hepatic background activity with MIBG.[8]

• Cervical neuroblastoma may be confusing clinically and is sometimes mistaken for an infectious mass with associated adenopathy, or branchial cleft cyst. Patients usually present with airway or swallowing dysfunction and/ or a dominant neck mass. At ultrasound, the dominant mass is identified, sometimes with calcifications, but frequently there is adjacent adenopathy that appears inflammatory. Often diagnosis is delayed because of the confusing ultrasound and clinical picture.[9]

CONTROVERSY

• The choice of imaging modality after initial screening ultrasound is controversial. Some authors advocate MRI because of its ability to visualize location of the tumor in multiple planes, extension through the neural foramina into the thecal sac, and the relationship to adjacent vascularity. However, CT is often the preferred imaging modality because of its visualization of tiny calcifications, its speed, and the fact that sedation is not usually required. Extension of tumor into the thecal sac can also be imaged with CT scan.[3,4]

Case 25

Clinical Presentation

Patient is a 28-day-old female infant, status postrepair of total anomalous pulmonary venous return, with increasing levels of BUN and creatinine.

Radiographic Studies

Longitudinal ultrasound of the left kidney (Fig. 25A) shows an enlarged kidney with loss of the corticomedullary differentiation, and linear streaking (arrowheads) in the distribution of the intralobar vessels. A longitudinal duplex Doppler image (Fig. 25B) shows lack of forward diastolic flow in the intralobar artery. This is a classic finding, but it is not always present, especially in the neonate. Normal renal waveform in the contralateral kidney is seen in Figure 25C with forward diastolic arterial flow. Longitudinal ultrasound (Fig. 25D) shows extension of the left renal vein mass (arrows) into the inferior vena cava.

Longitudinal ultrasound approximately one month later (Fig. 25E) shows interval decrease in renal size (caliper markers), persistent loss of the corticomedullary differentiation, and increased parenchymal echoes (arrows), probably secondary to developing fibrosis and atrophy. Figure 25F and Color Plate 6 show longitudinal color Doppler flow image of the normal contralateral kidney. A comparable longitudinal color image of the abnormal kidney (Fig. 25G, Color Plate 7), shows the decreased peripheral venous and arterial flow, renal enlargement, mottled echogenicity with loss of corticomedullary junction differentiation, and linear streaking (arrowheads) in the intralobar septa.

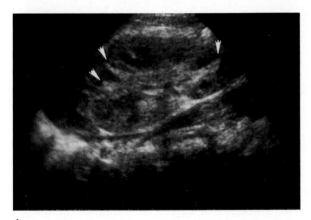

A

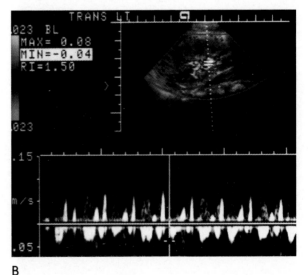

B

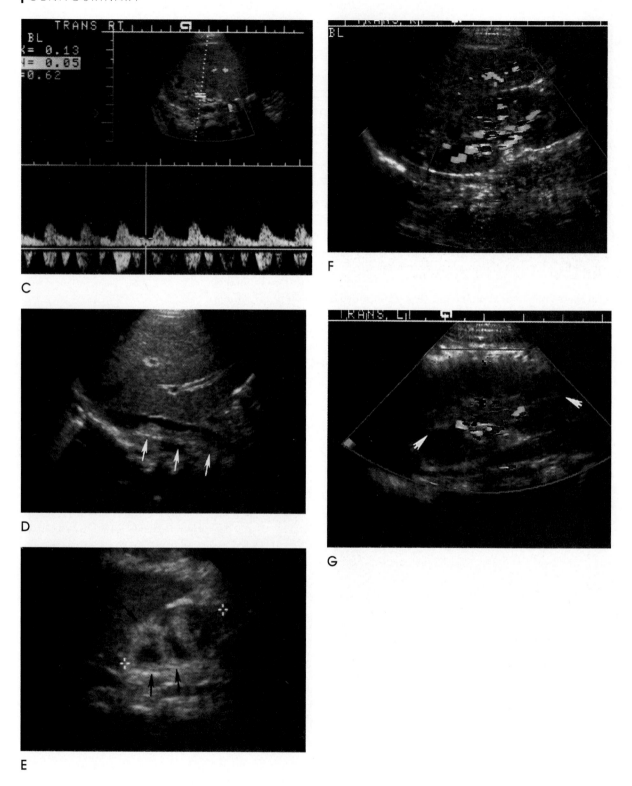

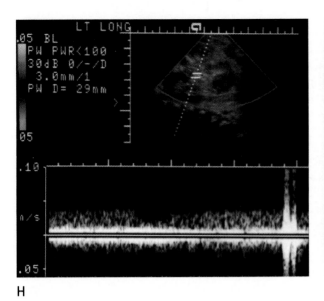

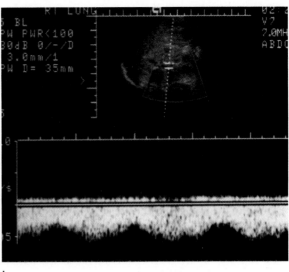

H

I

Diagnosis Renal Vein Thrombosis (RVT)

Discussion and Differential Diagnosis

Renal vein thrombosis has a variable clinical presentation, with an incidence between 1 in 150 and 1 in 250 among neonates at autopsy,[1] but may be even more common than recognized at autopsy. Ninety percent of RVT occurs in children younger than 1 year of age and 75% in children younger than 1 month of age.[2] Renal vein thrombosis may even occur prenatally.[3] The predisposing factor is usually some form of "renal shock," dehydration, or elevated hematocrit,[4] which leads to decreased arterial and subsequent decreased renal venous flow. The thrombosis begins in the intrarenal veins secondary to endothelial injury from decreased blood flow, extends into the intralobar veins and the main renal vein, and may extend into the inferior vena cava.[2,5] In older patients, RVT may be related to trauma, shock, hypovolemia, a thromboembolic state, nephrotic syndrome, systemic lupus erythematosus, or amyloidosis.[3] Sudden complete RVT presents with pain, nephromegaly, hematuria, proteinuria, flank mass, or elevation of blood pressure. Ultimately, RVT may lead to hemorrhagic renal infarction.[6] Chronic or gradual RVT may occur in patients with renal tumors, extrarenal tumors, lymphoma, or phlebitis of the inferior vena cava and renal veins.[6] In these patients, the indolent RVT presents with proteinuria, thrombocytopenia, and nonspecific clinical symptoms.[6] Renal vein thrombosis may occur in patients who are status postrenal transplant secondary to epithelial injury at the anastomosis of the renal vein, or secondary to extrinsic compression of the renal vein from hematoma, urinoma, or lymphocele.[5] These patients often have no pain at presentation, because the transplanted kidney is denervated. Renal vein thrombosis may originate in the inferior vena cava and spread peripherally into the renal vein in older patients.[7]

PEARLS

- The management of RVT is supportive therapy,[3] and patients may show spontaneous resolution or may progress to total renal atrophy on the affected side.[13] The survival rate is between 45% and 86%, with an increased incidence of renal failure and hypertension in survivors.[3]

- Serial ultrasound documents the evolution of RVT and confirms the diagnosis.[4]

- Associated adrenal hemorrhage is common in patients with left RVT because of the common venous drainage of the left adrenal gland and left kidney into the inferior vena cava.[7] If bilateral RVT is identified, thrombus or mass in the inferior vena cava proximal to the renal veins should be suspected.[7]

- The hyperechoic intralobar streaks secondary to hemorrhage, edema, or dystrophic calcifications in intralobar vessels are pathognomonic of RVT.[2,7,10–13]

- Absent transmitted right atrial pulsations in the intrarenal venous channels, or steady venous flow may be the earliest findings of RVT at Doppler ultrasound.[5] Later, as perfusion decreases, the renal vein waveform looks like the multiphasic hepatic vein waveform.[8,9]

- Main renal vein flow is usually present in the neonate with RVT but absent in renal transplant patients with renal vein thrombosis.[5]

- In the neonate with RVT, the diastolic flow is decreased, but not always reversed.[5] In the pediatric transplant kidney, there is usually a reversal of diastolic flow with RVT.

PITFALLS

- With subacute RVT, intrarenal venous flow returns secondary to collateral formation and flow around the clots; the resistive indices become normal secondary to

Diagnosis is usually made with ultrasound, including color Doppler imaging. In the neonate, the thrombosis begins in the intralobar and arcuate arteries; in the early stages, Doppler studies may show preserved intrarenal venous flow, but absent transmitted right atrial pulsations in the renal vein[5] (Fig. 25H). Figure 25I shows the normal contralateral kidney with normal pulsatile venous waveform. Later, as renal perfusion decreases, the renal vein Doppler pattern takes on the appearance of the hepatic vein, with a marked multiphasic wave form.[8,9] Arterial diastolic flow is decreased,[5] and there may be reversal of diastolic flow.[9] In the neonate, the resistive index (RI) is usually at least 10% higher in the thrombosed kidney than in the normal kidney. The classic adult patterns of absent renal vein flow and reversed diastolic renal arterial flow are usually not seen in the neonate with RVT but are seen in the child with acute RVT postrenal transplant.[5] Duplex ultrasound during the first week shows increased size, globular shape, increased echogenicity, and loss of corticomedullary differentiation of the thrombosed kidney.[4] Echogenic streaks radiating from the central renal sinus to the periphery of the kidney along the intralobar septa are pathognomonic of RVT and represent edema and hemorrhage along the course of the thrombosed intralobar veins.[2,7,10–13] This finding of echogenic streaks may be transitory, clearing with resolution of the edema and hemorrhage, or may become permanent if dystrophic calcifications develop at the site of the thrombosis and hemorrhage.[11] Occasionally, the calcifications are identified as linear or lacy calcifications on supine films of the abdomen.[11]

During the second week, there is interval decrease in renal size, with development of a mixed pattern of hyper- and hypoechogenicity of the central renal parenchyma.[18,12] Focal echolucencies may develop in the papilla and affected pyramids, probably secondary to renal tubular damage, destruction of the loop of Henley, and necrosis.[12] Early compensatory hypertrophy of the contralateral kidney may develop if it is nonthrombosed.[13] Ultrasound findings after the third or fourth week are variable. Echogenicity becomes more normal,[4,13] size may be normal, but focal scars, venous calcifications, or global atrophy may develop with loss of renal function.[4] Doppler studies may show return of venous flow in the intrarenal venous system secondary to collateral vessels forming around the clots; resistive indices may become normal.[5] At any time during the course of RVT, thrombus may be visualized in the renal veins, the inferior vena cava, or the iliac or femoral veins in renal transplant patients.[5] Nuclear medicine DMSA cortical imaging may be helpful during this stage in assessing renal viability.[13]

The differential diagnosis for an acutely enlarged kidney with decreased corticomedullary junction definition is usually between acute tubular necrosis (ATN) and RVT.[2] With ATN, the renal echogenicity is usually normal or increased.[9] With RVT, the renal echogenicity is inhomogeneous/blotchy, and hyperechoic intralobar streaks may develop in the renal parenchyma. Doppler findings may be similar in both ATN and RVT because the Doppler studies reflect poor perfusion to the kidney.[9] Serial ultrasound may show the typical evolution of RVT, including the development of renal scars or marked interval decrease in renal size from infarction.[4] DTPA renal scans are nonspecific.[2,3] CT and MRI are rarely indicated.

restoration of normal intrarenal arterial flow.[5] In these cases, it may be difficult to make the diagnosis of RVT if early examinations were not performed.[5]

- In renal transplant patients, intrarenal venous flow and normalization of intrarenal flow may occur much later and in a more limited sense because these patients do not have collateral pathways for renal venous drainage.[5]

CONTROVERSY

- Treatment with anticoagulant therapy is controversial for patients of all ages, but especially the neonate, because of the associated secondary risk of intracranial hemorrhage.[3]

Further Reading

1. Carty H, Brunelle F, Shaw D, Kendall B, eds. *Imaging Children.* New York: Churchill Livingstone; 1994:744–745.
2. Alexander AA, Merton DA, Mitchell DG, Gottlieb RP, Feld RI. Rapid diagnosis of neonatal renal vein thrombosis using color Doppler imaging. *J Clin Ultrasound* 21:468–471, 1993.
3. Kelalis PP, King LR, Belman AB. *Clinical Pediatric Urology, II.* 3rd ed. Philadelphia: WB Saunders Co; 1992: 1314–1323.
4. Cremin BJ, Davey H, Oleszczuk-Raszke K. Neonatal renal venous thrombosis: sequential ultrasonic appearances. *Clin Radiol* 44:52–55, 1991.
5. Laplante S, Patriquin HB, Robitaille P, Filiatrault D, Grignon A, Décarie J-C. Renal vein thrombosis in children: evidence of early flow recovery with Doppler US. *Radiology* 189:37–42, 1993.
6. Kirks DR, ed. *Practical Pediatric Imaging.* 2nd ed. Boston: Little, Brown & Co; 1991:1045–1048.
7. Orazi C, Fariello G, Malena S, Schingo P, Ferro F, Bagolan P. Renal vein thrombosis and adrenal hemorrhage in the newborn: ultrasound evaluation of 4 cases. *J Clin Ultrasound* 21:163–169, 1993.
8. Berland LL. Syllabus: The renal vasculature. In: *Color Doppler Ultrasonography Course.* Rockville, MD: AIUM; 1991:79–83.
9. Seibert JJ. Syllabus: Update in pediatric Doppler. In: *Update in Duplex, Power and Color Flow Imaging.* Laurel, MD: AIUM; 1996:93–100.
10. Errington ML, Hendry GMA. The rare association of right adrenal haemorrhage and renal vein thrombosis diagnosed with duplex ultrasound. *Pediatr Radiol* 25:157–158, 1995.
11. Lalmand B, Avni EF, Nasr A, Ketelbant P, Struyven J. Perinatal renal vein thrombosis. *J Ultrasound Med* 9:437–442, 1990.
12. Wright NB, Blanch G, Walkinshaw S, Pilling DW. Antenatal and neonatal renal vein thrombosis: new ultrasonic features with high frequency transducers. *Pediatr Radiol* 26:686–689, 1996.
13. Lin G-J, Yang P-H, Wang M-L. Neonatal renal venous thrombosis—a case report describing serial sonographic changes. *Pediatr Nephrol* 8:589–591, 1994.

Case 26

Clinical Presentation

A neonate with urinary sepsis.

Radiographic Studies

Longitudinal ultrasound of the right kidney (Fig. 26A) shows a primarily cystic mass with a thick echogenic rim (arrows), directly adjacent to the upper pole of the right kidney. Internal echoes are present, representing debris within the mass. Direct coronal CT scan (Fig. 26B) shows the cystic mass (arrows) distinct from the right kidney (arrowhead). A longitudinal ultrasound scan one week later (Fig. 26C) shows liquefaction into a relatively anechoic suprarenal mass (arrows), decreased in size. Caliper markers identify the right kidney. Transverse ultrasound at 4 weeks (Fig. 26D) shows decreased mass size (caliper markers) and increased echogenicity peripherally, probably secondary to calcification.

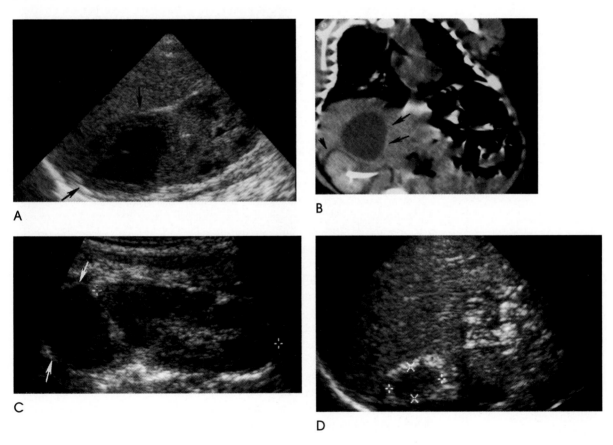

A

B

C

D

PEARLS

- Adrenal anomalies, including adrenal agenesis with ipsilateral renal agenesis, horseshoe adrenal gland with horseshoe kidneys, and adrenal ectopy can occur.[10]

- The most common cause of adrenal calcification on supine abdomen is previous adrenal hemorrhage in the neonate.[1]

- Ultrasound of the adrenal gland must always include evaluation of the ipsilateral kidney for morphology and vascularity. The left adrenal vein drains into the left renal vein; left renal vein thrombosis may cause secondary thrombosis of the left adrenal vein, and subsequent left adrenal hemorrhage.[11]

- Adrenal hemorrhage can occur in utero.

PITFALLS

- If sequential adrenal ultrasound does not show changing echogenicity and decreasing size of the suprarenal mass, then adrenal hemorrhage is not the diagnosis.[1,2]

- The right adrenal vein and right renal vein drain independently directly into the inferior vena cava. Right adrenal hemorrhage is rarely associated with right renal

Diagnosis Adrenal Hemorrhage

Discussion and Differential Diagnosis

Adrenal hemorrhage occurs almost exclusively in the newborn population[1]; the cause is unknown, but it is associated with birth trauma, stress, anoxia, and dehydration.[2] The newborn adrenal gland is large and hypervascular because during the third trimester of pregnancy, the fetal adrenal cortex completes the synthesis of maternally produced precursor steroids to estrogen and progesterone.[3] Three adrenal arteries supply dense arterioles in the medullary sinuses, with one central vein draining the gland.[4] Increases in adrenal arterial flow or venous pressure predispose to adrenal hemorrhage because of the gland's size and vascularity, and impaired autoregulation of circulation in the neonate.[4] The right adrenal is more susceptible to hemorrhage because of its direct drainage into the inferior vena cava (IVC); transient rises in venous pressure in the IVC are transmitted directly to the right adrenal vein and may cause medullary hemorrhage.[5] Newborn patients with adrenal hemorrhage present with flank mass, anemia, jaundice, or vomiting[6]; the hemorrhage may also be discovered as an incidental finding.[3] Occasionally, in the neonate, adrenal hemorrhage presents as falling hematocrit and scrotal swelling secondary to rupture of hemorrhage into the retroperitoneum and peritoneum, with passage of blood through the patent processus vaginalis into the scrotum.[6]

Adrenal hemorrhage is occasionally identified in older children who have experienced trauma or child abuse; in these patients, the hemorrhage may be secondary to rises in venous pressure in the inferior vena cava, or to shearing of small vessels from rapid deceleration.[7] In older patients with trauma, the hemorrhage is usually on the right, with associated ipsilateral rib fractures and intrathoracic or intra-abdominal visceral injury.[7] Adrenal hemorrhage is an uncommon complication of extracorporeal membrane oxygenation (ECMO), and may be secondary to heparin therapy, hypoxemia, or the previously existing condition that led to the ECMO therapy.[4] In older children, adrenal hemorrhage is also known complication of fulminant bacterial sepsis and disseminated intravascular coagulation (DIC) secondary to meningococcemia, the Waterhouse-Friderichsen syndrome.[8]

At ultrasound, the adrenal gland is triangular in shape, with two limbs forming a V or Y appearance[9]; the limbs are usually 1 to 2 cm in length (depending on the gestational age of the newborn).[10] The gland is uniformly thick, with a central linear hypoechoic area representing the adrenal medulla, and a peripheral hyperechoic zone representing the adrenal cortex.[10] Adrenal hemorrhage may obliterate the normal contours of the gland or may be focal, involving the medulla or either limb.[9] Ultrasound may initially show simply diffuse enlargement and decreased echogenicity of the adrenal cortex secondary to edema, prior to frank adrenal hemorrhage.[4] Immediately after the hemorrhage, the adrenal gland may be hyperechoic and look solid, secondary to dense echogenic blood.[2] As the hematoma resolves, the mass becomes smaller and more anechoic.[2] Later, the mass may become more echogenic secondary to clot, and ultimately calcification may develop in the suprarenal region.[2] The echogenicity of the hemorrhage depends on the ratio of clotted to nonclotted blood,[8] and sequential imaging over weeks to months shows a progressive decrease in size until the mass eventually disappears.[2] This sequential change in echogenicity

vein thrombosis, unless there is obstruction of the inferior vena cava cephalad to the adrenal gland or massive adrenal hemorrhage causing compression of the right renal hilum and obstruction of the renal vein.[11]

CONTROVERSY

- Although MRI can usually establish an immediate diagnosis, it is rarely indicated in the evaluation of adrenal hemorrhage because of the typical appearance and evolution of adrenal hemorrhage at ultrasound. The hemorrhage may be partial, unilateral, or bilateral, but it regresses over a series of weeks to months and may evolve into post-adrenal hemorrhage calcifications.[1,2]

- Duplex Doppler ultrasound can confirm the diagnosis of coexisting renal vein thrombosis; no other imaging studies are necessary.[11]

from solid to hypoechoic, and the progressive decrease in the size of the mass confirms the diagnosis. CT is usually not necessary.[3] MRI can be performed and demonstrates high signal on both T1- and T2-weighted images; it reduces the uncertainty of the diagnosis, but usually is not necessary.[3,6] Therapy consists of supportive measures with serial ultrasound exams to demonstrate resolution. Adrenal insufficiency usually does not occur, even if the hemorrhage is bilateral.[6]

The differential diagnosis includes adrenal cysts, neuroblastoma, exophytic Wilms' tumor, and renal duplication with obstruction of the upper pole.[2,6] Adrenal cysts are rare and do not change over time.[1] Adrenal neonatal neuroblastoma, rare and with an excellent prognosis,[2] is echogenic and vascular at Doppler ultrasound, compared with adrenal hemorrhage, which is avascular and becomes anechoic on serial ultrasound.[2] Exophytic Wilms tumor, upper pole hydronephrosis in a duplicated system, or retroperitoneal nodes should be considered in the older child and may be difficult to distinguish initially at ultrasound.[2] These entities do not show the serial changes or the decrease in size of adrenal hemorrhage. Rare adrenal neoplasms, including teratoma, dermoid, and pheochromocytoma, usually do not present in the neonate; in older children they can be differentiated using MRI.[2] Fungal opportunistic infections and granulomatous infections can also present as adrenal masses; these are extremely rare and do not follow the typical ultrasound course.[1]

Further Reading

1. Carty H, Brunelle F, Shaw D, Kendall B, eds. *Imaging Children.* New York: Churchill Livingstone; 1994:802–811.
2. Kirks DR, ed. *Practical Pediatric Imaging.* 2nd ed. Boston: Little, Brown & Co; 1991:1023–1026.
3. Westra SJ, Zaninovic AC, Hall TR, Kangarloo H, Boechat MI. Imaging of the adrenal gland in children. *Radiographics* 14:1323–1340, 1994.
4. Sivit CM, Short BL, Revenis ME, Rebolo LC, Brown-Jones C, Garin DB. Adrenal hemorrhage in infants undergoing ECMO: prevalence and clinical significance. *Pediatr Radiol* 23:519–521, 1993.
5. Sivit CJ, Ingram JD, Taylor GA, Bulas DI, Kushner DC, Eichelberger MR. Posttraumatic adrenal hemorrhage in children: CT findings in 34 patients. *Am J Roentgenol* 158:1299–1302, 1992.
6. Kelalis PP, King LR, Belman AB. *Clinical Pediatric Urology, II.* 3rd ed. Philadelphia: WB Saunders Co; 1992:1323–1325.
7. Nimkin K, Teeger S, Wallach MT, DuVally JC, Spevak MR, Kleinman PK. Adrenal hemorrhage in abused children: imaging and postmortem findings. *Am J Roentgenol* 162:661–663, 1994.
8. Sarnaik AP, Sanfilippo DJ, Slovis TL. Ultrasound diagnosis of adrenal hemorrhage in meningococcemia. *Pediatr Radiol* 18:427–428, 1988.

9. Cohen EK, Daneman A, Stringer DA, Soto G, Thorner P. Focal adrenal hemorrhage: a new US appearance. *Radiology* 161:631–633, 1986.

10. Burton EM, Strange ME, Edmonds DB. Sonography of the circumrenal and horseshoe adrenal gland in the newborn. *Pediatr Radiol* 23:362–364, 1993.

11. Errington ML, Hendry GMA. The rare association of right adrenal haemorrhage and renal vein thrombosis diagnosed with duplex ultrasound. *Pediatr Radiol* 25:157–158, 1995.

BONE

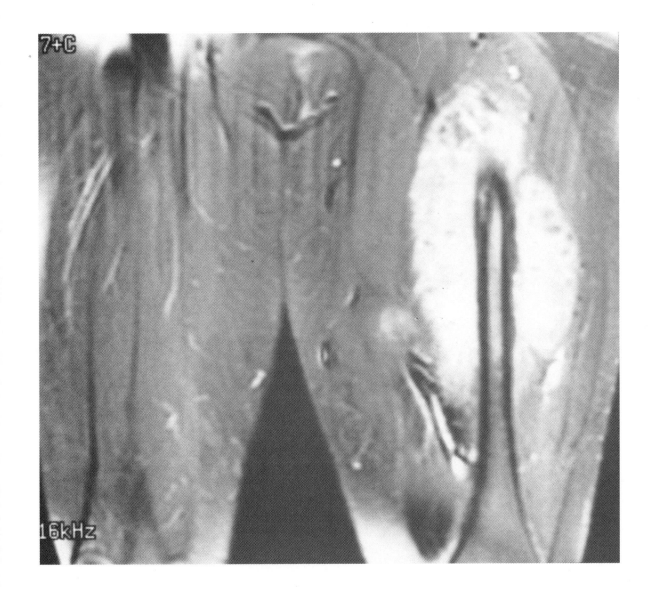

Case 1

Clinical Presentation

Painful left flat foot.

Radiographic Studies

Oblique radiopaque radiograph of the left foot (Fig. 1A) shows an osseous union of the calcaneus and navicular bones. Axial computed tomography (CT) of the feet (Fig. 1B) shows the osseous calcaneonavicular connection (arrowheads). Coronal CT of the feet (Fig. 1C) shows an associated union of the subtalar joint (arrow).

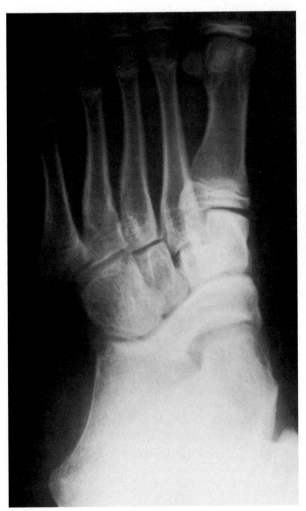

A

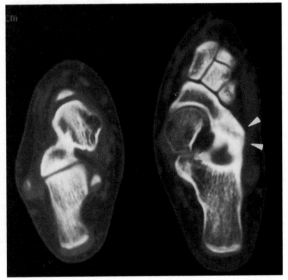

B

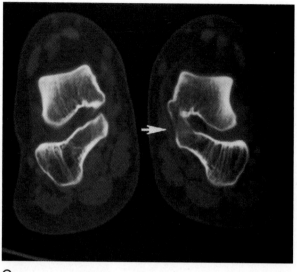

C

Diagnosis Tarsal Coalition

Discussion and Differential Diagnosis

Tarsal coalition involves an osseous or fibrocartilaginous union of two or more tarsal bones. Though tarsal coalition may be found incidentally in asymptomatic patients, adolescents commonly present with hindfoot abnormalities as tarsal ossification progresses.[1,2] The most common sites of tarsal coalition are the calcaneonavicular and talocalcaneal (subtalar) joint spaces. Bilateral tarsal coalitions are common, particularly at the calcaneonavicular site, and multiple sites of coalition within the same foot may occur.[1,3] A majority of patients present with a painful flat foot with decreased hindfoot motion on physical exam.[1] In some patients, associated peroneal muscle spasm or sensory alterations of the sole of the foot may be detected.[4] Though direct visualization of osseous calcaneonavicular coalition is common on plain radiographs, plain radiographic detection of subtalar coalition is more difficult. Radiographic findings of joint space narrowing, subchondral sclerosis, and findings assessing altered alignment of the talus and sustentaculum tali of the calcaneus have been described.[5] Coronal CT evaluation of the foot is performed to confirm the diagnosis, define extent of the tarsal coalition, assess for bilateral disease, and evaluate postoperative results.[2,4,5] A majority of subtalar coalitions involve the middle facet at or just posterior to the sustentaculum tali.[3,5] CT findings range from discrete osseous bridging across a joint space to more subtle joint space narrowing with marginal cortical irregularity seen in fibrocartilaginous coalitions.[3] If conservative treatment such as casting fails, surgical excision of the coalition with attempts to preserve joint motion is performed.[1,4]

Further Reading

1. Stormont DM, Peterson HA. The relative incidence of tarsal coalition. *Clin Orthop* 1983:183:28–36.
2. Deutsch AL, Resnick D, Campbell G. Computed tomography and bone scintigraphy in the evaluation of tarsal coalition. *Radiology* 1982:144(1):137–140.
3. Lee MS, Harcke HT, Kumar SJ, Bassett GS. Subtalar joint coalition in children: new observations. *Radiology* 1989:172:635–639.
4. Takakura Y, Sugimoto K, Tanaka Y, Tamai S. Symptomatic talocalcaneal coalition: its clinical significance and treatment. *Clin Orthop* 1991:269:249–256.
5. Lateur LM, Van Hoe LR, Van Ghillewe KV, Gryspeerdt SS, Baert AL, Dereymaeker GE. Subtalar coalition: diagnosis with the C sign on lateral radiographs of the ankle. *Radiology* 1994:193:847–851.

Case 2

Clinical Presentation

Refusal to walk.

Radiographic Studies

Longitudinal ultrasound of the right hip (Fig. 2A) shows convex distention of the hip joint capsule. Comparison image of the left hip (Fig. 2B) shows a concave, nondistended normal hip joint capsule. Upon needle aspiration of the right hip, 2 cc of cloudy joint fluid was obtained with a white blood cell count (WBC) of 90,000/mm^3.

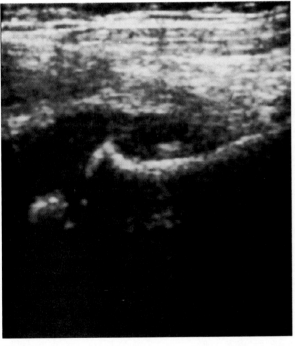

A

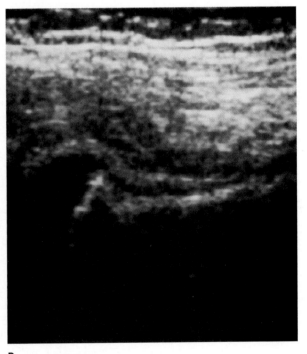

B

Diagnosis   Septic Arthritis

Discussion and Differential Diagnosis

During evaluation of the child with an irritable hip, prompt consideration and evaluation for septic arthritis is imperative to avoid long-term sequelae of suppurative infection of the hip joint. In children, acute presentation of hip joint pain, limp, and refusal to move the hip is generally found in conjunction with fever, elevated erythrocyte sedimentation rate, and elevated peripheral WBC.[1,2] Plain radiographic evaluation of the pelvis is inspected for the presence of joint fluid and for obliteration of soft tissue planes about the hip joint.[3] In addition, radiographic findings of fracture, avascular necrosis, or osteomyelitis are sought.[2,4] Accurate detection of hip joint effusion is provided by ultrasound imaging of the hip using an anterior parasagittal approach. Anechoic or echogenic displacement of the hip joint capsule from the proximal femoral cortex is found in both septic arthritis and toxic synovitis and compared to the contralateral hip joint.[2,4] Needle aspiration of hip joint fluid is performed and shows, on average, WBC greater than $50,000/mm^3$ in septic arthritis compared to less than $10,000/mm^3$ in toxic synovitis.[2] Adequate treatment of septic arthritis includes surgical drainage with antibiotic treatment whereas toxic synovitis resolves with bedrest and analgesic therapy. Prompt treatment reduces the likelihood of cartilage destruction, malalignment, and growth disturbance at the hip joint.[1,5] The differential diagnosis includes toxic synovitis, trauma, chronic synovial arthritis, and Legg-Perthes diseases. Associated intramedullary or intramuscular infection may be present.

Further Reading

1. Nade S. Acute septic arthritis in infancy and childhood. *J Bone Joint Surg Br* 1983:65(3):234–241
2. Zawin JK, Hoffer FA, Rand FF, Teele RL. Joint effusion in children with an irritable hip: US diagnosis and aspiration. *Radiology* 1993:187:459–463.
3. Hayden CK Jr, Swischuk LE. Periarticular soft-tissue changes in infections and trauma of the lower extremity in children. *Am J Roentgenol* 1980:134(2):307–311.
4. Marchal GJ, Van Holsbeeck MT, Raes M, et al. Transient synovitis of the hip in children: role of US. *Radiology* 1987:162(3):825–828.
5. Fabry G, Meire E. Septic arthritis of the hip in children: poor results after late and inadequate treatment. *J Pediatr Orthop* 1983:3(4):461–466.

Case 3

Clinical Presentation

Three infants with irritability and soft tissue swelling.

Radiographic Studies

Radiograph of the forearm (Fig. 3A) shows extensive periosteal new bone along the radius and ulna. A second patient with exuberant periosteal new bone involvement of the scapulae, clavicles, and ribs (Fig. 3B). A third patient with periosteal new bone involving the mandible (arrowheads, Fig. 3C).

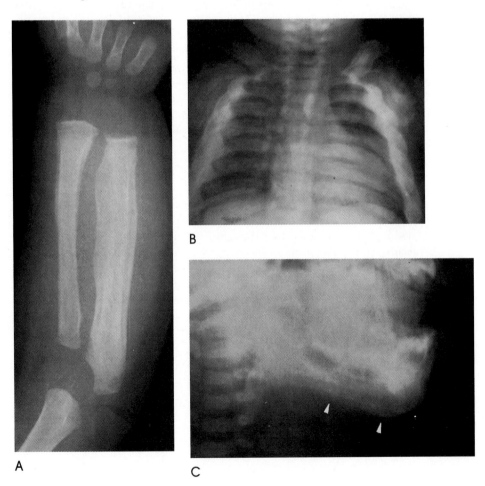

A

B

C

Diagnosis Caffey Disease

Discussion and Differential Diagnosis

Caffey disease (infantile cortical hyperostosis) is a rare disorder of unknown etiology generally presenting in the first 6 months of life. The usual presentation consists of irritability, firm deep soft tissue swellings, and scattered sites of cortical hyperostoses.[1,2] Frequently, fever, anemia, and elevated erythrocyte sedimentation rate are found.[1] Radiographic periosteal new bone is commonly found involving the mandible, clavicle, scapula, ribs, and tubular bones of the extremities.[1] Though nearly any bone can be involved, tarsal bone, carpal bone, or vertebral body involvement is particularly rare.[3] The clinical course is variable though a majority of cases show spontaneous resolution within weeks to months. Scattered lesions of differing stages of involvement and late recurrences of symptoms and hyperostoses have been reported.[2,4] Radiographically diaphyseal cortical thickening is detected and may be lamellated in appearance. Subsequent resorption of bone from within the medullary canal results in bone widening with cortical thinning.[2] Over time, remodeling and normalization of bone architecture generally occurs.[2] Biopsy shows thickening of lamellar cortical bone without inflammatory cellular infiltration or subperiosteal hemorrhage. Degenerative or fibrotic changes in the adjacent muscles may be found.[1,2,5] Infection, trauma, hypervitaminosis A, malignancy, and metabolic bone disease and prostaglandlin therapy should be considered in the differential diagnosis.

Further Reading

1. Caffey J. Infantile cortical hyperostoses. *J Pediatr* 1946:29(5):541–559.
2. Sherman MS, Hellyer DT. Infantile cortical hyperostosis: review of the literature and report of five cases. *Am J Roentgenol* 1950:63(2):212–222.
3. Harris VJ, Ramilo J. Caffey's disease: a case originating in the first metatarsal and review of a 12 year experience. *Am J Roentgenol* 1978:130(2):335–337.
4. Swerdloff BA, Ozonoff MB, Gyepes MT. Late recurrence of infantile cortical hyperostosis (Caffey's disease). *Am J Roentgenol Radium Ther Nucl Med* 1970:108(3):461–467.
5. Sanders DG, Weijers RE. MRI findings in Caffey's disease. *Pediatr Radiol* 1994:24:325–327.
6. Blank E. Recurrent Caffey's cortical hyperostosis and persistent deformity. *Pediatrics* 1975:55:856–860.

Case 4

Clinical Presentation

Shortened and bowed left thigh on physical exam.

Radiographic Studies

Pelvic radiograph (Fig. 4A) shows a markedly shortened left femur with absent left femoral head ossification, superolateral left hip subluxation, and a markedly dysplastic left acetabulum. Axial T1-weighted MRI of the pelvis (Fig. 4B) shows a markedly shortened left femur, a small left femoral head, and a shallow dysplastic left acetabulum.

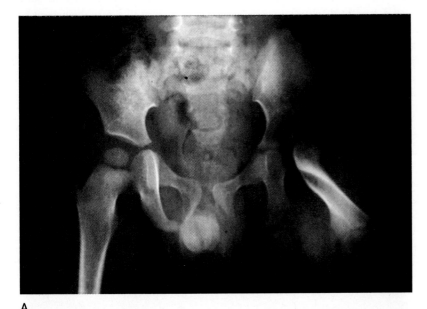

A

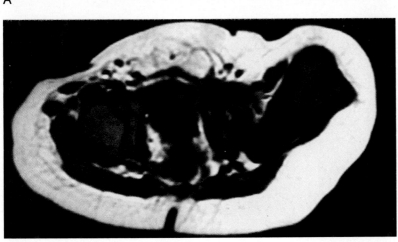

B

Diagnosis Proximal Femoral Focal Deficiency (PFFD)

Discussion and Differential Diagnosis

Proximal femoral focal deficiency is a rare congenital anomaly with varying degrees of absence of the proximal femur. In less severe cases, the femoral shortening is mild, osseous or cartilaginous continuity of the femoral neck and shaft is present, and the acetabulum is well developed or only moderately dysplastic.[1,2] Subtrochanteric varus deformity is characteristic, with the varus apex at or above the level of the acetabulum.[1] In more severe cases, the femoral shortening is greater and the acetabulum is severely dysplastic or absent. If present, the femoral head has no osseous connection to the femoral shaft.[2] Tapering of the proximal end of the femoral shaft may be found.[2] Clinically, a shortened thigh held in flexion, abduction, and external rotation is found.[3] Associated anomalies such as fibular hemimelia are frequent and bilateral involvement of femoral deficiency may occur.[1,2] MR imaging in selected cases to demonstrate cartilaginous components of the anomaly may be helpful and obviate need for arthrography.[2] Surgical procedures are aimed at treating varus alignment, leg length discrepancy, and hip joint instability. In some instances, congenital coxa vara must be considered in the differential diagnosis.

Further Reading

1. Levinson ED, Ozonoff MB, Royen PM. Proximal femoral focal deficiency (PPFD). *Radiology* 1977:125:197–203.
2. Hillmann JS, Mesgarzadeh M, Revesz G, Bonakdarpour A, Clancy M, Betz RR. Proximal femoral focal deficiency: radiologic analysis of 49 cases. *Radiology* 1987:165:769–773.
3. Pirani S, Beauchamp RD, Li D, Sawatzky B. Soft tissue anatomy of proximal femoral focal deficiency. *J Pediatr Orthop* 1991:11:563–570.
4. Sanpera I Jr, Sparks LT. Proximal femoral focal deficiency: does a radiologic classification exist? *J Pediatr Orthop* 1994:14:34–38.

Case 5

Clinical Presentation

A 5-year-old, status after motor vehicle accident.

Radiographic Studies

Radiograph of the knee shows fracture buckling the distal medial femoral cortex (Fig. 5A). Coronal gradient echo magnetic resonance image (MRI) sequence (Fig. 5B) shows extensive low signal intensity edema (arrowheads) involving both the medial metaphysis and medial epiphysis of the distal femur (Salter IV fracture). Coronal reconstruction image from a CT exam 6 months after the injury (Fig. 5C) shows a bony physeal bridge across the prior fracture site and varus alignment of the distal femoral epiphysis.

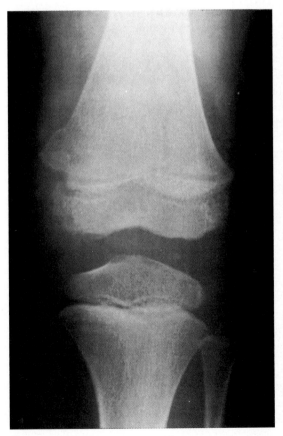

A

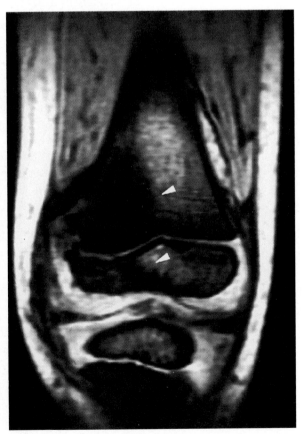

B

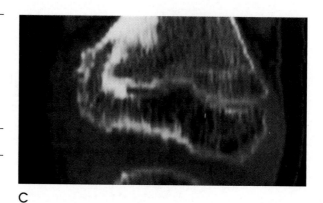

C

Diagnosis Growth Plate Arrest

Discussion and Differential Diagnosis

Direct traumatic injury of the growth plate or alteration of growth plate function by adjacent bone and joint infections may lead to subsequent growth plate arrest and resultant angular deformity or shortening of the involved bone. Though most traumatic physeal injuries heal without sequelae, significant growth impairment may result, depending on extent of physeal injury, years remaining to skeletal maturity, and amount of growth expected from the involved bone.[1,2] In patients at-high suspicion for growth plate arrest, detailed imaging of the growth plate and follow up of the patient to skeletal maturity are recommended.[1] Thin-section axial CT of the growth plate (with sagittal and coronal reconstructions) or direct coronal CT imaging of the growth plate has been utilized to detect partial growth plate arrest.[3] As the normal growth plate projects as low density soft tissue between the sclerotic epiphyseal and metaphyseal margins, CT findings of arrest include obliteration of the physeal space and bony trabeculae traversing the growth plate.[3] Limitations of CT imaging include difficulty of interpretation as the narrowing physis approaches maturity and underestimation of the extent of physeal bridging due to associated fibrous tissue.[3,4] In addition to accurately defining extent of both bony and fibrous physeal bridges, MRI has been advocated to detect earlier alterations of the growth plate allowing earlier intervention.[2] Surgical goals include osteotomy for angular deformity and minimizing limb length inequality. Surgical resection of localized physeal bridges with material interposition to prevent bridge recurrence may improve likelihood of subsequent longitudinal growth of the involved bone.[1,5]

Further Reading

1. Shapiro F. Epiphyseal disorders. *N Engl J Med* 1987:317(27):1702–1710.
2. Jaramillo D, Hoffer FA, Shapiro F, Rand F. MR imaging of fractures of the growth plate. *Am J Roentgenol* 1990:155:1261–1265.

3. DeCampo JF, Boldt DW. Computed tomography of partial growth plate arrest: initial experience. *Skeletal Radiol* 1986:15:526–529.
4. Peters W, Irving J, Letts M. Long-term effects on neonatal bone and joint infection on adjacent growth plates. *J Pediatr Orthop* 1992:12(6):806–810.
5. Lee EH, Gao GX, Bose K. Management of partial growth arrest: physis, fat or silastic? *J Pediatr Orthop* 1993:13:368–372.

Case 6

Clinical Presentation

Recurrent knee hemarthroses.

Radiographic Studies

Sagittal T2-weighted MR images (Fig. 6A) show a high signal knee joint effusion with low signal intensity synovial proliferation (arrow). A lateral radiograph of the elbow on subsequent presentation (Fig. 6B) shows a large dense elbow effusion secondary to hemarthrosis. Several years later, cartilage loss at the elbow joint is apparent (Fig. 6C).

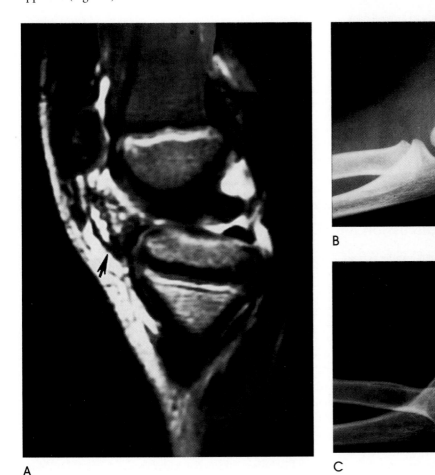

A

B

C

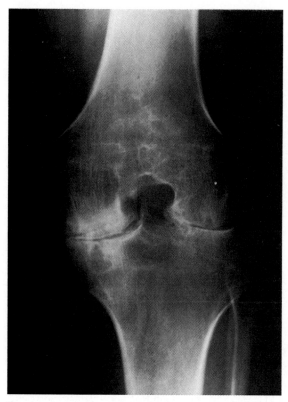

D

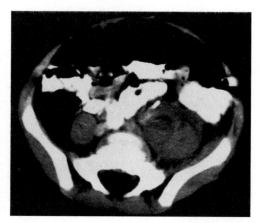

E

Diagnosis Hemophilia

Discussion and Differential Diagnosis

Hemophilia is a life-long bleeding disorder predominantly affecting male patients as an X-linked inherited trait. Hemophilia A (factor VIII deficiency) is much more common than hemophilia B (factor IX deficiency); and given a high mutation rate, a family history of the disease may be absent.[1] More frequent and earlier clinical presentations are expected in patients with more severe factor deficiencies (baseline factor level less than 1 to 2% of expected level).[1,2] Spontaneous or posttraumatic recurrent bleeding into a joint space or intramuscular compartment is commonly seen though intracranial hemorrhage or urinary tract hemorrhage may also be encountered.[1] Prompt treatment of acute hemarthroses is indicated to prevent a vicious circle of synovial proliferation, repetitive bleeding into the joint, and subsequent progressive cartilage loss.[1] Early radiographic findings characteristic of hemophilic arthropathy include osteopenia and epiphyseal enlargement.[2] Subsequent progressive findings include irregularity of the subchondral surface, cartilage space narrowing, subchondral cyst formation, and periarticular erosions (Fig. 6D). More advanced radiographic changes include incongruent articular surfaces, subluxation, or even ankylosis across the joint.[2] If conservative measures such as factor replacement,

PEARLS

- Aggressive treatment of hemarthroses may slow but generally does not halt progressive radiographic findings of hemophilic arthropathy.[3]

- Imaging may be particularly useful for iliopsoas intramuscular hemorrhage (Fig. 6E, large left psoas hematoma) as the clinical findings may suggest hip joint or other abdominal disorders.[1]

• Family history of disease may be absent.[1]

splinting, or physical therapy fail, then open or arthroscopic synovectomy may be attempted to reduce recurrent hemarthroses and to preserve or improve joint motion.[3] In some centers, outpatient synovectomy is performed by injecting a radionuclide into the affected joint under fluoroscopic control.[4] Extraarticular involvement may include an unresorbed intramuscular or subperiosteal hematoma resulting in a walled-off hemophilic pseudotumor. This may cause mass effect on surrounding neurovascular structures or chronic pressure erosion of adjacent bony structures. A majority of pseudotumors occur in the pelvis and lower extremities and radiographic findings include a soft tissue mass, periosteal new bone, and variable lytic destruction of the adjacent bone.[5] CT typically shows a large soft tissue lesion of near water attenuation enclosed by a thickened fibrous capsule.[6] CT may show coarse calcifications in the soft tissue lesion and is well suited to define the entire extent of the lesion, document involvement of neurovascular structures, and delineate associated bone destruction.[6]

Further Reading

1. Lusher JM, Warrier I. Hemophilia A. *Hematol Oncol Clin North Am* 1992: 6(5):1021–1033.
2. Pettersson H, Ahlberg A, Nilsson IM. A radiologic classification of hemophilic arthropathy. *Clin Orthop* 1980:149:153–159.
3. Triantafyllou SJ, Hanks GA, Handal JA, Greer RB III. Open and arthroscopic synovectomy in hemophilic arthropathy of the knee. *Clin Orthop* 1992: 283:196–204.
4. Siegel HJ, Luck JV Jr, Siegel ME, Quines C, Anderson E. Hemarthrosis and synovitis associated with hemophilia: clinical use of P-32 chromic phosphate synoviorthesis for treatment. *Radiology* 1994:190:257–261.
5. Brant EE, Jordan HH. Radiologic aspects of hemophilic pseudotumors in bone. *Am J Roentgenol Radium Ther Nucl Med* 1972:115(3):525–539.
6. Hermann G, Yeh HC, Gilbert MS. Computed tomography and ultrasonography of the hemophilic pseudotumor and their use in surgical planning. *Skeletal Radiol* 1986:15:123–128.

Case 7

Clinical Presentation

Refusal to walk.

Radiographic Studies

Radiograph of the right leg (Fig. 7A) shows an oblique lucency in the distal tibia. Lateral foot radiograph in another child refusing to bear weight (Fig. 7B) is unremarkable. Follow-up radiograph 1 week later (Fig. 7C) shows transverse sclerosis.

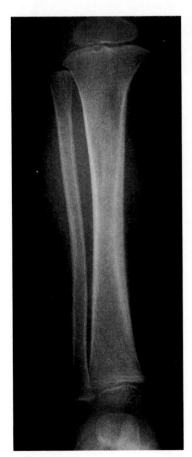

A

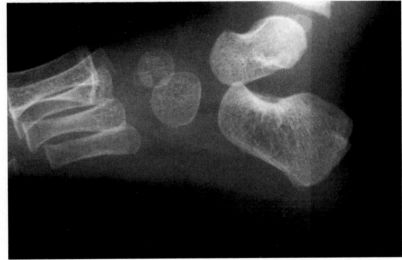

B

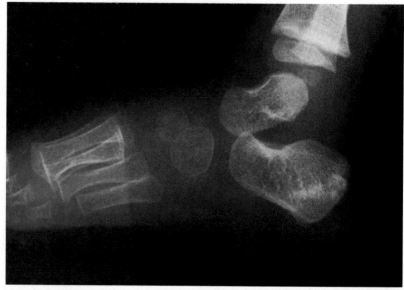

C

Diagnosis Toddler's Fracture

Discussion and Differential Diagnosis

When an ambulating infant presents with a new limp or refuses to bear weight, the diagnosis of a lower extremity toddler's fracture should be considered. A history of trauma may be well documented or absent in these irritable infants, and localizing findings on physical exam may be subtle. Sites of reported toddler's fractures include the distal tibial shaft, calcaneus, and cuboid bones, and subtle or absent initial radiographic findings of these fractures is the rule.[1-3] As these fractures are nondisplaced, additional views such as oblique views of the tibia or axial views of the calcaneus may be required to detect the fracture at presentation.[1,2] Follow-up radiographs are helpful with demonstration of sclerosis along the fracture line or demonstrating periosteal reaction.[1-3] If the diagnosis is not apparent and other causes such as infection are being considered, a bone scan will provide greater sensitivity in detecting focal or generalized tracer uptake at the site of fracture.[2,3] Uneventful healing of the toddler's fracture with immobilization or limited weight-bearing is expected.

Further Reading

1. Dunbar JS, Owen HF, Nogrady MB, McLeese R. Obscure tibial fracture of infants—the toddler's fracture. *J Can Assoc Radiol* 1964:15:136–144.
2. Starshak RJ, Simons GW, Sty JR. Occult fracture of the calcaneus—another toddler's fracture. *Pediatr Radiol* 1984:14:37–40.
3. Blumberg K, Patterson RJ. The toddler's cuboid fracture. *Radiology* 1991: 179:93–94.

Case 8

Clinical Presentation

Painful swelling of both knees.

Radiographic Studies

Radiograph of the knees (Fig. 8A) shows synovial-based swelling of the knees. Note prominent distal femoral epiphyses. Post-gadolinium T1-weighted MR image (Fig. 8B) shows thickened synovial enhancement of the hips. Radiograph of the wrist (Fig. 8C) at a more advanced stage of disease shows synovial-based swelling, generalized cartilage space narrowing, and extensive periarticular erosive changes.

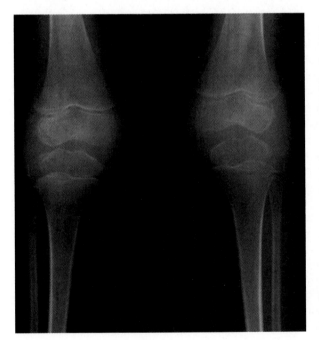

A

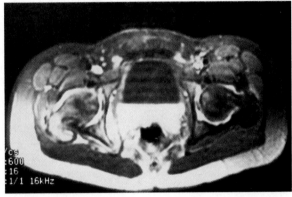

B

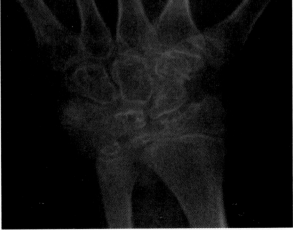

C

Diagnosis Juvenile Rheumatoid Arthritis

Discussion and Differential Diagnosis

Juvenile rheumatoid arthritis is the most common chronic synovial inflammatory disorder of childhood. Unlike those who suffer from adult rheumatoid arthritis, children are usually serologically negative for rheumatoid factor. In addition, children show greater involvement outside the hands and feet, are more likely than adults to have monoarticular disease, and are more likely to develop ankylosis across a joint space.[1,2] The child may present with signs of systemic illness (rash, pericarditis, splenomegaly, lymphadenopathy) with no early radiographic joint findings. Alternatively, a pauciarticular (four or fewer joints) or polyarticular presentation may be evident.[1,2] Common sites of disease onset include the knees, ankles, carpals, tarsals, and cervical spine. Synovial-based soft tissue swelling, adjacent periosteal new bone, and radiographic signs of growth disturbance precede the relatively late findings of cartilage loss or periarticular erosions.[1,2] Growth disturbance may be evident as epiphyseal overgrowth, early physeal fusion, shortened tubular bones, and decreased diaphyseal diameter.[1,2] In the cervical spine, ankylosis of the apophyseal joints, associated developmentally abnormal appearance of the cervical vertebral bodies, and atlanto-axial subluxation are frequent.[1,2] MR imaging with administration of gadolinium is capable of directly showing enhancement of the acutely inflamed synovium prior to radiographic abnormality.[3] In addition, MR imaging shows joint effusions, focal or generalized cartilage loss, and bone erosions to greater extent than do radiographs.[4] Though remission of active joint space inflammation may occur prior to adulthood, aggressive treatment with multiple medications is warranted given a significant percentage of patients with active synovial inflammation and progressive functional deterioration into adulthood.[5]

Further Reading

1. Martel W, Holt JF, Cassidy JT. Roentgenologic manifestations of juvenile rheumatoid arthritis. *Am J Roentgenol* 1962:88:400–423.
2. Ansell BM, Kent PA. Radiological changes in juvenile chronic polyarthritis. *Skeletal Radiol* 1977:1:129–144.
3. Gabriel H, Fitzgerald SW, Myers MT, Donaldson JS, Poznanski AK. MR imaging of hip disorders. *Radiographics* 1994:14:763–781.
4. Senac MO Jr, Deutsch D, Bernstein BH, et al. MR imaging in juvenile rheumatoid arthritis. *Am J Roentgenol* 1988:150:873–878.
5. Wallace CA, Levinson JE. Juvenile rheumatoid arthritis. Outcome and treatment for the 1990's. *Rheum Dis Clin North Am* 1991:17(4):891–905.

Case 9

Clinical Presentation

Subacute onset of limp.

Radiographic Studies

Frog-leg radiograph of the pelvis (Fig. 9A) shows a subchondral fracture of the left capital femoral epiphysis. In addition, sclerosis and loss of height of the epiphysis is apparent. Pelvic radiograph in another patient (Fig. 9B) shows loss of height, sclerosis, and fragmentation of the left femoral epiphysis. Abduction brace is applied to achieve femoral head containment in the acetabulum. Follow-up pelvic radiograph in this patient (Fig. 9C) shows some remodeling of the markedly flattened left femoral head and marked widening of the left femoral neck. Note lateral subluxation of the left hip, which is incompletely covered by the left acetabulum.

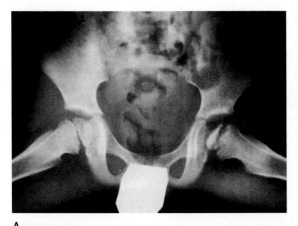

A

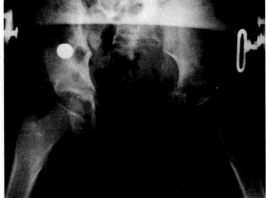

B

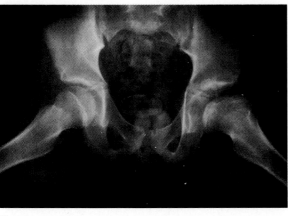

C

Diagnosis Legg-Calvé-Perthes Disease

Discussion and Differential Diagnosis

When a child presents with a limp or pain in the hip or knee, the diagnosis of Legg-Calvé-Perthes disease must be considered. In this condition, idiopathic avascular necrosis of the proximal femoral epiphysis occurs. Presentation is most common in children between the ages of 4 and 8 years and boys are affected four times more often than girls.[1,2] The presentation may be gradual; in some patients, a preceding history of trauma is obtained; and bilateral femoral epiphysis involvement occurs in approximately 10% of patients.[1] Initial radiographs may be normal or demonstrate localized epiphyseal demineralization, sclerosis, or a discrete subchondral fracture line. In more advanced cases, fragmentation and loss of height of the femoral epiphysis occurs, widening of the femoral neck is evident, and secondary metaphyseal changes are present.[1] Subsequent radiographs show reossification and remodeling of the fragmented femoral epiphysis. In mild cases, a nearly spherical femoral head contained within a normal acetabulum results. A flattened and deformed femoral head results in more severe cases. Restricted hip joint motion and joint pain can be expected when lateral subluxation of the femoral head and adaptive changes in the acetabulum alter congruity of the cartilage space of the hip joint.[1] A better prognosis is expected when the extent of femoral epiphysis is more localized at diagnosis, when the lateral pillar of the femoral epiphysis is spared, and in those patients who are younger at presentation.[1,2] MR imaging has been advocated to detect changes of ischemia prior to radiographic changes, to delineate the entire extent of epiphyseal involvement more accurately, and to better visualize healing changes prior to reossification.[3–5] Treatment consists of weight-relieving treatment and containment of the femoral epiphysis within the acetabulum. Conservative measures such as casting or abduction braces suffice in milder cases, but more severe cases require surgical procedures such as femoral varus osteotomy or shelf acetabuloplasty to decrease likelihood of long-term degenerative changes of the hip joint.[6,7] Differential diagnostic considerations include known causes of avascular necrosis such as Gaucher's disease or sickle cell disease, steroid therapy, hypothyroidism, trauma, or osteomyelitis.

Further Reading

1. Catterall A. The natural history of Perthes disease. *J Bone Joint Surg Br* 1971:53(1):37–53.
2. Farsetti P, Tudisco C, Caterini R, Potenza V, Ippolito E. The Herring lateral pillar classification for prognosis in Perthes disease: late results in 49 patients treated conservatively. *J Bone Joint Surg Br* 1995:77(5):739–742.
3. Bos CF, Bloem JL, Bloem RM. Sequential magnetic resonance imaging in Perthes disease. *J Bone Joint Surg Br* 1991:73(2):219–224.
4. Kaniklides C, Lonnerholm T, Moberg A, Sahlstedt B. Legg-Calvé-Perthes disease: comparison of conventional radiography, MR imaging, bone scintigraphy and arthrography. *Acta Radiol* 1995:36(4):434–439.

5. Ducou le Pointe H, Haddad S, Silberman B, Filipe G, Monroc M, Montagne JP. Legg-Perthes-Calvé disease: staging by MRI using gadolinium. *Pediatr Radiol* 1994:24(2):88–91.

6. Kruse RW, Guille JT, Bowen JR. Shelf arthroplasty in patients who have Legg-Calvé-Perthes disease. *J Bone Joint Surg Am* 1991:73(9):1338–1347.

7. Poussa M, Yrjonen T, Hoikka V, Osterman K. Prognosis after conservative and operative treatment in Perthes disease. *Clin Orthop* 1993:297:82–86.

Case 10

Clinical Presentation

Asymmetric calf size.

Radiographic Studies

Anteroposterior radiograph of the left leg (Fig. 10A) shows medial bowing of the distal tibia and fibula. Note thinning of the convex cortex of the bowed tibia and fibula. Lateral radiograph (Fig. 10B) shows posterior bowing of the distal tibia and fibula. Note marked cortical thickening of the concave tibial cortex.

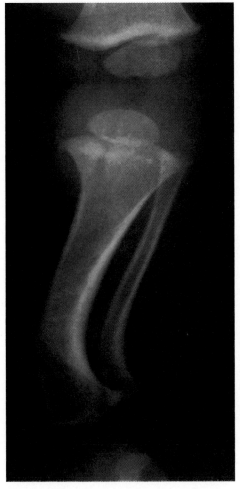
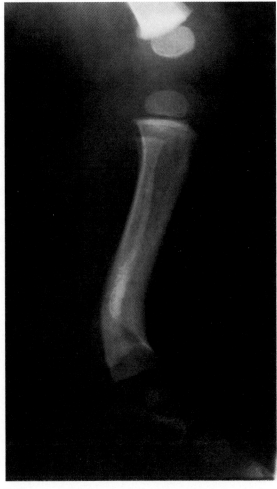

A   B

Diagnosis Tibial Bowing

Discussion and Differential Diagnosis

When tibial bowing is detected in the newborn period, distinction of a rather isolated abnormality of one lower extremity versus bowing of multiple long bones relating to a generalized skeletal dysplasia must be made. Posterior bowing of the tibia is encountered in an otherwise healthy newborn and is thought to be caused by external intrauterine compression.[1] Family history is absent, and an associated cutaneous dimple, smaller calf size, or ipsilateral foot anomalies may be found on physical exam.[1,2] The apex of posterior tibial bowing is usually bowed medially at the junction of the mid to distal third of the tibia.[1,2] Thickening of the concave cortex and thinning of the convex cortex of the bowed tibia is expected.[1] Although most cases of posteromedial bowing resolve without treatment, significant leg length discrepancy may be found on subsequent radiographs.[2] Anterior tibial bowing has a high association with neurofibromatosis and the development of tibial pseudarthroses. The apex of bowing in these cases is usually lateral, and cystic or sclerotic changes in the medullary canal may be found prior to fracture and pseudarthrosis formation.[3] Tibial bowing associated with a generalized skeletal dysplasia is generally evident following a thorough family history, physical examination, and detection of multiple radiographic findings throughout the skeleton.

Further Reading

1. Thompson W, Oliphant M, Grossman H. Bowed limbs in the neonate: significance and approach to diagnosis. *Pediatr Ann* 1976:5(1):50–62.
2. Hofmann A, Wenger DR. Posteromedial bowing of the tibia: progression of discrepancy in leg lengths. *J Bone Joint Surg Am* 1981:63(3):384–388.
3. Andersen KS. Radiological classification of congenital pseudarthrosis of the tibia. *Acta Orthop Scand* 1973:44:719–727.

Case 11

Clinical Presentation

Bruises of varying ages.

Radiographic Studies

Bone scintigraphy (Fig. 11A) shows abnormal uptake in multiple left posteromedial ribs and abnormal uptake in the left scapula (arrow). No periosteal new bone or callus was detected on radiographic evaluation of the ribs. Radiograph of the left shoulder shows angulation of the left scapula (arrow, Fig. 11B) at acute fracture site. Scintigraphic images of the lower extremities (Fig. 11C) show abnormal uptake throughout the left tibia and increased activity in both proximal tibias (rounded rather than oval metaphyses). Radiographs of the legs (Fig. 11D) show a focal buckle fracture (arrow) of the proximal left tibial metaphysis without radiographic signs of healing. Note transverse sclerosis of the proximal right tibial metaphysis consistent with healing fracture from an earlier traumatic event.

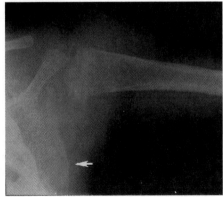

B

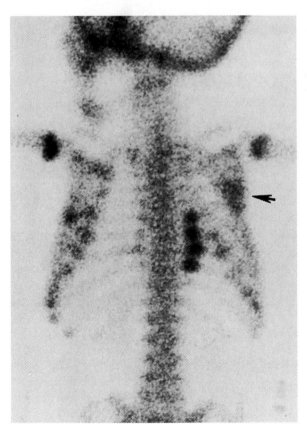

A

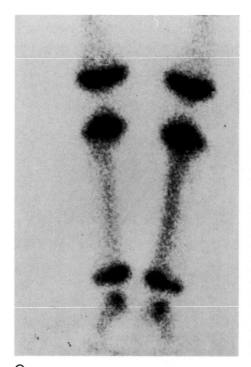

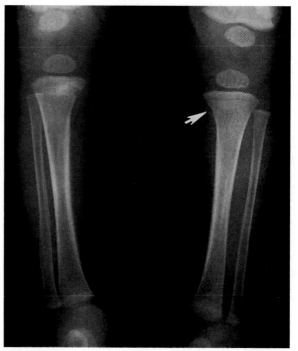

C   D

Diagnosis Child Abuse

Discussions and Differential Diagnosis

When multiple fractures are noted throughout the skeleton in differing stages of healing, or when fractures are detected in locations generally not injured in childhood accidental trauma, then the diagnosis of child abuse (nonaccidental trauma, battered child syndrome) must be considered. A majority of cases of child abuse occur in children younger than two years of age.[1] Shaking of an infant plays an important role in both cerebral and skeletal injuries, particularly in children under 1 year of age.[2,3] A thorough clinical search for bruises, retinal hemorrhages, or burns is important in the workup but may be absent in the presence of suspicious radiographic findings. Skeletal imaging options include radiographic skeletal survey and bone scintigraphy. The skeletal survey should include anteroposterior images throughout the skeleton and lateral views of the spine and skull with images coned down to the region of interest.[3] Advantages of the skeletal survey include more accurate aging of fractures, increased detection of skull fractures, and detection of possible underlying metabolic bone disease not possible on bone scintigraphy. Bone scintigraphy is more sensitive in detecting sites of skeletal trauma unrecognized on the radiographic skeletal survey, particularly in the demonstration of rib fractures.[4] Common sites of fracture highly suggestive of abuse include a transverse fracture of the metaphysis or a posteromedial rib fracture at the costovertebral junction.[3] Though less commonly encountered, fractures of the sternum, scapula, and spinous processes are highly suggestive of nonaccidental trauma.[1,5] Non-metaphyseal fractures of the long bones are frequently found but are less specific for the diagnosis of nonaccidental trauma.[1] CT or MR imaging of the head is indicated to detect intracranial injuries, which account for most of the fatal cases and long-term disability of child abuse.[3] Abdominal imaging is performed when directed by clinical or laboratory findings. The differential diagnosis of the skeletal findings of nonaccidental trauma includes many conditions that cause fractures, metaphyseal irregularities, or periosteal reaction. These entities, which include disorders such as osteogenesis imperfecta, infection, leukemia, or vitamin A intoxication, can usually be distinguished from child abuse on the basis of other radiographic bone findings or extraskeletal radiographic findings.[6] In addition, clinical and laboratory findings suggestive of other skeletal disease processes are usually apparent.

Further Reading

1. Kogutt MS, Swischuk LE, Fagan CJ. Patterns of injury and significance of uncommon fractures in the battered child syndrome. *Am J Roentgenol* 1974: 121(1):143–149.
2. Caffey J. The parent-infant traumatic stress syndrome; (Caffey-Kempe syndrome), battered babe syndrome). *Am J Roentgenol* 1972:114(2):217–229.
3. Kleinman PK. Diagnostic imaging in infant abuse. *Am J Roentgenol* 1990: 155(4):703–712.
4. Sty JR, Starshak RJ. The role of bone scintigraphy in the evaluation of the suspected abused child. *Radiology* 1983:146(2):369–375.
5. Kleinman PK, Zito JL. Avulsion of the spinous processes caused by infant abuse. *Radiology* 1984:151(2):389–391.
6. Brill PW, Winchester P. Differential diagnosis of child abuse. In: Kleinman PK, ed. *Diagnostic of Child Abuse*. Baltimore: Williams & Wilkins; 1987:11:221–241.

Case 12

Clinical Presentation

One month of left thigh pain.

Radiographic Studies

Anteroposterior radiograph of the pelvis (Fig. 12A) shows a medially placed left capital femoral epiphysis. Frog-leg radiograph of the pelvis following surgical fixation (Fig. 12B) shows reduction. Subsequent follow-up frog-leg pelvic radiograph (Fig. 12C) shows abnormal sclerosis of the mid and posterior left femoral head. Anteroposterior pelvic radiograph at a later follow-up (Fig. 12D) shows progressive findings with fragmentation of the central left femoral head. In addition, cartilage space narrowing has developed.

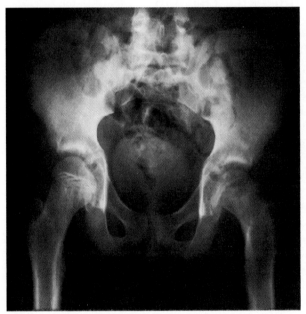

A

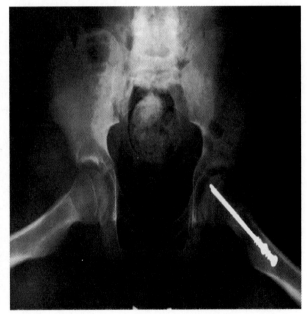

B

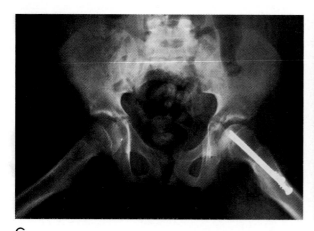

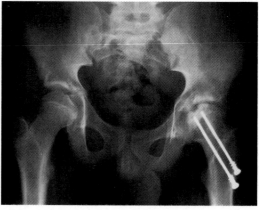

C

D

PEARLS

- SCFE relating to endocrine disease presents at a wider age range and most commonly is caused by hypothyroidism or growth hormone deficiency.[4]

PITFALLS

- Delayed diagnosis is more common when hip pain is absent or when thigh or knee pain is found on exam.[2]

CONTROVERSY

- The exact role between timing of surgical treatment and development of subsequent avascular necrosis is uncertain.

Diagnosis Slipped Capital Femoral Epiphysis (SCFE)

Discussion and Differential Diagnosis

Slipped capital femoral epiphysis involves displacement of the capital femoral epiphysis relative to the proximal femoral metaphysis. The disorder occurs in adolescence, is more likely to occur in obese patients, and may be preceded by a known traumatic event.[1] Though hip pain, limp, and decreased internal rotation on physical exam constitute the typical presentation, a significant number of cases have vague findings clinically (thigh or knee pain) resulting in a delay in diagnosis.[2] SCFE has traditionally been categorized as acute, chronic (over 2 to 3 weeks of symptoms), or acute-on-chronic. More recently, classification of SCFE into stable (able to bear weight with or without crutches) and unstable (unable to bear weight even with crutches) categories has been proposed.[3] Initial radiographic assessment includes anteroposterior and frog-leg lateral views of the pelvis to detect physeal widening, epiphyseal displacement, and alteration of the femoral head-shaft angle. Inspection of the opposite hip is imperative given a high incidence of bilateral SCFE particularly in patients with underlying endocrine or metabolic disease.[4] Ultrasound has been advocated for visualization of the slipped epiphysis and evaluation of an associated joint effusion, which may indicate instability in SCFE.[5] Treatment options include preoperative traction, maneuvers attempting reduction of the displaced epiphysis, and surgical fixating procedures (pins or cannulated screws). Follow-up radiographs are useful for displaying posttreatment reduction of the epiphysis, adjacent bony remodeling, and alignment of orthopedic hardware, and for monitoring the known complications of avascular necrosis and chondrolysis (Fig. 12D).

Further Reading

1. Aronson DD, Peterson DA, Miller DV. Slipped capital femoral epiphysis: the case for internal fixation in situ. *Clin Orthop* 1992:281:115–122.
2. Ledwith CA, Fleisher GR. Slipped capital femoral epiphysis without hip pain leads to missed diagnosis. *Pediatrics* 1992:89(4 pt 1):660–662.

3. Loder RT, Richards BS, Shapiro PS, Reznick LR, Aronson DD. Acute slipped capital femoral epiphysis: the importance of physeal stability. *J Bone Joint Surg Am* 1993:75(8):1134–1140.
4. Loder RT, Wittenberg B, deSilva G. Slipped capital femoral epiphysis associated with endocrine disorders. *J Pediatr Orthop* 1995:15:349–356.
5. Castriota-Scanderbeg A, Orsi E. Slipped capital femoral epiphysis: ultrasonographic findings. *Skeletal Radiol* 1993:22:191–193.

Case 13

Clinical Presentation

A 15-year-old boy with shoulder pain.

Radiographic Studies

Left shoulder radiograph (Fig. 13A) shows a well-defined, mildly expansile lytic lesion adjacent to the proximal humeral physis. Axial noncontrast CT exam (Fig. 13B) shows the well-defined lytic lesion with a small amount of internal calcified matrix (arrow) identified suggesting cartilaginous nature of the lesion. Sagittal CT reconstruction image (Fig. 13C) shows both metaphyseal and epiphyseal extent of the lytic lesion.

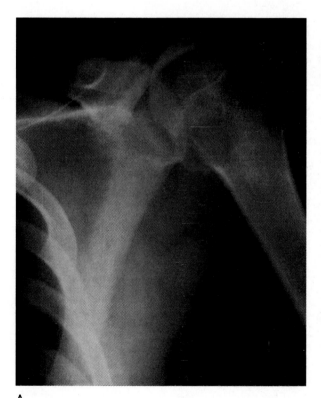

A

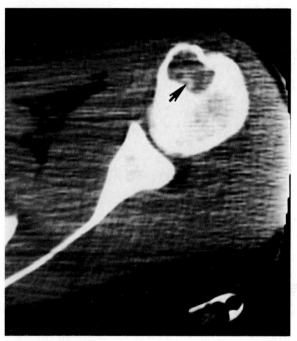

B

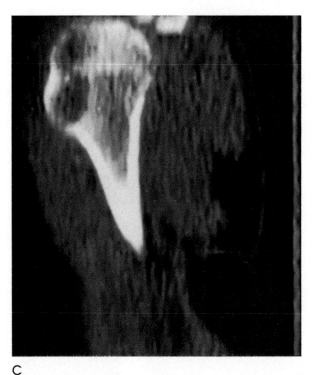

C

Diagnosis   Chondroblastoma

Discussion and Differential Diagnosis

Chondroblastoma is a generally benign chondroid lesion of bone that presents most often in mid to late adolescence adjacent to an active growth plate. A majority of these lesions occur in the long bones and present as localized pain. Less commonly, decreased range of motion of an adjacent joint or associated muscle wasting is detected clinically.[1] Common sites of involvement include the distal femur, proximal tibia, proximal humerus, and proximal femur.[1,2] Within a long tubular bone, chondroblastoma is nearly always within the epiphysis, though the lesion frequently extends into the metaphysis. Lesions are less commonly found in an apophysis or entirely within the metaphysis.[1] Radiographs most often show an eccentric lytic lesion with a thin sclerotic margin. Solid or layered periosteal reaction is shown in over half of long bone chondroblastomas.[2] Increased detection of intrinsic calcification and cortical destruction can be expected on CT evaluation whereas MRI is superior at demonstrating adjacent soft tissue or bone marrow edema.[3] If the lesion is entirely epiphyseal, the differential diagnosis includes subchondral bone cyst, infection, and histiocytosis. When the lesion extends into the metaphysis, additional causes such as enchondroma, osteoblastoma, or aneurysmal bone cyst must be considered.[1] Treatment generally consists of surgical curettage and bone grafting.

Further Reading

1. Bloem JL, Mulder JD. Chondroblastoma: a clinical and radiological study of 104 cases. *Skeletal Radiol* 1985:14:1–9.
2. Brower AC, Moser RP, Kransdorf MJ. The frequency and diagnostic significance of periostitis in chondroblastoma. *Am J Roentgenol* 1990:154:309–314.
3. Weatherall PT, Maale GE, Mendelsohn DB, Sherry CS, Erdman WE, Pascoe HR. Chondroblastoma: classic and confusing appearance at MR imaging. *Radiology* 1994:190:467–474.

Case 14

Clinical Presentation

A 15-year-old girl with left thigh mass.

Radiographic Studies

Left femur radiograph (Fig. 14A) shows cortical irregularity of the mid femoral shaft with a large associated soft tissue mass. Bone windows from axial CT exam show the cortical irregularity to better advantage (arrowheads, Fig. 14B). Axial T2-weighted MR sequence (Fig. 14C) shows abnormal intramedullary high-signal intensity. Contrast between the high signal lobular soft tissue mass and thigh musculature is shown to better advantage than on the CT exam. Coronal post-gadolinium T1-weighted imaging with fat suppression (Fig. 14D) shows abnormal intramedullary enhancement and enhancement of the large associated soft tissue mass.

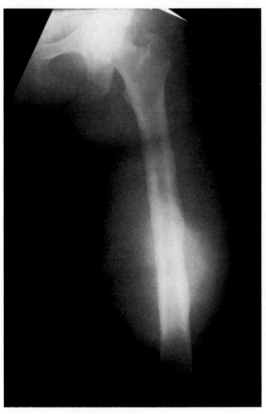

A

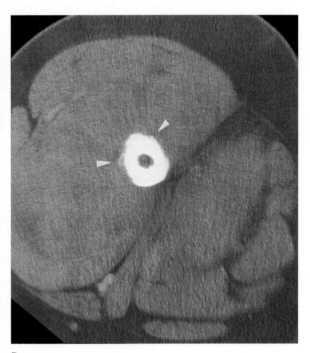

B

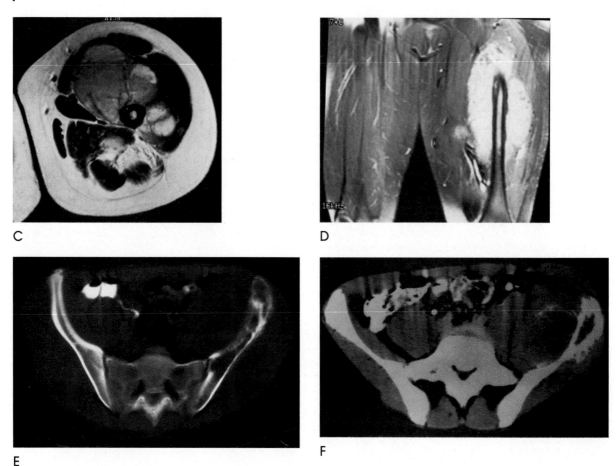

C

D

E

F

Diagnosis Ewing Sarcoma

Discussion and Differential Diagnosis

Ewing sarcoma is an aggressive round cell tumor generally arising within bone in the second decade of life. Patients generally present with localized pain and swelling, and associated fever and leukocytosis are common.[1] Though diaphyseal origin of Ewing sarcoma occurs more commonly than in osteosarcoma, a majority of Ewing sarcomas originate in the metadiaphyseal region when long bones are involved.[1,2] Involvement of flat bones and the axial skeleton is much more frequent in Ewing sarcoma than in osteosarcoma.[1–3] Figures 14E, F shows an aggressive left ileal lytic Ewing sarcoma with associated periosteal reaction and a large associated soft tissue mass. The radiographic findings are variable and include permeative ill-defined lytic destruction, a well-defined purely lytic lesion, a mixed lytic/sclerotic pattern, or a honeycomb appearance of the bone. Rarely, a purely sclerotic radiographic finding is encountered, particularly in the pelvis and spine, and distinction from osteomyelitis and osteosarcoma may be difficult.[4] Periosteal reaction may be laminated, spiculated, or solid.[4] An associated soft tissue mass is present in most cases, is often bulky, and may extend much greater than extent of the intraosseous abnormality.[2] Complete intraosseous and soft tissue extent are provided by CT or MR imaging. Metastatic disease is present in up to one third of patients at presentation and usually involves the lungs or other bones.[5] Treatment generally includes a combination of chemotherapy and radiation treatment of the primary tumor.[5] Surgical excision is attempted in selected cases but often involves a difficult surgical approach depending on location of the tumor. Poorer prognosis is expected with metastases at presentation, larger tumor volume, and axial skeleton location of the primary lesion.[3,5]

Further Reading

1. Dahlin DC, Coventry MB, Scanlon PW. Ewing's sarcoma. *J Bone Joint Surg Am* 1961:43(2):185–192.
2. Vohra VG. Roentgen manifestations in Ewing's sarcoma: a study of 156 cases. *Cancer* 1967:20:727–733.
3. Kissane JM, Askin FB, Foulkes M, Stratton LB, Shirley SF. Ewing's sarcoma of bone: clinicopathologic aspects of 303 cases from the Intergroup Ewing's Sarcoma Study. *Hum Pathol* 1983:14(9):773–779.
4. Shirley SK, Gilula LA, Seigal GP, Foulkes MA, Kissane JM, Askin FB. Roentgenographic-pathologic correlation of diffuse sclerosis in Ewing sarcoma of bone. *Skeletal Radiol* 1984:12:67–78.
5. Hayes FA, Thompson EI, Parvey L, et al. Metastatic Ewing's sarcoma: remission induction and survival. *J Clin Oncol* 1987:5(8):1199–1204.
6. O'Keeffe F, Lorigan JG, Wallace S. Radiological feature of extraskeletal Ewing sarcoma. *Br J Radiol* 1990:63:456–460.

Case 15

Clinical Presentation

A 7-year-old boy with left knee pain.

Radiographic Studies

Anteroposterior radiograph (Fig. 15A) shows mixed lytic and sclerotic lesion of the proximal tibial metaphysis with signs of periosteal new bone formation and periosteal elevation. Coronal T1-weighted MR image (Fig. 15B) shows low signal replacement of the normal fatty marrow in the proximal left tibial metaphysis. No epiphyseal involvement was seen on MR. Bone window image from CT exam (Fig. 15C) shows intramedullary sclerosis, cortical breakthrough, and periosteal new bone. Soft tissue window CT image (Fig. 15D) shows abnormal intramedullary soft tissue and sclerosis and an associated soft tissue mass (arrowheads). CT scan following chemotherapy (Fig. 15E) shows posttreatment healing ossification (arrowheads) within the soft tissue mass.

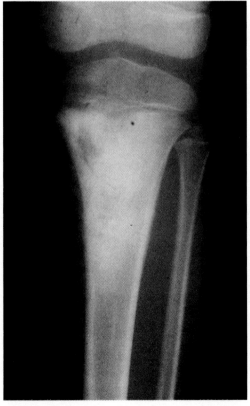

A

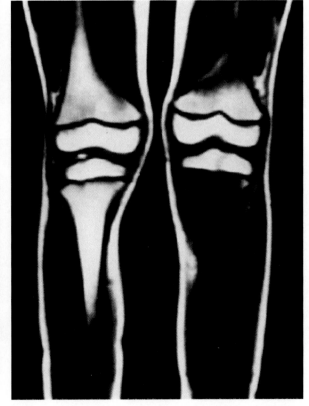

B

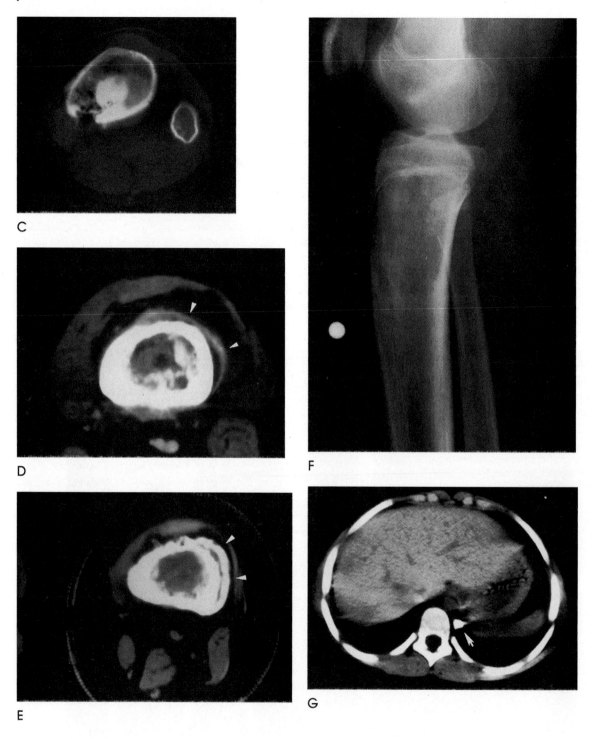

C

D

E

F

G

Diagnosis Osteogenic Sarcoma

Discussion and Differential Diagnosis

Osteogenic sarcoma (osteosarcoma) is the most common primary bone malignancy of pediatrics. A majority of lesions present during the adolescent growth spurt with localized pain and a palpable mass.[1,2] Conventional osteosarcoma has an intramedullary origin, and—depending on predominant tissue—histologically is classified into osteoblastic, fibroblastic, or chondroblastic varieties.[1]

Classically, osteosarcoma presents radiographically as an ill-defined lytic lesion mixed with patchy sclerosis within a metaphysis about the knee joint. Cortical breakthrough, an associated soft tissue mass with cloud-like osteoid matrix and aggressive spiculated periosteal reaction, is evident in most. Less commonly, osteosarcoma may present radiographically as purely sclerotic or purely lytic lesion in the metaphysis.[3,4] The classic radiographic appearance is characteristic, but the purely lytic variety of osteosarcoma (Fig. 15F) may be difficult to distinguish from aggressive lesions such as metastatic disease, Ewing sarcoma, or malignant fibrous histiocytoma or from benign lesions such as aneurysmal bone cyst or giant cell tumor.[4] "Skip" metastases occurring as a separate lesion in the same bone as the primary tumor are found in up to one fifth of patients.[1,3] Occasionally, a patient will present with osteosarcomatosis where multifocal, rapidly appearing, usually symmetric, sclerotic metaphyseal lesions are detected at or soon after diagnosis.[5]

Metastatic disease in osteosarcoma most frequently involves the lungs and skeleton, though pleural, lymph node, pericardial, kidney, and brain metastases may be found.[1] MR imaging is the most accurate in the demonstration of complete intraosseous extent of tumor and for imaging the extraosseous extent and relationship to the adjacent joint space and neuro-vascular structures.[6] CT and bone scan are indicated to detect pulmonary and skeletal metastases. Initial treatment in osteosarcoma is chemotherapy, which has improved survival and increases the possibility of limb salvage surgery. In addition, a high percentage of tumor necrosis at histology following preoperative chemotherapy correlates with improved long-term survival.[7] Radiographic indicators of a good response to chemotherapy include decreased tumor bulk, increased ossification of the soft tissue mass, increased medullary canal sclerosis, and a more well defined periosteal response.[2] If limb salvage surgery is not feasible, surgical amputation of the primary tumor may be required. Aggressive surgical resection of pulmonary metastases has proved beneficial in osteosarcoma.[8]

Further Reading

1. Tebbi CK, Gaeta J. Osteosarcoma. *Pediatr Ann* 1988:17:285–300.
2. Smithe J, Heelan RT, Huvos AG, et al. Radiographic changes in primary osteogenic sarcoma following intensive chemotherapy. Radiological-pathological correlation in 63 patients. *Radiology* 1982:143:355–360.
3. Kumar R, David R, Madewell JE, Lindell MM Jr. Radiographic spectrum of osteogenic sarcoma. *Am J Roentgenol* 1987:148:767–772.
4. deSantos LA, Edeiken B. Purely lytic osteosarcoma. *Skeletal Radiol* 1982:9:1–7.

- Lung involvement in osteosarcoma may result in pneumothorax.[1]

PITFALLS
- Lung parenchymal and lymph node metastases may ossify (arrow, Fig. 15G) and must be distinguished from calcified granulomatous disease.

CONTROVERSY
- Some authors believe osteosarcomatosis represents aggressive metastatic spread of disease; others believe this represents multifocal primary sites of osteosarcoma throughout the skeleton.[5]

5. Hopper KD, Moser RP Jr, Haseman DB, Sweet DE, Madewell JE, Kransdorf MJ. Osteosarcomatosis. *Radiology* 1990:175:233–239.

6. Gillespy T III, Manfrini M, Ruggieri P, Spanier SS, Pettersson H, Springfield DS. Staging of intraosseous extent of osteosarcoma: correlation of preoperative CT and MR imaging with pathologic macroslides. *Radiology* 1988:167:765–767.

7. Hudson M, Jaffe MR, Jaffe N, et al. Pediatric osteosarcoma: therapeutic strategies, results, and prognostic factors derived from a 10-year experience. *J Clin Oncol* 1998:(12):1988–1997.

8. Han MT, Telander RL, Pairolero PC, et al. Aggressive thoracotomy for pulmonary metastatic osteogenic sarcoma in children and young adolescents. *J Pediatr Surg* 1981:16(6):928–933.

Case 16

Clinical Presentation

A 4-year-old girl with left hip pain and elevated erythrocyte sedimentation rate (ESR).

Radiographic Studies

Radiograph of the proximal left femur (Fig. 16A) shows an oval metaphyseal lytic lesion. Post-gadolinium coronal T1-weighted image with fat suppression (Fig. 16B) shows intense intramedullary enhancement of the proximal left femoral metaphysis and diaphysis. Intense adjacent soft tissue enhancement is noted. A more posterior image (Fig. 16C) shows an oval intramedullary lesion (arrow).

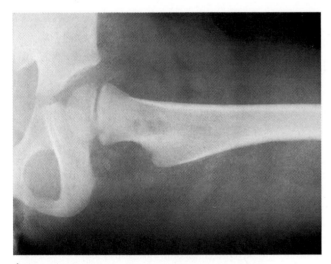

A

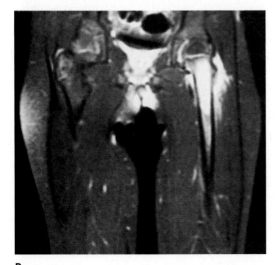

B

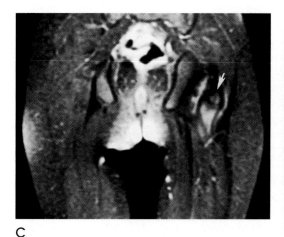

C

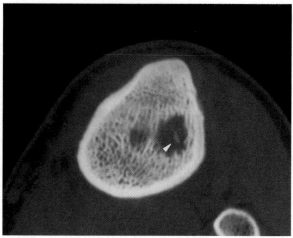

D

Diagnosis Osteomyelitis

Discussion and Differential Diagnosis

Based on the blood supply to growing bones, the metaphyses of long bones are the most common site of acute hematogenous osteomyelitis in pediatrics. The child usually presents with fever, localized bone tenderness, leukocytosis, and elevated ESR. When the disease is at a more advanced stage, swelling, erythema, and decreased range of motion at the adjacent joint may be found.[1] Though the long bones are the most common site of involvement, pelvic and spine presentation of osteomyelitis is frequent in children. In neonates, localizing clinical findings are often absent, multifocal lesions are common, and epiphyseal involvement occurs, making radiologic detection critical.[1–3] Radiographic findings include deep soft tissue swelling, lytic bone destruction, and periosteal new bone formation. Bone scintigraphy is more sensitive for detection of osteomyelitis in most instances and may demonstrate additional lesions more accessible to biopsy or culture.[3] Common organisms isolated include *Staphylococcus aureus* and streptococcal species. If patients are appropriately treated with antibiotics, morbidity is low. If inadequately treated, increased extent of involvement in the form of subperiosteal fluid collections, adjacent soft tissue fluid collections, and transphyseal spread may occur and growth disturbances may result. Associated septic arthritis may ensue, particularly when osteomyelitis occurs near the hip or shoulder joint.[1] Given the ischemia and thrombosis associated with the inflammatory process, a sequestrum of dead bone (arrowhead, Fig. 16D) may result and provide a source of prolonged or recurrent infection.[1] In such instances, imaging with CT or MR may be necessary to demonstrate soft tissue or subperiosteal fluid collections to be drained or sequestra to be resected. Post-gadolinium MR imaging is particularly useful for demonstrating noncontiguous sites of active inflammation and complete intramedullary extent and for detecting presence and extent of physeal involvement.[4,5]

PEARLS

• Pelvic osteomyelitis may be difficult to detect radiographically and may clinically simulate hip joint disease, discitis, or abdominal pathology.[1,6]

• Osteomyelitis in sickle cell disease often involves the diaphysis, multiple locations are common, and distinction from bone infarction on clinical grounds is difficult.[7]

PITFALLS

• Without high-resolution imaging equipment and magnification views, distinction of metaphyseal osteomyelitis from the active physis on bone scintigraphy may be difficult.[3]

Further Reading

1. Nade S. Acute haematogenous osteomyelitis in infancy and childhood. *J Bone Joint Surg Br* 1983:65(2):109–119.
2. Brill PW, Winchester P, Krauss AN, Symchych P. Osteomyelitis in a neonatal intensive care unit. *Radiology* 1979:131:83–87.
3. Bressler EL, Conway JJ, Weiss SC. Neonatal osteomyelitis examined by bone scintigraphy. *Radiology* 1984:152:685–688.
4. Dangman BC, Hoffer FA, Rand FF, O'Rourke EJ. Osteomyelitis in children: gadolinium-enhanced MR imaging. *Radiology* 1992:182:743–747.
5. Jaramillo D, Treves ST, Kasser JR, et al. Osteomyelitis and septic arthritis in children: appropriate use of imaging to guide treatment. *Am J Roentgenol* 1995:165:399–403.
6. Mah ET, LeQuesne GW, Gent RJ, Paterson DC. Ultrasonic signs of pelvic osteomyelitis in children. *Pediatr Radiol* 1994:24:484–487.
7. Stark JE, Glasier CM, Blasier RD, Aronson J, Seibert JJ. Osteomyelitis in children with sickle cell disease: early diagnosis with contrast-enhanced CT. *Radiology* 1991:179:731–733.

Case 17

Clinical Presentation

Abnormal foot on physical exam.

Radiographic Studies

Lateral simulated weight-bearing radiograph (Fig. 17A) shows talocalcaneal alignment suggesting hindfoot varus. The lateral talocalcaneal angle was decreased, measuring 20°. The anteroposterior (AP) view (Fig. 17B) shows a nearly parallel alignment of the talus and calcaneus consistent with hindfoot varus. Marked forefoot varus is noted.

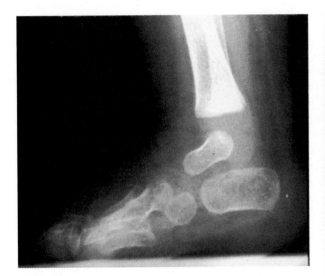

A

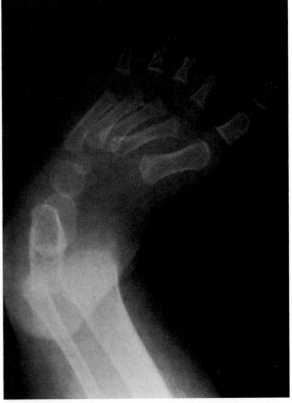

B

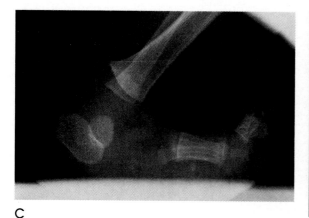

C

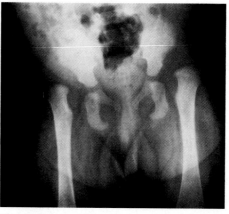

D

PEARLS

• In calcaneus alignment of the ankle, excessive dorsiflexion is present, the calcaneus is more vertically aligned, and the angle between the midcalcaneus and mid tibia on lateral radiographs is decreased.[1,2]

• Though a congenital foot deformity may be detected as an isolated finding, association with generalized skeletal dysplasias, metabolic disorders, and neuromuscular conditions must be considered in some patients (Fig. 17D, same patient as Fig. 17C. Patient with bilateral vertical talus has associated bilateral hip dislocations).[3]

PITFALLS

• Numerous varied ranges of "normal" talocalcaneal

Diagnosis Congenital Foot Anomalies

Discussion and Differential Diagnosis

When evaluating an infant or child with a congenital foot deformity, thorough clinical assessment of abnormal position or motion at the ankle joint, subtalar joint, and the midtarsal joint is required. The radiologic evaluation requires careful positioning of the feet with AP and lateral views of the foot taken with the patient standing or in a simulated weight-bearing position in which maximum dorsiflexion of the foot is obtained.[1,2] In a normal foot, the midtalar and midcalcaneal longitudinal axes are divergent, and in the AP view, the midtalar line points toward the head of the first metatarsal while the midcalcaneal line points toward the head of the fourth metatarsal. The most commonly encountered foot deformity is congenital clubfoot or talipes equinovarus. Talipes refers to the congenital nature of the abnormality; equinus refers to excessive plantar flexion at the ankle joint with abnormal elevation of the posterior aspect of the calcaneus.[1,2] Varus of the hindfoot is suggested on radiographs when the longitudinal axes of the talus and calcaneus become less divergent and approach a parallel alignment on both AP and lateral projections. Varus of the forefoot is displayed by metatarsus adductus seen on the AP view as the midshaft metatarsal axes are angled toward the midline of the body. In distinction to clubfoot, the less common deformity of congenital vertical talus has valgus of the hindfoot in which the axes of the talus and calcaneus become more divergent, evidenced by a more vertically oriented talus on the lateral view (Fig. 17C). Resultant talonavicular dislocation and a rigid flatfoot ensue.[1,2]

Further Reading

1. Ritchie GW, Deim HA. Major foot deformities: their classification and x-ray analysis. *J Can Assoc Radiol* 1968:19:155–166.

angles have been reported, and age-dependent changes in these "normal" ranges have been documented.[4]

2. Templeton AW, McAlister WH, Zim ID. Standardization of terminology and evaluation of osseous relationships in congenitally abnormal feet. *Am J Roentgenol* 1965:93(2):374–381.

3. Taybi H, Lachman RS. *Radiology of Syndromes, Metabolic Disorders, and Skeletal Dysplasias,* 4th ed. St. Louis: Mosby; 1996:1025–1026, 1044.

4. Vanderwilde R, Staheli LT, Chew DE, Malagon V. Measurements on radiographs of the foot in normal infants and children. *J Bone Joint Surg Am* 1988: 70(3):407–415.

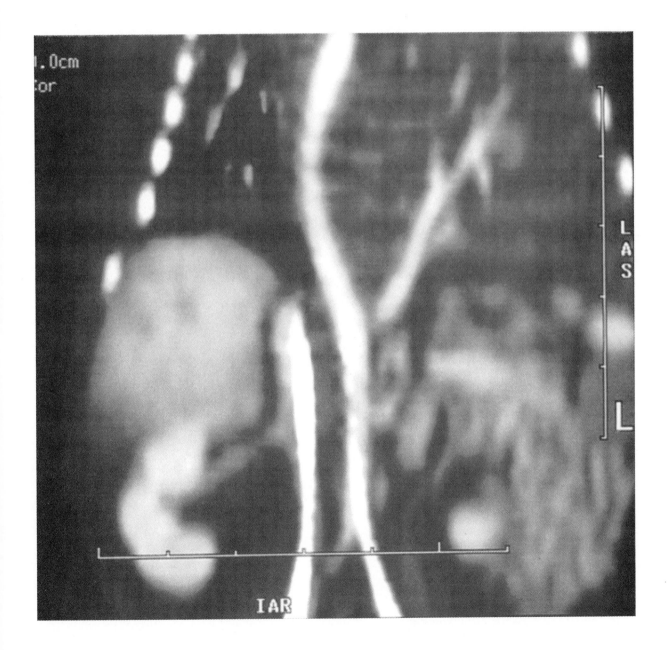

Case 1

Clinical Presentation

Heart murmur noted on school physical.

Radiographic Studies

Posteroanterior (Fig. 1A) and lateral (Fig. 1B) views of chest reveal a smoothly contoured mass in the anterior mediastinum; a curvilinear rim of calcification (arrowheads, Fig. 1B) is noted superiorly. This is confirmed on noncontrast CT scan (Fig. 1C) which demonstrates rim calcification and water attenuation cysts within the mass, which originates from the right lobe of the thymus. Post-contrast CT image (Fig. 1D) shows cystic, soft tissue and fatty attenuation components of this rim-enhancing mediastinal mass.

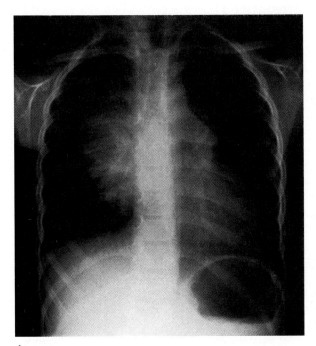

A

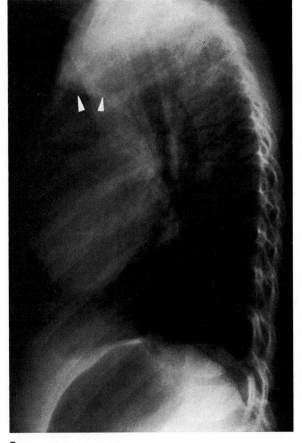

B

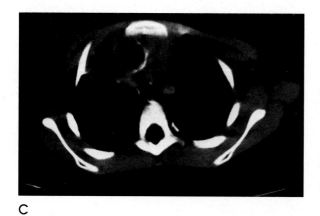

C

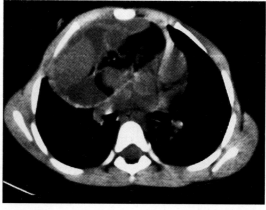

D

Diagnosis Mediastinal Germ Cell Tumor (Teratoma)

Discussion and Differential Diagnosis

Roughly one third of all mediastinal tumors in children are located in the anterior mediastinum, and teratomas account for approximately 20% of all mediastinal masses in infants and young children.[1] In the anterior mediastinum, lymphoma, leukemia, teratomas, and dermoids are the most frequently encountered tumors. In the pediatric age group, thymomas are uncommon and tumors of thymus gland origin are rare. For practical purposes, the primary differential considerations for anterior mediastinal masses in the pediatric age range are lymphoma and teratoma, with lymphoma more common in the older pediatric patient and teratoma more common in the younger child.

Teratomas fall in the category of germ cell tumors (GCTs) and contain elements of at least two of the three embryonic layers.[2] They typically consist of multilocular cysts mixed with solid elements, but may be mostly solid or have a unilocular cystic appearance. If soft tissue, fat, and calcification are demonstrated in an anterior mediastinal mass, the diagnosis of teratoma can be established on the basis of imaging.[3] The presence of teeth is pathognomonic.[2] In young infants, the tumor is nearly always benign. Other GCTs that may present in the mediastinum are teratocarcinoma, choriocarcinoma, seminoma, endodermal sinus (yolk sac) tumor, and mixed germ cell tumor.[4] In the case of a solid germ cell tumor, it may not be possible to differentiate it from lymphoma or thymoma. Differential considerations for cystic anterior mediastinal masses include teratoma (GCT), cystic hygroma, thymic cyst, thymoma (cysts related to hemorrhage and necrosis), and lymphoma with cystic degeneration.

Most patients with mediastinal teratoma are asymptomatic but those with larger tumors may present with chest pain, dyspnea, respiratory distress, cough, pneumonia, or heart murmur. The severity of symptoms depends on the degree of airway compression.

Further Reading

1. Swischuk LE. *Imaging of the Newborn, Infant and Young Child,* 3rd ed. Baltimore: Williams & Wilkins; 1989:189, 191–192.
2. Rosado-de-Christenson ML, Templeton PA, Moran CA. Mediastinal germ cell tumors: radiologic and pathologic correlation. *Radiographics* 12(5):1013–1030, 1992.
3. Levitt RG, Husband JE, Glazer HS. CT of primary germ-cell tumors of the mediastinum. *Am J Roentgenol* 142:73–78, 1984.
4. Hedlund GL, Kirks DR, Respiratory system. In: Kirks DR, ed. *Practical Pediatric Imaging: Diagnostic Radiology of Infants and Children,* 2nd ed. Boston: Little Brown & Co; 1991: 659.
5. Derenoncourt AN, Castro-Magana M, Jones KL. Mediastinal teratoma and precocious puberty in a boy with mosaic Klinefelter syndrome. *Am J Med Genet* 55:38–42, 1995.
6. Fulcher AS, Proto AV, Jolles H. Cystic teratoma of the mediastinum: demonstration of fat/fluid level. *Am J Roentgenol* 154:259–260, 1990.

Case 2

Clinical Presentation

A 14-year-old patient who presented with complaints of shortness of breath, fatigue, and recent weight loss.

Radiographic Studies

Anterior (Fig. 2A) and lateral (Fig. 2B) radiographs of the chest show a large mass in the anterior mediastinum, which is more prominent on the right than the left. Also visible are bilateral hilar adenopathy, extensive subcarinal adenopathy, narrowing of left mainstem bronchus, and patchy infiltrates, well seen on the lateral projection but made nearly invisible on the posteroanterior view by overpenetration. These infiltrates were located in right middle and left lower lobes. Selected CT images show multiple nodular infiltrates in right middle and left lower lobes (Fig. 2C) and subcarinal nodes (Fig. 2D), and a large solid anterior mediastinal mass causing posterior displacement and compression of the carina (Fig. 2E). The area of low attenuation (arrow) probably represents focal necrosis.

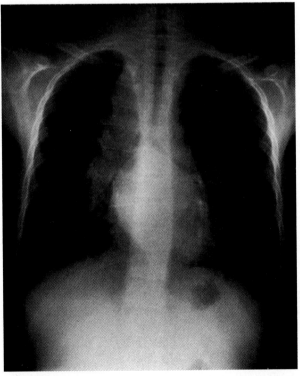

A

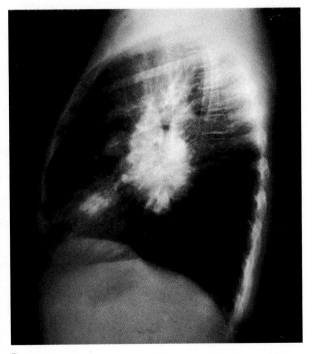

B

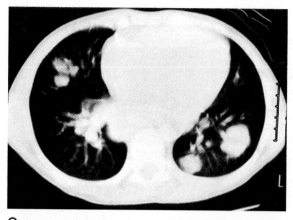

C

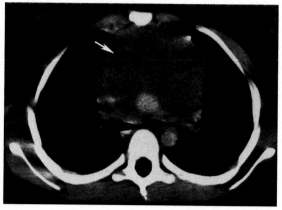

E

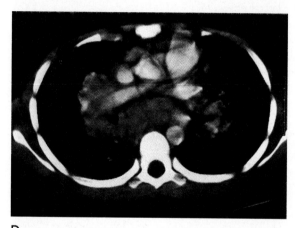

D

Diagnosis Lymphoma

Discussion and Differential Diagnosis

Lymphoma is the third most common of all childhood malignancies, accounting for 13% of cancers; leukemia and CNS tumors represent 30% and 19%, respectively. In children under age 10 years, non-Hodgkin lymphoma is more common than Hodgkin lymphoma. Together, these lymphomas represent 23% of all mediastinal masses in children and they are the most common cause for an anterior mediastinal mass in childhood.[1]

Of childhood chest masses, those in the mediastinum are the most common. Mediastinal masses occur with roughly equal frequency in anterior (30 to 40%), middle (30%), and posterior (30 to 40%) mediastinum.[2] Eighty-five percent of all anterior mediastinal masses in children are caused by malignant lymphoma, benign thymic enlargement, or teratomas.[1] Differential diagnoses include germ cell tumors other than teratoma (i.e., endodermal sinus tumor, seminoma, embryonal cell carcinoma, and seminoma), thymoma, thymic cyst, cystic hygroma, and ectopic thyroid

PEARLS

- Non-Hodgkin lymphoma is the most common AIDS-related neoplasm in children.[5]

- Pleural effusions are encountered in 5% of patients with mediastinal lymphoma, possibly related to venous or lymphatic compression. Pericardial fluid is almost always related to direct tumor extension.[1]

- Necrotic nodes are not uncommon following treatment. Node necrosis at presentation may be seen in nodular sclerosing Hodgkin disease.[4]

- Enhancing nodes are classically present in Castleman disease.

- Most commonly involved lymph nodes in intrathoracic lymphoma are in the anterior mediastinal, pretracheal, and hilar chains. Not to be overlooked are nodes in axillary, subcarinal, paracardiac, internal mammary chains, and superior diaphragmatic chains. Many of these nodes will not be detectable by plain radiographs, and careful CT evaluation is essential.

- Patients may develop second neoplasms following treatment for lymphoma. Leukemia develops in up to 5% of patients with Hodgkin disease who are treated with chemotherapy.[3]

- Recurrence usually develops within 2 years following completion of treatments. CT scan or chest radiograph reveals the recurrent disease in most cases.

PITFALLS

- Residual disease following treatment remains difficult to evaluate as CT evaluation may not be able to distinguish between posttreatment fibrosis and remaining tumor.

gland. For practical purposes, however, anterior mediastinal masses in children represent lymphoma arising in lymph nodes and/or thymus (70% in one large series) or teratoma (10% in the same series).[2] Similarly, the most common masses in the middle mediastinum are of nodal origin and relate to lymphoma or inflammatory node involvement. Bronchopulmonary foregut malformations account for most of the other middle mediastinal masses in children.

Hodgkin lymphoma tends to involve lymph nodes and most commonly presents with cervical adenopathy. The disease spreads by involvement of adjacent nodal groups, and up to 85% of patients have mediastinal involvement at the time of presentation, with thymic infiltration in approximately 30%.[1,2] It should be noted that CT more accurately detects intrathoracic disease than do plain chest radiographs.[2] Approximately one third of patients with Hodgkin lymphoma have hilar lymphadenopathy. Parenchymal disease is present in 5 to 12% of patients; it does not occur without mediastinal node involvement.

Hodgkin disease has two peaks of age distribution, one in teenagers and young adults, and one in patients 55 years and older. The incidence in the younger age group has been increasing as a result of an increased incidence of the nodular sclerosis subtype.[3] Four histologic subtypes of Hodgkin disease are recognized. In decreasing order of incidence, these are nodular sclerosis (58%), mixed cellularity (23%), lymphocyte predominance (6%), and lymphocyte depletion (4%). Nine percent of Hodgkin lymphomas cannot be classified and fall into a miscellaneous category.[3] Mediastinal involvement is more common in the nodular sclerosing subtype. Airway compression is present in 55% of patients with mediastinal lymphoma[1] and may be life threatening, particularly in a sedated, supine patient. Compression of the tracheobronchial tree is more accurately evaluated by CT than by plain films.[1]

Cystic changes can be seen in the thymus at the initial presentation with Hodgkin lymphoma as well as after radiation treatment. Nodal calcification may develop after treatment; it is rarely detected at the time of presentation.[1]

Non-Hodgkin lymphoma represents 7% of all childhood malignancies, compared to 5% for Hodgkin lymphoma. Both types have a male predominance, which is as high as 3 to 1 with Hodgkin disease in children younger than 12 years.[2] Non-Hodgkin lymphoma typically presents with extranodal disease. A mediastinal mass is found at time of presentation in 25 to 30% of patients.[2] Non-Hodgkin lymphomas are histologically classified as low, intermediate, and high grade.[4] Lymphoblastic lymphoma is one of the high-grade non-Hodgkin lymphomas that presents in the anterior mediastinum. It is usually of T-cell origin and typically occurs in the adolescent to young adult age group. It constitutes 40% of all childhood lymphomas. The other non-Hodgkin lymphoma typically seen in the mediastinum is a large B-cell lymphoma generally seen in women in their thirties. Primary non-Hodgkin lymphoma is rare in the lung, but pulmonary parenchymal involvement can occur in disseminated disease.

Differential considerations for mediastinal mass with parenchymal infiltrate include sarcoidosis, tuberculosis, histoplasmosis, and angioimmunoblastic lymphadenopathy. In the differential diagnosis for mediastinal adenopathy or mass, consider adenopathy from infectious mononucleosis, sarcoidosis, Castleman disease, and primitive neuroectodermal tumors.

Further Reading

1. Merten DF. Diagnostic imaging of mediastinal masses in children. *Am J Roentgenol* 158:832, 1991.
2. Siegel BA, Proto AV, eds. *Pediatric Disease (Fourth Series) Test and Syllabus.* Reston, VA: American College of Radiology; 1993: 131–164, 593.
3. Murray KA, Chor PJ, Turner JF Jr. Intrathoracic lymphoproliferative disorders and lymphoma. *Curr Prob Diagn Radiol* 25(3):78–106, 1996.
4. Fishman EK, Kuhlman JE, Jones RJ. CT of lymphoma: spectrum of disease. *Radiographics* 11:647–669, 1991.
5. Siskin GP, Haller JO, Miller S, Sundaram R. AIDS-related lymphoma: radiologic features in pediatric patients. *Radiology* 196:63–66, 1995.

Case 3

Clinical Presentation

Two newborn infants with severe respiratory distress.

Radiographic Studies

Anterior (Fig. 3A) and lateral (Fig. 3B) chest radiographs of the first patient show an enlarged left lower lobe containing variable-sized cysts. There is compression of the left upper lobe and the mediastinum is markedly shifted to the right. The chest radiograph of the second patient (Fig. 3C) shows a large left pleural effusion and mass effect creating rightward mediastinal shift. Ultrasound examination (Fig. 3D) of the lower left hemithorax reveals a small amount of fluid surrounding an echogenic, solid-appearing mass. The lower contour of this thoracic mass is indicated by arrowheads. The mass filled the lower half of the left hemithorax. Below the diaphragm, ascites can be seen around the spleen.

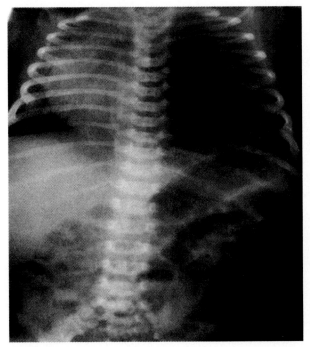

A

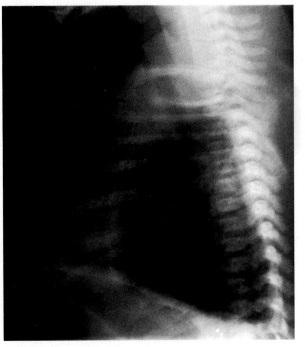

B

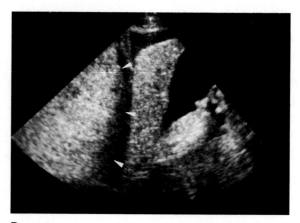

D

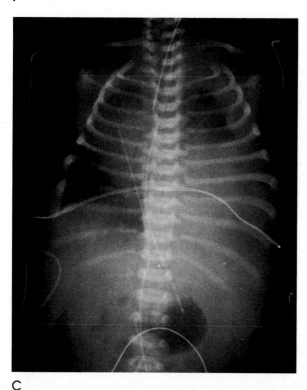

C

Diagnosis Congenital Cystic Adenomatoid Malformation (CCAM)

Discussion and Differential Diagnosis

Congenital cystic adenomatoid malformation of the lung is a hamartomatous multicystic mass of disorganized lung tissue with terminal bronchiole proliferation.[1] The involved lobe is enlarged, has normal pulmonary vascular supply and drainage, lacks cartilage at microscopic study, and communicates with the bronchial tree, although the bronchial connections may be altered. Aeration also occurs through the pores of Kohn.[1] The typical presentation is that of a near-term infant with marked respiratory distress. There may be fetal hydrops and maternal polyhydramnios. Patients presenting in the first 6 months of life usually exhibit respiratory distress.[2] Those older than 6 months at time of presentation usually have symptoms of infection.[2]

Three different types of CCAM have been described:

A. Approximately 50% of CCAM are of *macrocystic* variety (type I), containing variable-sized cysts with at least one large cyst (>2 cm in size).[2] This type offers the best prognosis. Other congenital anomalies are found in 5%.[2]

B. Roughly 40% of CCAM are *microcystic* (type II), the mass consisting of multiple, small (1 to 10 cm), evenly spaced, thin-walled cysts. Other congenital abnormalities are frequently found (55%)[2] and may involve the heart, kidneys,

period and present later with symptoms of infection.

- The cysts of CCAM may be fluid-filled at birth and the chest radiograph in that case shows a mass or opaque hemithorax.[5]

- Sonography of the opaque hemithorax allows delineation of pleural effusion, fluid-filled cysts, as well as differentiation between macrocystic and microcystic lesions.

- A classification based on prenatal ultrasound distinguishes just two types of CCAM: microcystic (cysts <5 mm in diameter) and macrocystic (cysts >5 mm in diameter).

- Adzick et al. suggest an association between poor neonatal outcome and the presence of fetal hydrops rather than a relationship to histologic type.[6]

- CT may be helpful, as it accurately depicts the internal architecture of the various types of CCAM.[7]

PITFALLS
- More than one lobe may be involved with CCAM, and features of both type I and type II CCAM may be present in the same patient.[7]

skeletal system, or gastrointestinal tract. Patients with type II CCAM have a poor prognosis.[2]

C. The remaining approximately 10% of CCAM *appear grossly solid* (type III) but contain a myriad of tiny cysts. Prognosis is poorer in patients with this lesion.[2]

There is no gender predilection, nor predilection for side of abnormality.[2] The lesion is slightly more common in the upper lobes[1] and bilateral involvement is rare. In utero diagnosis allows for early surgical intervention. The differential diagnosis includes congenital lobar emphysema, diaphragmatic hernia, and bronchopulmonary foregut malformation. Diaphragmatic hernia is diagnosed by its scaphoid abdomen and decreased bowel gas in the abdomen.

Further Reading

1. Kuhn JP, Slovis TL, Silverman FN, Kuhns LR. The neck and respiratory system. In: Silverman FN, ed. *Caffey's Pediatric X-ray Diagnosis.* 9th ed. Chicago: Yearbook Medical Publishers; 1993: 453–455.
2. Siegel BA, Proto AV, eds. *Pediatric Disease (Fourth Series) Test and Syllabus.* Reston, VA: American College of Radiology; 1993: 102–106.
3. Johnson JA, Rumack CM, Johnson ML, Shikes R, Appareti K, Rees G. Cystic adenomatoid malformation: antenatal demonstration. *Am J Roentgenol* 142:483–484, 1984.
4. Mashiach R, Hod M, Friedman S, Schoenfeld A, Ovadia J, Merlob P. Antenatal ultrasound diagnosis of congenital cystic adenomatoid malformation of the lung: spontaneous resolution in utero. *J Clin Ultrasound* 21:453–457, 1993.
5. Alford BA, McIlhenny J, Jones JE, et al. Asymmetric radiographic findings in the pediatric chest: approach to early diagnosis. *Radiographics* 13(1):77–93, 1993.
6. Adzick NS, Harrison MR, Glick PL, et al. Fetal cystic adenomatoid malformation: prenatal diagnosis and natural history. *J Pediatr Surg* 20(5):483–488, 1985.
7. Kim WS, Lee KS, Kim I-O, et al. Congenital cystic adenomatoid malformation of the lung: CT-pathologic correlation. *Am J Roentgenol* 168:47–53, 1997.

Case 4

Clinical Presentation

A newborn with respiratory distress.

Radiographic Studies

Chest radiograph (Fig. 4A) obtained a few hours after birth shows an enlarged centrally dense right lung with shift of mediastinum to the left. Chest radiograph obtained the next day (Fig. 4B) shows a hyperlucent, enlarged right middle lobe with compression atelectasis of the right upper lobe and right lower lobe.

Figure 4C is the chest radiograph of a different patient who presented with mild respiratory symptoms at 3 months of age. There is a hyperlucent left upper lobe with increased volume creating mediastinal shift to the right and a component of compression atelectasis in the left lower lobe, manifested by crowding of vessels. The presence of vascular structures in the hyperinflated left upper lobe is well demonstrated by CT (Fig. 4D).

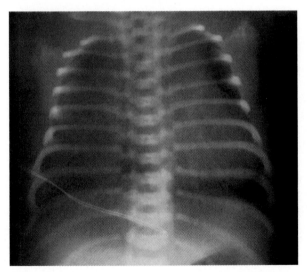

A

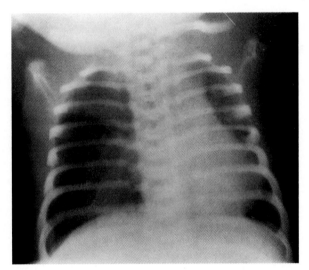

B

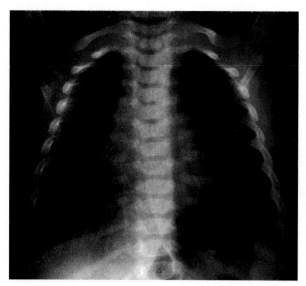

C

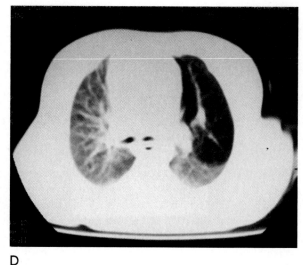

D

Diagnosis Congenital Lobar Emphysema (CLE)

Discussion and Differential Diagnosis

Overinflation, at birth, of one or more lobes in either lung is known as congenital lobar emphysema. The condition is seen more frequently in males than females, with a ratio of 3 to 1.[1] Involvement of left upper lobe is reported in 43% of cases, of right middle lobe in 32%, right upper lobe in 20%, and of two lobes in 5%.[1] Symptoms usually are present at birth or appear within the first few months of life and include cough, wheezing, tachypnea, cyanosis, and respiratory distress. Diminished breath sounds may be encountered over the affected lobe. Eighty percent of patients present within the first 6 months of life.[2] Congenital lobar emphysema is treated by surgical resection, and prognosis is excellent.

There is no single cause of CLE. Suggested causes include bronchial obstruction, bronchomalacia, postinflammatory alveolar damage, or developmental change in the alveoli.[3] A definite bronchial abnormality has been described in less than 50% of patients, including focal bronchial cartilage underdevelopment, intrinsic bronchial stenosis, intraluminal web, inspissated secretions or exudate, and extrinsic compression by a mass or vessel.[2] On histologic study, some of the hyperinflated lobes are found to be polyalveolar, containing an increased number of normal-sized alveoli, as opposed to having a normal number of enlarged alveoli as in other cases of CLE.

The hyperinflated lobe may be opaque on initial early films secondary to prolonged retention of fetal lung liquid. As this fluid is slowly cleared from the lobe, hyperaeration will become obvious. In one study, only polyalveolar lobes (PAL) demonstrated prolonged retention of fetal lung liquid on early films.[3] Patients with PAL also tended to be symptomatic earlier in life than those who had CLE without polyalveolar lobe.

PEARLS

- During the fluid-filled, opacified phase of CLE, ultrasound examination may help in differentiating this entity from congenital cystic adenomatoid malformation, bronchopulmonary foregut malformation, cystic hygroma, and solid masses.

- Association with congenital heart disease is seen in 15 to 30% of patients, most often patent ductus arteriosus or ventricular septal defect.[2]

PITFALLS

- A case of hyperinflation of the entire left lung has been reported by Wadsworth and

McAlister caused by an intraluminal mass at the takeoff of the left mainstem bronchus.[4] Abnormal aeration of an entire lung indicates a problem with the mainstem bronchus and is to be differentiated from the typical *lobar* distribution of abnormal aeration seen in CLE.[4]

- Lower lobe overinflation has been reported in a patient with acute respiratory syncytial virus infection.[5] It is also described as a postoperative phenomenon in patients following repair of diaphragmatic hernia.[6]

The hyperinflated lobe of CLE has visible, although attenuated vessels, out to its periphery and lacks septations. This allows differentiation from cystic adenomatoid malformation.

Further Reading

1. Hedlund GL, Kirks DR. Respiratory system. In: Kirks DR, ed. *Practical Pediatric Imaging. Diagnostic Radiology of Infants and Children,* 2nd ed. Boston: Little, Brown & Co; 1991: 579.
2. Siegel BA, Proto AV, eds. *Pediatric Disease (Fourth Series) Test and Syllabus.* Reston, VA: American College of Radiology; 1993: 98, 119.
3. Cleveland RH, Weber B. Retained fetal lung liquid in congenital lobar emphysema: a possible predictor of polyalveolar lobe. *Pediatr Radiol* 23:291–295, 1993.
4. Wadsworth DT, McAlister WH. Congenital intraluminal tracheal cyst causing an obstructed left lung in a newborn. *Pediatr Radiol* 25:478–479, 1995.
5. Newman B, Yunis E. Lobar emphysema associated with respiratory syncytial virus pneumonia. *Pediatr Radiol* 25:646–648, 1995.
6. Swischuk LE. *Imaging of the Newborn, Infant and Young Child,* 3rd ed. Baltimore: Williams & Wilkins; 1989: 100–106.

Case 5

Clinical Presentation

The patient had repeated infections. Presentation with hemoptysis and congestive heart failure has also been described.[1]

Radiographic Studies

Anterior radiograph of the chest shows a small, patchy area of air space consolidation in the right lower lobe near the medial cardiophrenic angle (Fig. 5A). Pulmonary artery branches to the right lower lobe are slightly laterally draped. A prior chest radiograph (Fig. 5B) shows a large triangular area of consolidation in the same location. CT scan (Fig. 5C) shows a well-demarcated right lower lobe cystic lesion (arrowheads) distorting normal lung architecture. Post-contrast CT image (Fig. 5D) reveals the takeoff of the systemic artery (arrow) to the right lower lobe from the upper abdominal aorta. (Case courtesy Marilyn Siegel, MD, Mallinckrodt Institute of Radiology.)

In a different patient, the systemic feeding artery and draining pulmonary vein to a left lower lobe mass are well demonstrated by spiral CT. Coronal reconstruction from post-contrast spiral CT (Fig. 5E) shows a large abdominal aortic feeding artery (arrow) supplying the large left-sided mass. Note midline shift of the thoracic aorta due to this mass lesion. Axial reconstruction image from the same exam (Fig. 5F) displays the venous drainage into the left atrium. (Case courtesy Steven Sargent, MD, Dartmouth-Hitchcock Medical Center.)

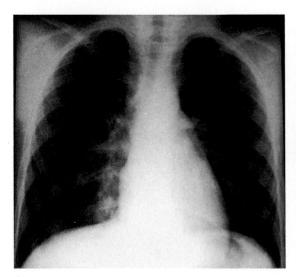

A

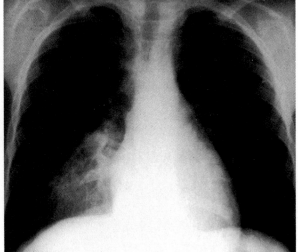

B

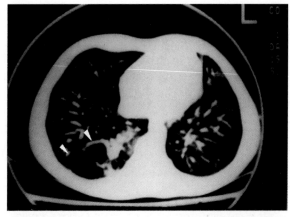

C

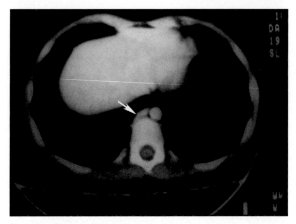

D

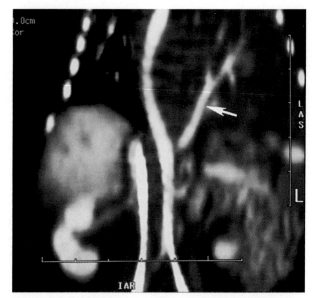

E

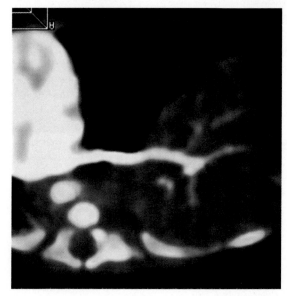

F

Diagnosis Pulmonary Sequestration

Discussion and Differential Diagnosis

Pulmonary sequestration is described as "a congenital mass of nonfunctioning pulmonary tissue that has no normal connection with the bronchial tree or the pulmonary arteries."[1] The arterial supply to the sequestered lung usually arises from the abdominal aorta. The venous drainage pattern is variable to either pulmonary or systemic veins, with intralobar sequestration usually draining to pulmonary veins and extralobar sequestration usually draining to systemic veins. Aeration may occur through collateral channels or abnormal connections to the tracheobronchial tree, or may be the result of chronic infection. Precisely how a sequestration develops is not completely understood but it falls, along with bronchogenic cysts, esophageal duplication cysts, neurenteric cysts, and esophageal bronchus, in the broader category of bronchopulmonary foregut malformations.[2]

Communication with either the supra- or infradiaphragmatic gastrointestinal tract may be present.[2,3] Contrast examination of the upper GI tract is indicated as part of the workup. Angiography best outlines the anomalous blood supply but is infrequently performed. MRI or spiral CT may identify the anomalous feeding vessel; in the infant, color Doppler ultrasound may be useful.

Two types of sequestration are described, intralobar and extralobar. There is considerable overlap between these two types, particularly in patterns of vascular supply and venous drainage, and the distinction may be somewhat artificial. The typical features of these sequestration types are described.

Intralobar sequestration (75 to 85% of all pulmonary sequestrations).[4]

- Two thirds are located on the left in the paravertebral gutter (one third on the right). Sequestrations may rarely occur in the upper lung or bilaterally.
- The sequestered lung is covered by the pleura of the adjacent normal lung.
- Other congenital anomalies are rare, as opposed to the frequent association with extralobar sequestrations.
- When the sequestered lung is homogeneously dense, it can mimic bronchogenic cyst, volume loss, pneumonia, or a pulmonary mass.
- When the sequestered lung is irregularly aerated, it may resemble a cystic mass such as congenital cystic adenomatoid malformation (CCAM).[1]

Extralobar sequestration (15 to 25% of all pulmonary sequestrations).

- Usually located in the left paravertebral gutter (at, in, or below diaphragm), and discovered as an incidental mass-like density in approximately 10%[4] of patients. More than half are diagnosed in symptomatic infants 0 to 6 months old who may present with cyanosis, respiratory distress, or difficulty with feeding.[5]
- The sequestered lung is separated from the adjacent normal lung and has its own separate pleural covering; superimposed infection is less common than in intralobar sequestration.
- More common in male patients, with a 4 to 1 male-to-female ratio.[4]
- Associated congenital anomalies are common—congenital cardiac abnormalities, bronchopulmonary foregut cysts, pulmonary vascular anomalies, and diaphragmatic hernia (30%).[1] Association with type 2 CCAM has also been reported.[6]

PEARLS

- CT and/or MRI allows accurate evaluation of any infradiaphragmatic extension of an extralobar sequestration.
- In the case of subdiaphragmatic location of extralobar pulmonary sequestration, the differential diagnosis includes neuroblastoma, teratoma, foregut cysts, and renal or adrenal masses or hemorrhage.[4,7]
- Association between nonimmune fetal hydrops and extralobar sequestration has been reported as has an association between extralobar sequestration and tension hydrothorax.[8]
- Torsion of the sequestration with consequent obstruction of draining veins and lymphatics is suggested as a cause of the hydrothoraces seen in association with some extralobar sequestrations.[9]

PITFALLS

- Areas of chronic pulmonary inflammation and bronchiectasis may have systemic arterial blood supply. This does not represent a classic sequestration, as the affected area has a normally branching bronchial tree,[1] and is known as a pseudosequestration.[5]

CONTROVERSY
• Some suggest that most intralobar sequestrations are acquired rather than congenital.[4]

• Differential diagnosis includes posterior mediastinal masses.

Further Reading

1. Kuhn JP, Slovis TL, Silverman FN, Kuhns LR. The neck and respiratory system. In: Silverman FN, ed. *Caffey's Pediatric X-ray Diagnosis.* 9th ed. Chicago: Yearbook Medical Publishers; 1993: 455–459.

2. Leithiser RE Jr, Capitanio MA, Macpherson RI, Wood BP. Communicating bronchopulmonary foregut malformations. *Am J Roentgenol* 146:227–231, 1986.

3. Jamieson DH, Fisher RM. Communicating bronchopulmonary foregut malformation associated with esophageal atresia and tracheoesophageal fistula. *Pediatr Radiol* 23:557–558, 1993.

4. Rosado-de-Christenson ML, Frazier AA, Stocker JT, Templeton PA. Extralobar sequestration: radiologic-pathologic correlation. *Radiographics* 13(2):425–441, 1993.

5. Felker RE, Tonkin ILD. Imaging of pulmonary sequestration. *Am J Roentgenol* 154:241–249, 1990.

6. Benya EC, Bulas DI, Selby DM, Rosenbaum KN. Cystic sonographic appearance of extralobar pulmonary sequestration. *Pediatr Radiol* 26:605–607, 1993.

7. Matzinger MAE, Matzinger FR, Matzinger KE, Black MD. Antenatal and postnatal findings in intraabdominal pulmonary sequestration. *Can Assoc Radiol J* 43(3):212–214, 1992.

8. Romero R, Chervenak FA, Kotzen J, Berkowitz RL, Hobbins JC. Antenatal sonographic findings of extralobar pulmonary sequestration. *J Ultrasound Med* 1:131–132, 1982.

9. Hernanz-Schulman M, Stein SM, Neblett WW, et al. Pulmonary sequestration: diagnosis with color Doppler sonography and a new theory of associated hydrothorax. *Radiology* 180:817–821, 1991.

Case 6

Clinical Presentation

Asymptomatic teenage patient assessed for scoliosis (Figs. 6A, 6B, 6C).

A 2-month-old infant presented with stridor, wheezing, and chronic cough (Figs. 6D, 6E, 6F). Hemoptysis may be the presenting complaint, as well as symptoms of pneumonia.

Radiographic Studies

Chest radiographs of the asymptomatic teenager (Figs. 6A, 6B) show a round, smoothly contoured middle mediastinal mass arising from the right retrocardiac mediastinum. The patient has a right convex thoracic scoliosis; the chest radiographs are otherwise unremarkable. Postcontrast CT image (Fig. 6C) shows a well-defined homogeneous oval mass. Attenuation values were higher than water, consistent with mucoid content. There were no calcifications.

The symptomatic infant has a mass between the trachea and esophagus (Fig. 6D) displacing the trachea anteriorly and the barium-filled esophagus posteriorly. Post-gadolinium sagittal T1-weighted MR image (Fig. 6E) shows a nonenhancing oval cystic lesion causing anterior displacement of the trachea. Axial T2-weighted MR image (Fig. 6F) shows high signal intensity fluid in this mediastinal mass.

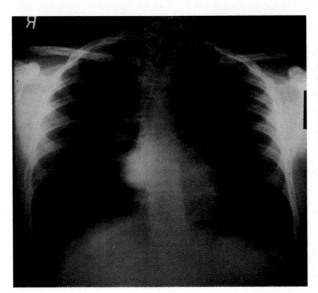

A

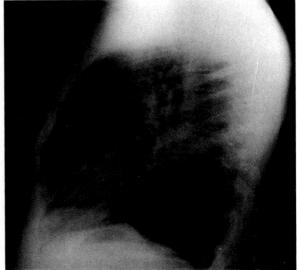

B

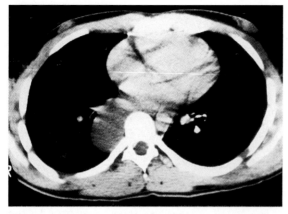

C

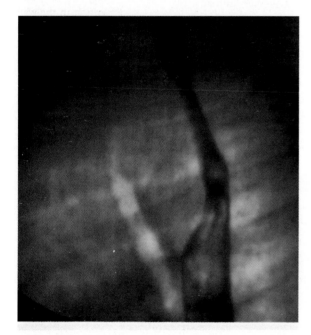

D

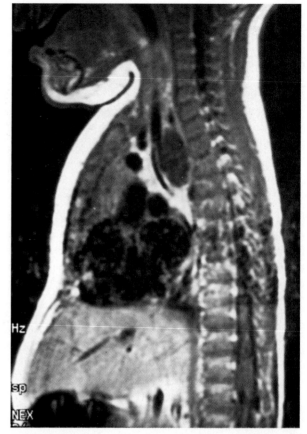

E

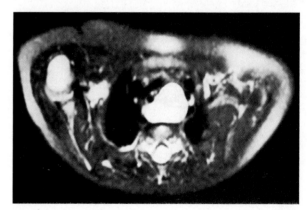

F

Diagnosis Bronchogenic Cyst

Discussion and Differential Diagnosis

Bronchogenic cysts may present in the mediastinum or in the lung parenchyma. Mediastinal cysts typically are located near the carina, behind the trachea, or along the mainstem bronchi. They usually do not communicate with the airway and consequently appear as solid masses. The intrapulmonary bronchogenic cyst typically *does* communicate with the airway and will appear as a solitary round or oval thin-walled, air-containing cyst.[1] An air-fluid level signifies infection. Air trapping may be present if one of the major bronchi is compressed by a centrally located bronchogenic cyst.[1]

Attenuation values on CT are variable, approaching those of water if the cyst content is serous and those of soft tissue if the cyst content is more mucoid. The avascular nature of these cysts is well demonstrated by CT. Calcification in the wall is rare.[1]

Bronchogenic cysts are thought to develop as the result of an abnormality in the lung budding process that follows the initial separation of the primitive foregut into esophagus and trachea, and they fall in the spectrum of bronchopulmonary foregut malformations. A ventral lung bud arises from the primitive trachea and undergoes a process of repetitive branching to form the tracheobronchial tree. An abnormality in the early phases of this budding process is thought to lead to mediastinal location of bronchogenic cyst, whereas a later event leads to intrapulmonary location of the cyst.[1]

The differential diagnosis for an air-filled cyst (or a cyst with an air fluid level) includes congenital cystic adenomatoid malformation, lung abscess, pneumatocele, and cavitating lesions such as laryngeal papilloma. For a fluid-containing cyst, the differential diagnosis includes lung neoplasm (primary or metastatic) and round pneumonia.[2] Matzinger et al.[3] reported a teenager with an intrapulmonary subpleural bronchogenic cyst, who presented with a tension pneumothorax related to cyst rupture following blunt chest trauma.

PEARLS

PITFALLS

- Adults with bronchogenic cysts tend to be more frequently symptomatic—67% with mediastinal cysts and 90% with lung cysts, as reported by St.-Georges et al.[5] Complicated cysts were present in over one third of patients, and the following complications were encountered: fistulization, cyst wall ulceration, hemorrhage, infection, and secondary bronchial atresia.

CONTROVERSY

- No clear-cut predilection for intrapulmonary or mediastinal location has been demonstrated, with one series reporting 14% intrapulmonary location and another reporting 70% of bronchogenic cysts in pulmonary location.[1]

Further Reading

1. Siegel BA, Proto AV, eds. *Pediatric Disease (Fourth Series) Test and Syllabus.* Reston, VA: American College of Radiology; 1993: 98, 100, 108.
2. Kuhn JP, Slovis TL, Silverman FN, Kuhns LR. The neck and respiratory system. In: Silverman FN, ed. *Caffey's Pediatric X-ray Diagnosis.* 9th ed. Chicago: Yearbook Medical Publishers; 1993: 452–453.
3. Matzinger MA, Matzinger FR, Sachs HJ. Intrapulmonary bronchogenic cyst: spontaneous pneumothorax as the presenting symptom. *Am J Roentgenol* 158: 987–988, 1992.

4. Swischuk LE. *Imaging of the Newborn, Infant and Young Child,* 3rd ed. Baltimore: Williams & Wilkins; 1989: 129.

5. St-Georges R, Deslauriers J, Duranceau A, et al. Clinical spectrum of bronchogenic cysts of the mediastinum and lung in the adult. *Ann Thorac Surg* 52:6–13, 1991. Abstract.

Case 7

Clinical Presentation

This patient was found to have an incidental "murmur" over her left lateral chest. She had no clubbing, but hypoxemia was present by pulse oximetry.

Radiographic Studies

A well-defined nodule is present peripherally in the left lower lung (Fig. 7A). A tubular structure extends from the nodule medially toward the left pulmonary hilum. CT scan (Fig. 7B) shows a prominent vessel coursing to the pleural-based nodule. The left pulmonary artery angiogram (Fig. 7C) and segmental lower lobe pulmonary artery contrast injection (Fig. 7D) demonstrate a single artery supplying the tortuous, ectatic nidus. A single markedly enlarged early draining vein is seen.

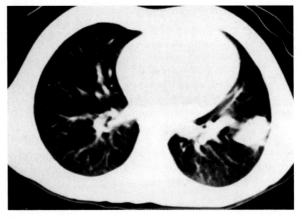

B

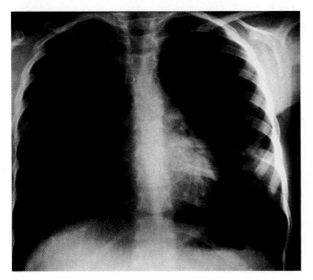

A

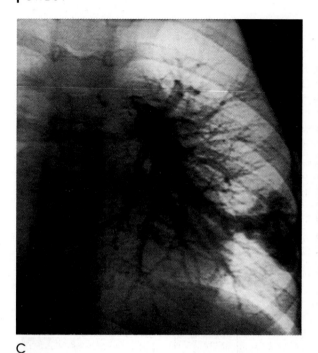

C

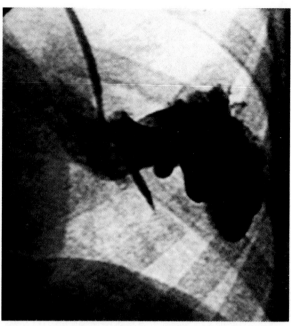

D

Diagnosis   Pulmonary Arteriovenous Malformation (PAVM)

Discussion and Differential Diagnosis

PEARLS

● PAVMs are more frequent in the lower lungs, in a subpleural location.[4]

● Risk of paradoxical embolization is higher with PAVMs located in the lower lung because of the preferentially increased flow of blood to these portions of the lung when the patient is upright.[1]

● The vascular nature of the nodular densities of the AVM as seen on plain films is usually demonstrable by CT. MRI has been shown to be helpful in distinguishing a solid lung nodule from an AVM.[5]

A PAVM is an abnormal connection between a pulmonary artery and a pulmonary vein. The abnormal connection between the artery and vein is at the capillary level. These abnormal vessels dilate over time, eventually creating the typical dilated, tortuous vascular channels. The feeding artery is a pulmonary arterial branch in most cases, but it may be a systemic artery branch. PAVMs can be seen as sporadic abnormalities, but nearly half of patients with PAVMs have Rendu-Osler-Weber syndrome, also known as hereditary hemorrhagic telangiectasis.[1] PAVMs also can be acquired, resulting from infections, trauma, or malignancy, or associated with cirrhosis of the liver.

Patients with PAVM may be asymptomatic. When the lesion creates symptoms and physical findings, these relate to right-to-left shunting through the AVM (hypoxemia, clubbing of fingers and toes, dyspnea, polycythemia). Less frequently, paradoxical embolization (transient ischemic attack, stroke, brain abscess) or hemorrhagic complications (hemoptysis, hemothorax) occur. Hewes et al.[1] reported four adult patients (ages 21 to 35 years) with hereditary hemorrhagic telangiectasis and PAVM in whom a cerebrovascular accident was the first symptom of the underlying condition. White et al.[2] found a risk of paradoxical CNS embolization in 10% of patients with multiple PAVMs and recommend balloon embolotheraphy of any PAVM that "lower[s] the arterial blood gas" or is large enough to be visible on a chest film.[2]

- In order to exclude multiple lesions, the pulmonary angiogram in a patient with a pulmonary AVM should include both lungs in their entirety.

- Uncovering the familial presence of epistaxis, GI bleeding, and/or CNS catastrophes in the course of obtaining a detailed history in patients with pulmonary AVM may be the clue to the diagnosis of Rendu-Osler-Weber syndrome.

Pulmonary angiography is the examination of choice for detailed evaluation of PAVM.[3] The most common PAVM has a single feeding branch off the pulmonary artery, a single draining vein with an intervening bulbous, nonseptated connecting channel. This so-called simple type of AVM was found in 79% of all PAVMs. Twenty-one percent were of the complex type, with two or more feeding arteries and at least two draining veins connected by a tortuous dilated and septated vascular channel. Both types can be present in the same patient.

Plain film differential considerations are those of pulmonary nodules (coin lesions): granuloma, plasma cell granuloma, mucoid impaction of bronchus, hematoma, sequestration, bronchopulmonary foregut malformation, round pneumonia/round atelectasis, chest wall masses, abdominal organ ectopy.

Further Reading

1. Hewes RC, Auster M, White RI Jr. Cerebral embolism—first manifestation of pulmonary arteriovenous malformation in patients with hereditary hemorrhagic telangiectasia. *Cardiovasc Intervent Radiol* 8:151–155, 1985.
2. White RI Jr, Mitchell SE, Kan J. Interventional procedures in congenital heart disease. *Cardiovasc Intervent Radiol* 9:286–298, 1996.
3. White RI Jr, Mitchell SE, Barth KH, et al. Angioarchitecture of pulmonary arteriovenous malformations: an important consideration before embolotherapy. *Am J Roentgenol* 140:681–868, 1983.
4. Barth KH, White RI Jr, Kaufman SL, Terry PB, Roland J-M. Embolotherapy of pulmonary arteriovenous malformations with detachable balloons. *Radiology* 142:599–606, 1982.
5. Dinsmore BJ, Gefter WB, Hatabu H, Kressel HY. Pulmonary arteriovenous malformations: diagnosis by gradient-refocused MR imaging. *J Comput Assist Tomogr* 14(6):918–923, 1990.

Case 8

Clinical Presentation

A 6-week-old patient presented with cough and a history of conjunctivitis.

Radiographic Studies

Anterior (Fig. 8A) and lateral (Fig. 8B) radiographs reveal symmetrically overexpanded lungs with diffuse linear peribronchial interstitial infiltrates. Scattered alveolar densities reflect focal patchy atelectasis or infiltrates.

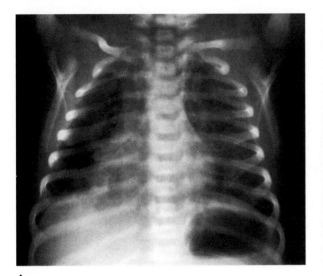

A

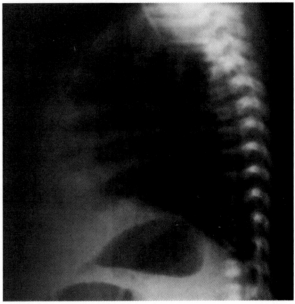

B

Diagnosis Chlamydia Pneumonia

Discussion and Differential Diagnosis

Neonatal chlamydia pneumonia is a birth-acquired infection with *Chlamydia trachomatis,* an obligate intracellular organism that has both viral and bacterial features. The typical patient is between 2 weeks and 3 months of age, has eosinophilia, elevated immunoglobulins, conjunctivitis, otitis media, tachypnea, a staccato cough, no or (at most) low grade fever, and moderate respiratory symptoms.[1-3] *Chlamydia trachomatis* causes cervicitis in women. It is estimated that conjunctivitis and eosinophilia develop in 50% of infected infants[1,3] and pneumonia in approximately 10%. Conjunctivitis is present in up to half of the infants with pneumonia.[3]

The typical radiographic findings consist of symmetric pulmonary overinflation, parahilar, peribronchial linear, or reticulonodular infiltrates, and patches of focal air space densities. Differential considerations include viral pneumonia (respiratory syncytial virus, adenovirus, cytomegalovirus), bronchopulmonary dysplasia, repeated aspiration, cystic fibrosis, and immune deficiency, but the clinical course, physical findings, and immunoglobulin increase allow an accurate diagnosis in the majority of cases.[1]

Further Reading

1. Radkowski MA, Kranzler JK, Beem MO, Tipple MA. Chlamydia pneumonia in infants: radiography in 125 cases. *Am J Roentgenol* 137:703–706, 1981.
2. Swischuk LE. *Imaging of the Newborn, Infant and Young Child,* 3rd ed. Baltimore: Williams & Wilkins; 1989: 167–170.
3. Siegel BA, Proto AV, eds. *Pediatric Disease (Fourth Series) Test and Syllabus.* Reston, VA: American College of Radiology; 1993: 277, 298–299.

Case 9

Clinical Presentation

This 6-month-old boy presented with a history of recent cold symptoms, increasing cough, abdominal pain, and a fever (temperature, 104°F). His white blood cell count was elevated with an increased polymorphonuclear count.

Radiographic Studies

Anterior (Fig. 9A) and lateral (Fig. 9B) radiographs of the chest reveal a round soft tissue density in the left lower lobe.

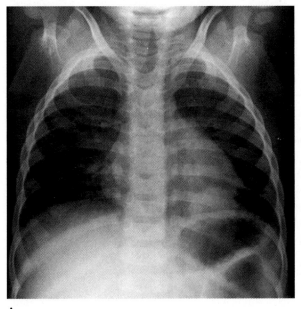

A

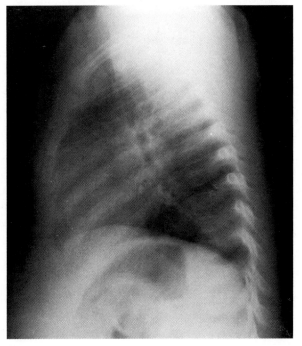

B

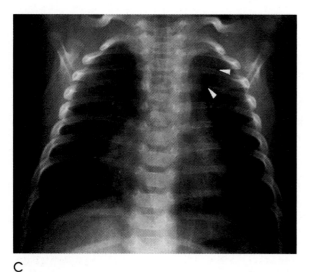

C

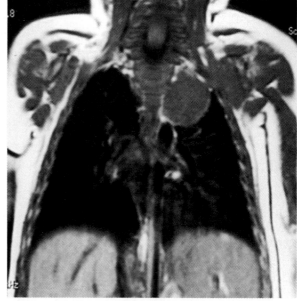

D

Diagnosis Round Pneumonia

Discussion and Differential Diagnosis

Round pneumonia is a not uncommon manifestation of bacterial pulmonary infection in young children. The pneumonia manifests itself as a round, sharply margin-ated, soft tissue density mimicking a pulmonary mass. This so-called round pneumonia falls under the broad category of pulmonary pseudotumor. Usually, round pneumonia is pleural based, and it predominates in the lower lobes.[1] The round pneumonia responds rapidly to antibiotics and becomes ill-defined during early resolution. According to Hedlund and Kirks,[1] air bronchograms are visible "in approximately 20% of round pneumonias."

Most bacterial pneumonia in children is caused by *Streptococcus pneumoniae,* group A *Streptococcus,* or *Staphylococcus. Hemophilus influenzae, Klebsiella,* and *Pseudomonas* are less common causes for pneumonia in children.[1] Most cases of round pneumonia are caused by pneumococcal infections.

The history and physical findings usually allow an accurate diagnosis of round pneumonia in a young child with a pulmonary mass. Differential considerations include round atelectasis, plasma cell granuloma (post-inflammatory pseudotumor), bronchogenic cyst, sequestration, pulmonary blastoma or hamartoma, metastasis, pulmonary arteriovenous malformation, hematoma, intrathoracic kidney, and chest wall masses. When the round density abuts the mediastinum, the differential diagno-sis additionally includes a possible posterior mediastinal mass, as was the case in the 3-month-old infant whose chest radiograph is shown in Figure 9C. There is a rounded medial left upper chest opacity without obvious air bronchograms (arrowheads). A posterior mediastinal mass was confirmed on MR imaging (Fig. 9D, coronal T1-

weighted image), which shows a solid mass without air bronchograms (neuroblastoma at pathology).

If the pneumonia does not clear in the usual time frame (2 to 4 weeks), the possibility of an underlying process should be kept in mind.[1] For example, sequestration, bronchopulmonary foregut cyst, endobronchial foreign body or granuloma, adenopathy causing bronchial compression, or nonbacterial cause of infection such as tuberculosis or fungal infection must be considered.[1] Fungal infection is also considered if an older (>8 years old) patient presents with a round pneumonia.

Further Reading

1. Hedlund GL, Kirks DR. Respiratory system. In: Kirks DR, ed. *Practical Pediatric Imaging. Diagnostic Radiology of Infants and Children,* 2nd ed. Boston: Little Brown & Co; 1991: 543, 629.
2. Kuhn JP, Slovis TL, Silverman FN, Kuhns LR. The neck and respiratory system. In: Silverman FN, ed. *Caffey's Pediatric X-ray Diagnosis.* 9th ed. Chicago: Yearbook Medical Publishers; 1993: 526.

Case 10

Clinical Presentation

A term newborn infant presents with moderate respiratory distress.

Radiographic Studies

The left hemithorax is opaque and smaller than the right. The right lung is hyperaerated, herniates across midline, and has increased vascularity. The cardiac silhouette is deviated to the left, and left-sided ribs one through three are anomalous (Fig. 10).

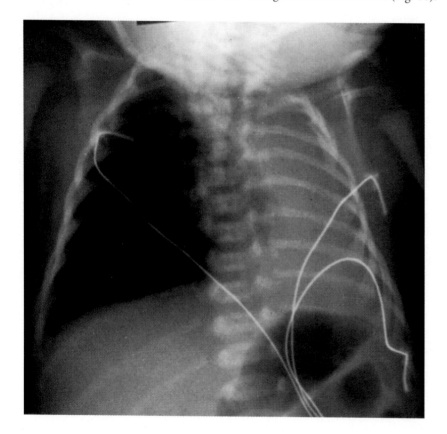

Diagnosis Pulmonary Agenesis

Discussion and Differential Diagnosis

Absence of lung parenchymal tissue is a feature of both pulmonary agenesis and pulmonary aplasia. Differentiation depends on development of the bronchus. In aplasia, there is a blind-ending bronchus, whereas in agenesis, the bronchus is absent starting at the carina. Also absent in pulmonary agenesis are the pulmonary artery and vein.[1] Absence of a bronchus can be verified with bronchoscopy or with cross-sectional imaging. MRI or contrast enhanced CT is helpful in assessing the pulmonary artery for presence and size. There is no predilection for right- or left-sided absence, and the incidence is the same in both sexes. With right-sided agenesis, however, the rightward displacement of the arch, descending aorta, left pulmonary artery, and the heart along with cardiac rotation may lead to entrapment of the left mainstem bronchus, which in turn causes severe hyperinflation of the left lung.[2] Similar clinical and radiographic findings are described with the right pneumonectomy syndrome.[3]

Patients with right-sided pulmonary agenesis tend to be more symptomatic, and they have a worse clinical outcome than those with left-sided pulmonary agenesis.[2]

Anomalies of the skeleton (ipsilateral hemivertebra or skeletal anomalies), genitourinary and gastrointestinal tracts (tracheoesophageal fistula),[4] as well as the cardiovascular system (tetralogy of Fallot, patent ductus arteriosus) are seen in approximately half the patients.[1] Agenesis of one or more lobes of lung can occur. According to Hedlund and Kirks, this always occurs on the right (as do lobar hypoplasia and aplasia).[5] Bilateral pulmonary agenesis is a very rare fatal anomaly in which the respiratory tract terminates in a blind-ending trachea. Other severe anomalies are usually present.

Further Reading

1. Kuhn JP, Slovis TL, Silverman FN, Kuhns LR. Normal lung and anomalies. In: Silverman FN, ed. *Caffey's Pediatric X-ray Diagnosis.* 9th ed. Chicago: Yearbook Medical Publishers; 1993: 448–450.
2. Newman B, Gondor M. MR evaluation of right pulmonary agenesis and vascular airway compression in pediatric patients. *Am J Roentgenol* 168:55–58, 1997.
3. Shepard JO, Grillo HC, McLoud TC, Dedrick CG, Spizarny DL. Right-pneumonectomy syndrome: radiologic findings and CT correlation. *Radiology* 161:661–664, 1986.
4. Kitagawa H, Nakada K, Fujioka T, et al. Unilateral pulmonary agenesis with tracheoesophageal fistula: a case report. *J Pediatr Surg* 30(10):1523–1525, 1995.
5. Hedlund GL, Kirks DR. Respiratory system. In: Kirks DR, ed. *Practical Pediatric Imaging. Diagnostic Radiology of Infants and Children,* 2nd ed. Boston: Little Brown & Co; 1991; 6:608–612.
6. Swischuk LE. *Imaging of the Newborn, Infant and Young Child,* 3rd ed. Baltimore: Williams & Wilkins; 1989: 1:79–89.

Case 11

Clinical Presentation

This 6-year-old patient had a cold approximately 1 week prior to admission. After 3 to 4 days, her cough worsened and she developed spiking fevers (temperatures to 104°F). On admission, she was tachypneic with nasal flaring. The left hemithorax was dull to percussion, heart sounds were displaced to the right, and breath sounds were absent on the left.

Radiographic Studies

The anterior chest radiograph (Fig. 11A) shows an opacified left hemithorax, rightward displacement of the mediastinum, and widening of the left intercostal spaces. Except for the proximal left mainstem bronchus, there are no air bronchograms on the left. Ultrasound of the left chest in this patient shows extensive echogenic pleural fluid (Fig. 11B). The echogenic fluid surrounds the collapsed left lung. An air bronchogram is visible in the atelectatic lung (arrow).

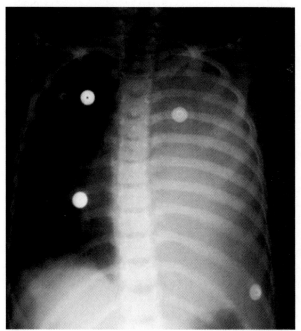

A

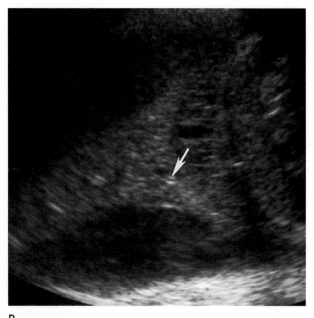

B

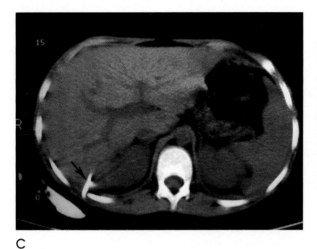

C

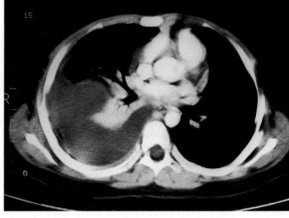

D

Diagnosis Empyema

Discussion and Differential Diagnosis

The presence of fluid in the pleural space is most often obvious on conventional anterior and lateral chest radiographs. Additional decubitus films help determine whether the pleural fluid flows freely or is loculated. If the pleural fluid is mobile, decubitus films also allow evaluation of the ipsilateral lower lung, which is often obscured by the fluid on the upright radiographs.

Pleural space infection is usually related to underlying pneumonia. It may also be the result of chest trauma, septic embolization to the lungs, or extension of infectious processes in the retropharyngeal space, subphrenic area, liver, pancreas, or bony thoracic cage.[1,2] Empyema can also develop following percutaneous drainage of upper abdominal abscesses if the pleural space is contaminated during the procedure. In children, pleural fluid related to underlying pneumonia (parapneumonic effusion) usually occurs with bacterial infections. The most commonly encountered organisms are *Streptococcus pneumoniae* and *Staphylococcus aureus.* Also to be considered are infections with *Haemophilus influenzae, Klebsiella,* tuberculosis, and anaerobic organisms.[1,3]

Parapneumonic effusions are said to undergo three stages of evolution: exudative, fibrinopurulent, and organized.[1,2] Some exudative effusions resolve with antibiotic treatment. Those with low pH (<7.20), elevated lactic dehydrogenase, or low glucose are likely to progress through the next two stages if not treated. Definitive treatment for these so-called complicated parapneumonic effusions includes some type of drainage. Empyema is a form of complicated parapneumonic effusion characterized by pus or by positive culture or positive Gram stain in the pleural fluid.[2]

Both ultrasonography and CT are helpful in further assessment of pleural fluid accumulations. Initial use of ultrasonography is preferred in the workup of children with pleural fluid accumulation as it does not involve the use of ionizing radiation. Exudative effusions tend to be sonolucent. The fibrinopurulent and organized stages of parapneumonic effusions correlate with echogenic fluid (Fig. 11B) and the presence of septations. Loculation of fluid usually is seen with a purulent exudate.[1]

PITFALLS

- Atelectasis in the upper lobe may mimic an apical pleural fluid collection on plain film.[6]

CT accurately detects fluids in the pleural space. It also usually allows one to distinguish parenchymal from pleural abnormalities, something which can be impossible on plain films. Multiple fluid loculations and abnormalities in the chest wall are also well demonstrated on CT, as are other complications of pneumonia such as pneumatoceles, abscess cavities, and bronchopleural fistula. In addition, CT accurately images the occasional large mass with or without associated pleural effusion, which may mimic a large complex pleural fluid collection. The CT images seen in Figures 11C and 11D are those of a patient referred to our institution with a right empyema after percutaneous liver abscess drainage. The percutaneous liver drainage catheter (arrow, Fig. 11C) crosses the right posterior pleural gutter. The more cephalad right pleural fluid collection (Fig. 11D) surrounds an atelectatic right lower lobe. Note convex anterior and medial margins of the pleural collection characteristic of empyemas.

If an empyema or complicated parapneumonic effusion is suspected based on the clinical picture, the plain films, ultrasonography, or CT, a diagnostic thoracentesis is indicated. Sonography may help in directing the thoracentesis. Along with antibiotics, treatment of an empyema includes drainage. There are multiple options, including thoracentesis, radiologic catheter placement, and various surgical approaches[2,3] among which is thoracoscopic decortication. Some surgeons find that patients who undergo this procedure recover more rapidly. In addition, intrapleural fibrinolytic therapy has been helpful in managing loculated empyema via percutaneous approach.[2,4]

Further Reading

1. Kuhn JP, Slovis TL, Silverman FN, Kuhns LR. The neck and respiratory system. In: Silverman FN, ed. *Caffey's Pediatric X-ray Diagnosis.* 9th ed. Chicago: Yearbook Medical Publishers; 1993: 422–441.
2. Klein JS, Schultz S, Heffner JE. Interventional radiology of the chest: image-guided percutaneous drainage of pleural effusions, lung abscess, and pneumothorax. *Am J Roentgenol* 164:581–588, 1995.
3. Hedlund GL, Kirks DR. Respiratory system. In: Kirks DR, ed. *Practical Pediatric Imaging. Diagnostic Radiology of Infants and Children,* 2nd ed. Boston: Little Brown & Co; 1991; 6:552, 632–633, 629.
4. Ryan JM, Boland GW, Lee MJ, Mueller PR. Intracavitary urokinase therapy as an adjunct to percutaneous drainage in a patient with a multiloculated empyema. *Am J Roentgenol* 167:643–647, 1996.
5. Seibert JJ, Glasier CM, Leithiser RL, Jr. The pediatric chest. In: Rumack CM, Wilson SR, Charboneau JW, eds. *Diagnostic Ultrasound.* St. Louis: Mosby; 1991[1]: 1099–1123.
6. Tamaki Y, Pandit R, Gooding CA. Neonatal atypical peripheral atelectasis. *Pediatr Radiol* 24:589–591, 1994.

Case 12

Clinical Presentation

Prenatal ultrasound had established an abnormality in this near-term infant with severe respiratory distress. Her chest was asymmetrical, with the right side more prominent than the left; the abdomen was scaphoid; heart sounds were heard laterally on the left; and breath sounds were absent on the right.

Radiographic Studies

Figures 12A and 12B are the anterior and lateral radiographs of our index patient. The abdomen is scaphoid, there is a paucity of intraabdominal bowel gas, air-filled structures are present over the right upper quadrant, and the normal liver shadow is missing. The right hemithorax is large and filled with multiple cystic lucencies. The mediastinum is deviated toward the left and the left lung is partially atelectatic. The gastric tube courses along a left deviated and air-distended esophagus. The stomach is slightly medial in position.

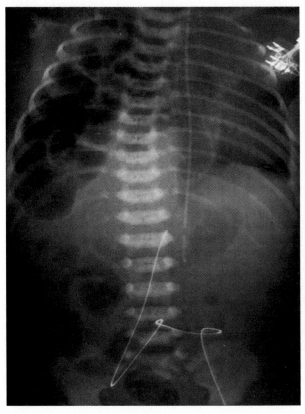

A

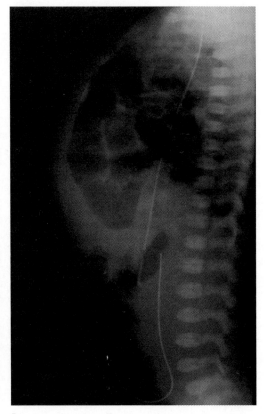

B

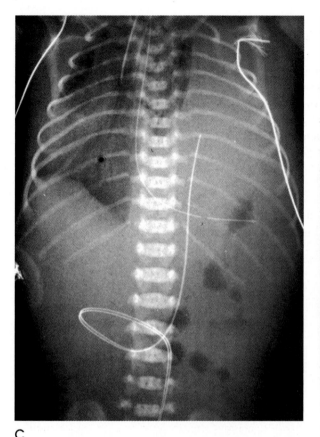

C

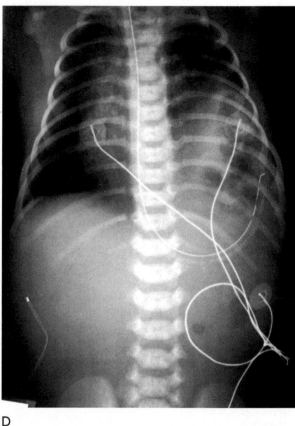

D

PEARLS

• Injection of a small amount of air through the gastric tube will outline the position of the GI tract. This can be helpful in the case of a hernia containing non–air-filled bowel loops (as in the patient shown in Figure 12C).

• Midline hernias occur but are rare. These develop through a centrally located diaphragmatic defect. Herniated GI tract can be encountered in the

Diagnosis Congenital Diaphragmatic Hernia

Discussion and Differential Diagnosis

In congenital diaphragmatic hernia, abdominal contents invaginate into the chest cavity through anterior or posterior developmental defects in the diaphragm. Herniation through the posterolateral foramen of Bochdalek is more common than herniation through the anterior and medial foramen of Morgagni. Herniation through a central defect is rare. Bochdalek hernia occurs in 1 in 2,000 to 12,500 live births[1] and has a left-over-right predominance as high as 9:1.[1] Bilateral diaphragmatic hernias occur infrequently.[2] Associated anomalies may be present in the ipsilateral upper extremity.[3] Abdominal renal ectopy[1] may be seen and congenital heart defects are frequently present.[4]

Development of the fetal lung is adversely affected by the intrathoracic herniated abdominal contents, resulting in pulmonary hypoplasia. The larger the mass effect exerted by the hernia and the earlier it occurs, the more severe the pulmonary hypoplasia and the respiratory distress. These patients also have the worst prognosis. Both the ipsilateral lung and the contralateral lung may be hypoplastic. The status

retrosternal space or inside the pericardial sac.

• The herniated intrathoracic stomach is prone to volvulus and may perforate.

• Delayed development of diaphragmatic hernia has been observed in neonates with group B streptococcal infection. The delayed herniation usually occurs on the right. This possibility should be considered when right lower lung density develops and the liver shadow migrates cephalad after initial normal appearance. Pleural effusion may also be present.[6]

• Torsion and infarction of the spleen may be a complication in Bochdalek hernia. Splenic infarction has also been reported in one patient after repair of a Bochdalek hernia that was diagnosed and repaired when the patient was 7 years old.[7]

• Despite the lack of normal mesenteric fixation in patients with repaired congenital diaphragmatic hernias, the risk for midgut volvulus is reported to be low.[8]

PITFALLS

• Appearance of a mass above the repaired diaphragm may signal recurrence of the diaphragmatic hernia. This

of the contralateral lung determines the clinical presentation and outcome, which are also greatly affected by the occurrence of persistent fetal circulation. While an accurate diagnosis of diaphragmatic hernia can be made by prenatal ultrasound, the degree of associated pulmonary hypoplasia is more difficult to predict. The size of the contralateral lung can be measured sonographically by utilizing a four-chamber view as demonstrated by Guibaud et al.[4] On postnatal radiographs, the herniated bowel loops create a solid-appearing space-occupying mass until such time as swallowed air starts outlining the lumen of the GI tract. Figure 12C is an anterior radiograph of a patient with a left Bochdalek hernia that occupies virtually the entire left hemithorax. Because the radiograph was obtained shortly after birth and the infant had not yet swallowed much air, the herniated loops are still airless, simulating a solid mass. The high stomach (inferred by the position of the gastric tube) and the leftward as well as upward displacement of the umbilical vein catheter indicate that the stomach and liver are displaced into the left chest. An additional example of upward displacement of the gastric tube is shown in Figure 12D. This is a different patient with a left Bochdalek hernia containing stomach, multiple air-filled bowel loops, and left lobe of liver. At surgery, the spleen was also located in the chest.

The classic plain film findings are:

• Chest cavity (usually the left) filled with multiple cystic lucencies
• Contralateral mediastinal shift
• Scaphoid abdomen with paucity of intraabdominal GI tract air.

Differential considerations for a cystic-appearing hemithorax include congenital cystic adenomatoid malformation, bronchogenic cyst, lobar emphysema, and postinfectious pneumatoceles.[5] In these conditions, the aerated GI tract is in the normal abdominal location. Pneumonia with pneumatoceles is not likely to present at birth but is in the differential diagnosis for the patient with a late presentation of diaphragmatic hernia.

For the solid-appearing hemithorax seen with lack of air in the herniated GI tract, the following differential applies:

• Herniation of solid organ only (such as liver)
• Chylothorax
• Empyema
• Fluid-filled anomalous lung such as congenital cystic adenomatoid malformation, congenital lobar emphysema, or pulmonary sequestration
• Other chest masses[3]

Ultrasound examination is very helpful in assessment of the opaque, increased-volume hemithorax as it allows one to assess for accumulated pleural fluid, possible underlying mass, or herniated abdominal organs. Pleural fluid occurs more frequently with a right-sided hernia.[3] Patients with large congenital diaphragmatic hernias present with acute, severe respiratory distress at the time of birth. Those with small or late-developing hernias have milder symptoms, which may include vomiting and pain in addition to respiratory symptoms. Morgagni hernias usually do not create respiratory distress but may, on occasion, have an acute presentation with cyanosis and severe respiratory symptoms.[3]

mass may contain fluid or air. Similar radiographic findings are created by the presence of a residual hernia sac.

- Herniation of abdominal contents through an anterior and central diaphragmatic defect may create a picture of pronounced cardiomegaly either by elevation of the heart or by extension of the hernia into the pericardial sac. Central hernias can be demonstrated by both prenatal and postnatal ultrasonography.[3,9]

- Differentiation between Morgagni hernia and diaphragmatic eventration can be difficult. Ultrasonography is helpful in distinguishing these entities.[5]

- Because of the lung hypoplasia, normally a pneumothorax is present in the postoperative period. The hypoplastic lung should slowly reexpand.

CONTROVERSY

- Conventional wisdom[3] has it that the prognosis is worse with right-sided congenital diaphragmatic hernia than with left. The recent study by Guibaud et al.[4] did not confirm this association. Similarly, in this same series of 43 patients, the presence of hydramnios and early in utero diagnosis did not have a statistically significant association with poor postnatal outcome.

Further Reading

1. Kuhn JP, Slovis TL, Silverman FN, Kuhns LR. The neck and respiratory system. In: Silverman FN, ed. *Caffey's Pediatric X-ray Diagnosis.* 9th ed. Chicago: Yearbook Medical Publishers; 1993: 415–420, 2002–2006.
2. Siegel BA, Proto AV, eds. *Pediatric Disease (Fourth Series) Test and Syllabus.* Reston, VA: American College of Radiology; 1993: 123–125, 127.
3. Swischuk LE. *Imaging of the Newborn, Infant and Young Child,* 3rd ed. Baltimore: Williams & Wilkins; 1989; 1: 100–106.
4. Guibaud L, Filiatrault D, Garel L, et al. Fetal congenital diaphragmatic hernia: accuracy of sonography in the diagnosis and prediction of the outcome after birth. *Am J Roentgenol* 166:1195–1202, 1996.
5. Kirks DR, Caron KH. Gastrointestinal tract. In: Kirks DR, ed. *Practical Pediatric Imaging. Diagnostic Radiology of Infants and Children,* 2nd ed. Boston: Little Brown & Co; 1991:581.
6. McCarten KM, Rosenberg HK, Borden S IV, Mandell GA. Delayed appearance of right diaphragmatic hernia associated with group B streptococcal infection in newborns. *Radiology* 139:385–389, 1981.
7. De Foer B, Breysem L, Smet M-H, Baert AL. Late-onset Bochdalek hernia with a rare postoperative complication: case report. *Pediatr Radiol* 24:306–307, 1994.
8. Levin TL, Liebling MS, Ruzal-Shapiro C, Berdon WE, Stolar CJH. Midgut malfixation in patients with congenital diaphragmatic hernia: what is the risk of midgut volvulus? *Pediatr Radiol* 25:259–261, 1995.
9. Gross BR, D'Agostino C, Coren CV, Petrikovsky BP. Prenatal and neonatal sonographic imaging of a central diaphragmatic hernia. *Pediatr Radiol* 26:395–397, 1996.

Case 13

Clinical Presentation

This 18-hour-old infant developed mild respiratory distress approximately 6 hours after being delivered by cesarean section.

Radiographic Studies

Anterior (Fig. 13A) and lateral (Fig. 13B) chest radiographs show mildly prominent streaky perihilar interstitial markings, thick fissures, heart size at the upper limits of normal, and symmetrically moderately overinflated lungs. Chest radiograph was clear 24 hours later.

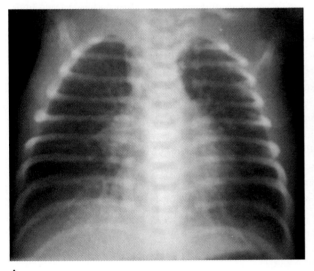

A

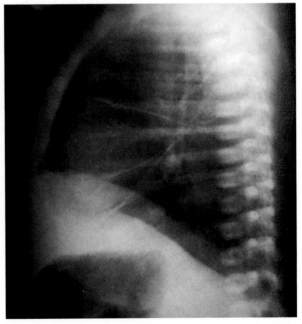

B

Diagnosis Transient Tachypnea of Newborn (TTN)

Discussion and Differential Diagnosis

Prolonged retention of fetal lung liquid is thought to be the cause of transient tachypnea of the newborn, which has also been referred to as transient respiratory distress of the newborn, wet lung disease, or neonatal retained fluid syndrome.[1,2] Prolonged fluid retention may result when there is lack of the thoracic cage squeeze that normally occurs with vaginal delivery. This mechanism typically clears 30% of the normal fetal lung fluid.[2] The condition is therefore more common in patients who are premature, were delivered by cesarean section, or experienced a precipitous delivery. An association with maternal diabetes, maternal fluid overload, hypoproteinemia, hyponatremia, and erythrocythemia is also described.[1,2] The pulmonary capillaries clear 40% of the normal fetal lung liquid and 30% is cleared by the pulmonary lymphatics.[2] In the setting of prolonged retention of fetal lung liquid, these lymphatics become overdistended, pulmonary compliance changes, the lungs become hyperinflated, and the patient develops respiratory distress.[1,2]

The clinical findings of nasal flaring, retractions, grunting, tachypnea and occasional mild cyanosis usually develop during the first few hours after birth, peak before 24 hours of age, and then improve rapidly.[1,2] Patients usually are asymptomatic by 2 to 3 days of age, most as early as 24 hours. The clinical course correlates well with the radiographic changes,[1] which classically consist of symmetric perihilar streaky densities with vascular congestion, fluid in the fissures, mild to moderate pulmonary hyperinflation, and small pleural effusions. The heart may be slightly prominent but true cardiomegaly is not a feature of TTN. Alveolar density patterns can be seen in the early phases of TTN. The more alveolar pattern mimics the changes of hyaline membrane disease (HMD), but the hyperinflation seen with TTN helps in differentiation as the lungs are small in HMD. Additional differential considerations include:

- Clear amniotic fluid aspiration
- Pneumonia
- Mild meconium aspiration
- Pulmonary edema (secondary to obstruction of pulmonary venous drainage)
- Heart failure
- Pulmonary lymphangiectasia (pleural effusions tend to be larger).

Further Reading

1. Swischuk LE. *Imaging of the Newborn, Infant and Young Child,* 3rd ed. Baltimore: Williams & Wilkins; 1989; 1: 50–54.
2. Hedlund GL, Kirks DR. Respiratory system. In: Kirks DR, ed. *Practical Pediatric Imaging. Diagnostic Radiology of Infants and Children,* 2nd ed. Boston: Little Brown & Co; 1991; 6: 599–601.
3. Cleveland RH. A radiologic update on medical diseases of the newborn chest. *Pediatr Radiol* 25:631–637, 1995.

PEARLS

- The lung densities may be asymmetric and more pronounced on the right side.[1]

- The densities of TTN tend to develop in the dependent portions of the lungs, i.e., in the posterior lower lobes.[2]

- Lungs are hyperaerated.

- Pulmonary hyperaeration may persist longer after clear amniotic fluid aspiration, with clearing after 4 to 5 days.[2]

- The polyalveolar lobe type of congenital lobar emphysema causes focal retention of fetal lung liquid.[3]

Case 14

Clinical Presentation

A 14-month-old girl with recent onset of cough and wheezing.

Radiographic Studies

Chest radiograph (Fig. 14A) shows an overinflated left lung creating mediastinal shift to the right. A radiograph obtained during expiration (Fig. 14B) reveals normal egress of air on the right, increasing right mediastinal shift, and persistent hyperexpansion of the left lung, confirming air trapping on the left side. Figure 14C is a high kilovolt peak (kVp) view of the airway in anterior projection. It shows poor definition and narrowing of the mid left mainstem bronchus.

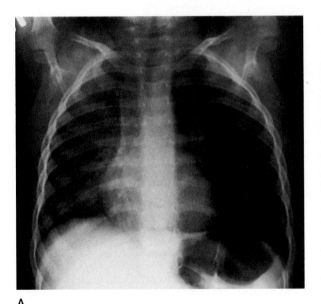

A

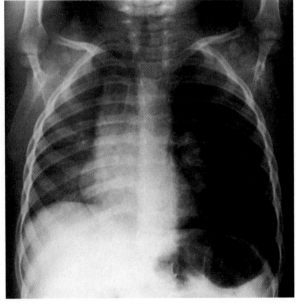

B

PEARLS

• A high kVp film of the airway may reveal a change in airway caliber or increased density over the airway as a reflection of a nonopaque endobronchial foreign body as illustrated in Figure 14C.

• CT is the most sensitive imaging procedure for diagnosing endobronchial foreign bodies. It readily depicts differences in aeration, and with the use of contiguous thin slices, the foreign body is nearly always demonstrable. CT is reserved for difficult cases.

• Manual pressure applied to the patient's upper abdomen may help to achieve a good exhalation during chest fluoroscopy or expiration filming.

• Decubitus or expiratory films are not helpful after the foreign body has produced complete obstruction with atelectasis. They are only helpful when air trapping is present.

• Potential complications related to an unrecognized endobronchial foreign body include:
—asthma-like illness
—chronic pneumonia
—bronchiectasis
—lung abscess
—sepsis.

• Ernst and Mahmud described a pattern of peripheral airway

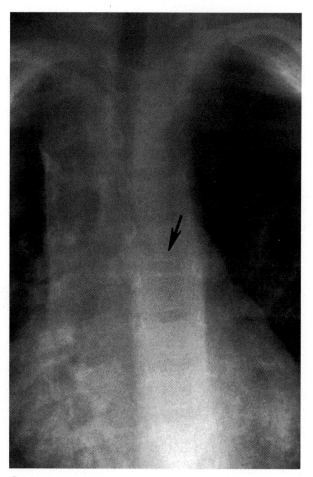

C

Diagnosis Foreign Body Aspiration

Discussion and Differential Diagnosis

Aspiration of foreign material is a common occurrence in infants between ages 6 months and 3 years, and the possibility of an aspirated foreign body should be kept in mind any time a young patient presents with unexplained respiratory symptoms. A foreign body lodged in the subglottic trachea may create symptoms more suggestive of a lower rather than an upper respiratory tract problem. Therefore, this portion of the airway should be carefully assessed when included on the chest radiograph. Additional upper airway studies may be indicated in the appropriate clinical setting. This case study concerns foreign body aspiration into the lower airway, where aeration distal to the foreign body is affected depending on the degree of airway obstruction. Total obstruction leads to atelectasis or consolidation (20% of foreign body inhalations)[1]; high grade but incomplete obstruction leads to so-called obstructive emphy-

dilatation that simulated the presence of multiple cysts in a patient with an endobronchial foreign body. The airway reverted to normal appearance after the foreign body was removed.[3]

PITFALLS
- The inspiration chest radiograph is normal in 20% of patients with an endobronchial foreign body, and in 30% of these patients, all radiographs are normal.[1]

- An ingested foreign body lodged in the upper esophagus may induce tracheospasm or create tracheal compression.[2]

sema or air trapping on the side of the foreign body, best confirmed by filming in expiration or with patient in decubitus position or by chest fluoroscopy.

Because the majority (at least 90%) of inhaled foreign bodies are nonopaque, the radiographic diagnosis depends on the recognition of aeration abnormalities. Unilateral obstructive emphysema is the most common manifestation of an endobronchial foreign body.[2] If the foreign body lodges at the carina, both lungs may show overinflation or volume loss. Foreign bodies tend to be right-sided in 55%, left-sided in 33%, bilateral in 7%, and in the trachea in 5%.[1] The importance of the patient's history and clinical presentation cannot be stressed enough. The possibility of an airway foreign body should be considered when

- The patient has wheezing without underlying lung disease.[1]
- The patient is less than 3 years old and has pneumonia or suspected pneumonia.[1]
- The patient has a pneumomediastinum or pneumothorax (with or without airspace consolidation).[1]
- The patient has hemoptysis and air space consolidation unresponsive to treatment.[2]
- There is a convincing history, even if all films are normal.[1]
- "Pneumonia" is present with volume loss.

Differential considerations in unilateral air trapping include (in addition to foreign bodies), intrinsic bronchial lesions, such as mucous plug, bronchial adenoma, and bronchial stenosis/atresia; and extrinsic lesions, such as compression from vascular abnormalities, adenopathy, or mediastinal masses, pulmonary vascular asymmetry (as in, for example, absence of left pulmonary artery associated with tetralogy of Fallot), primary parenchymal disease (as in Swyer-James-Macleod syndrome), or pulmonary hypoplasia.[2]

Further Reading

1. Hedlund GL, Kirks DR. Respiratory system. In: Kirks DR, ed. *Practical Pediatric Imaging. Diagnostic Radiology of Infants and Children,* 2nd ed. Boston: Little Brown & Co; 1991: 683, 686–689.
2. Leonidas JC, Berdon W. The neck and respiratory system, part 2. In: Silverman FN, ed. *Caffey's Pediatric X-ray Diagnosis.* 9th ed. Chicago: Yearbook Medical Publishers; 1993: 480, 482–483, 485.
3. Ernst KD, Mahmud F. Reversible cystic dilatation of distal airways due to foreign body. *South Med J* 87(3):404–406, 1994.

Case 15

Clinical Presentation

A 1400-gram premature infant was born at 34 weeks' gestation. Severe respiratory distress at birth was manifested by tachypnea, subxiphoid retractions, grunting, and cyanosis.

Radiographic Studies

Diffuse, finely granular opacities in both lungs create homogeneous and symmetric increased density with peripheral air bronchograms (Fig. 15A). In this intubated infant, the typical decreased lung volume is best demonstrated by exaggerated upward bowing of the diaphragm on the lateral radiograph (Fig. 15B). Lateral radiograph in another premature infant (Fig. 15C) shows subxiphoid retraction (arrow) indicating decreased lung volume.

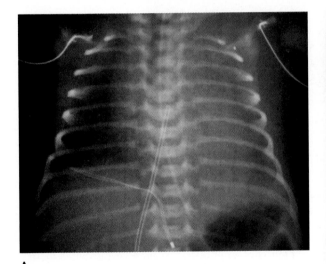

A

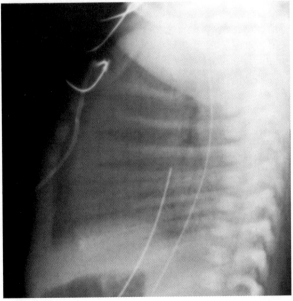

B

- HMD lungs are underaerated, with domed-up diaphragms and sternal retraction. HMD lungs have symmetrical alveolar disease. With any asymmetry, suspect superimposed pneumonia.

- Maternal administration of steroids for at least 24 hours prior to birth helps to mature the neonatal lungs and modifies the classic radiographic pattern of hyaline membrane disease.[4]

- Intrauterine stress also may cause outpouring of steroids, maturing the type 2 alveolar lining cells. This steroid output also "shrinks" the thymus. A premature infant with no thymus usually will not have HMD.

- HMD is commonly seen in infants of diabetic mothers. These newborns, though large, are immature. HMD is rarely seen in an infant born at term.[2]

- Inherited deficiency of pulmonary surfactant does occur and should be considered when a term infant presents with a clinical and radiographic picture of HMD.[6]

- Group B streptococcal infection can closely mimic the clinical and radiographic findings of HMD. The presence

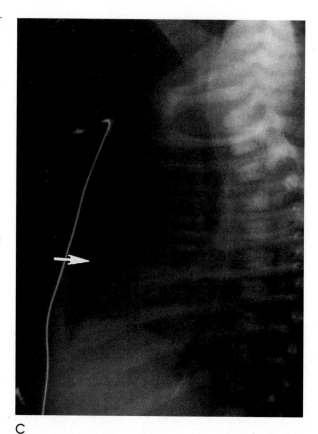

C

Diagnosis   Hyaline Membrane Disease (HMD)

Discussion and Differential Diagnosis

Hyaline membrane disease is seen most often in low-birthweight (less than 2500 grams) premature infants born earlier than 36 to 38 weeks of gestation.[1] The typical small and opaque lungs are a reflection of diffuse alveolar atelectasis caused by lack of surfactant in the premature infant lung.[2–4] The peripheral air bronchograms are created by the contrast between the air-containing peripheral bronchial tree and the nonaerated surrounding acini. Hyaline membranes develop from capillary leak and cellular debris[4] and are the result of the underlying lung disease rather than the cause of the problem, as might be suggested by the term "hyaline membrane disease." Other terms used to describe this condition are respiratory distress syndrome or idiopathic respiratory distress syndrome. Both of these describe the patient's clinical presentation and do not address the underlying cause. Swischuk and John[5] have suggested the use of "surfactant deficiency disease" instead of hyaline membrane disease. Respiratory distress related to underlying hyaline membrane disease typically starts immediately after birth or within the course of the next few hours. Respiratory

of pleural effusions may be the only distinguishing feature. They are not a feature of uncomplicated HMD and are present in up to two thirds of patients with pneumonia. The two conditions may coexist.[1]

● Administration of exogenous surfactant may result in nonuniform asymmetric clearing. The residual areas of opacity may resemble changes of pneumonia.[2]

● Development of pulmonary interstitial emphysema after surfactant treatment has a grave prognosis.[7]

● Subxiphoid chest wall retraction can create a rounded lucency over the low mid chest on the anterior chest radiograph. This may mimic a pneumomediastinum.

symptoms starting after 8 hours of age are unlikely to be the result of hyaline membrane disease.

Surfactant production returns by age 5 to 7 days[4] and pulmonary aeration improves at that time, with clearing in a predictable pattern from upper lobe caudad and from lateral to medial.[3] The use of exogenous surfactant shortens the time for radiographic clearing, allows easier ventilation, and decreases complicating air leak. No definite impact has been shown on the development of intracranial hemorrhage, chronic lung disease, or shunting through the patent ductus arteriosus.[2]

There are many potential complications of HMD. Quite a few are iatrogenic in nature, involving air block related to positive pressure ventilation. Differential considerations for the fine granular densities of hyaline membrane disease include the following:

● Pneumonia
   —group B streptococus, cytomegalovirus, *Listeria monocytogenes*
● Pulmonary edema
   —patent ductus arteriosus
   —obstruction to pulmonary venous drainage
   —hypoplastic left heart
   —neurogenic pulmonary edema secondary to intracranial hemorrhage
● Wet lung disease
● Sepsis
● Pulmonary hemorrhage.

In most of these conditions, the lung volumes are not as diminished as they are in HMD.[3,4] Also, they often have asymmetrical infiltrates.

Further Reading

1. Cleveland RH. A radiologic update on medical diseases of the newborn chest. *Pediatr Radiol* 25:631–637, 1995.
2. Leonidas JC, Berdon W. The neck and respiratory system, part 7. In: Silverman FN, ed. *Caffey's Pediatric X-ray Diagnosis.* 9th ed. Chicago: Yearbook Medical Publishers; 1993; 2:1969–1978, 1982–1984.
3. Hedlund GL, Kirks DR. Respiratory system. In: Kirks DR, ed. *Practical Pediatric Imaging. Diagnostic Radiology of Infants and Children,* 2nd ed. Boston: Little Brown & Co; 1991; 6: 585–589, 595.
4. Swischuk LE. *Imaging of the Newborn, Infant and Young Child,* 3rd ed. Baltimore: Williams & Wilkins; 1989; 1: 28–49.
5. Swischuk LE, John SD. Immature lung problems: can our nomenclature be more specific? *Am J Roentgenol* 166:917–918, 1996.
6. Ballard PL, Nogee LM, Beers MF, et al. Partial deficiency of surfactant protein B in an infant with chronic lung disease. *Pediatrics* 96:1046–1052, 1995. Abstract.
7. Dinger J, Schwarze R, Rupprecht E. Radiological changes after therapeutic use of surfactant in infants with respiratory distress syndrome. *Pediatr Radiol* 27:26–31, 1997.

Case 16

Clinical Presentation

Four different infants are depicted in this case study. All were meconium stained and had meconium suctioned from below the vocal cords at birth. Severe respiratory distress was present in each case. All four were postmature.

Radiographic Studies

The ossification centers for the humeral head epiphyses or the coracoid process are visible in each patient, consistent with the clinical postmaturity (see straight white arrow over the left shoulder in Fig. 16A, 16B, 16E). Extensive patchy airspace densities are intermingled with foci of hyperaeration creating a pattern of coarse, diffuse but nonuniform and asymmetric infiltrates. The infiltrates are more prominent centrally in the patient in Figure 16B, whose lungs are also markedly hyperinflated with flattening of the diaphragm. On the lateral view in this patient (Fig. 16C), signs of hyperinflation include anterior rounding of the sternum, the prominent retrosternal clear space, and increased anteroposterior (AP) dimension of chest.

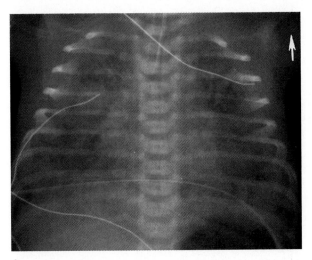

A

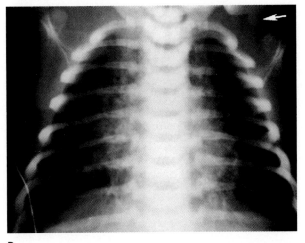

B

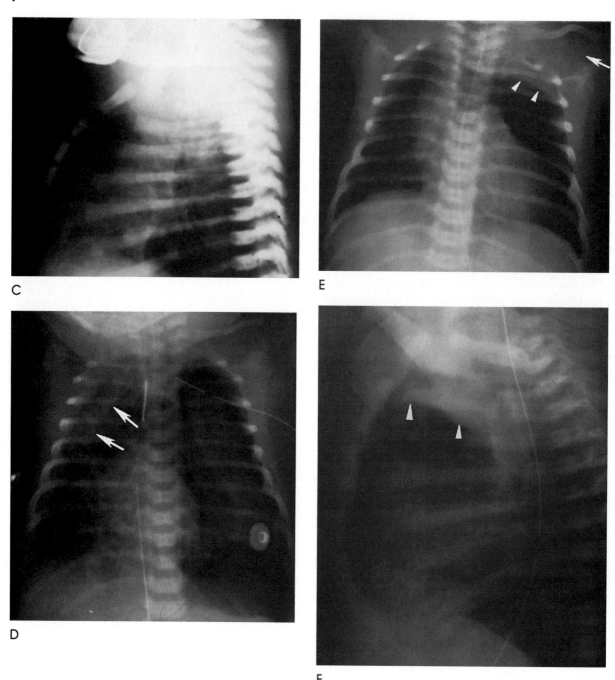

Diagnosis Meconium Aspiration

Discussion and Differential Diagnosis

Fetal distress may lead to in utero fetal gasping, which then results in aspiration of amniotic fluid. If the fetal distress also causes evacuation of meconium, the amniotic fluid will be laden with this thick, tenacious material. Radiographic changes related to meconium aspiration vary depending on the amount of meconium in the fluid and the extent of the aspiration. Chest radiographs may be normal or show extensive bilateral infiltrates and air trapping. Meconium aspiration generally occurs in postmature infants. These infants typically have proximal humeral and/or coracoid epiphyses.[1] Meconium-stained amniotic fluid is observed in 10 to 15% of all live births[2]; actual meconium aspiration (i.e., meconium found below the vocal cords) occurs in 1 to 5% of live births.[2,3] Affected infants experience severe respiratory distress immediately after birth, manifested by retractions, grunting, tachypnea, and cyanosis. Most aspiration of meconium occurs at delivery when the meconium in the hypopharynx is aspirated into the lungs after the chest has been compressed by the vagina and reexpands. Immediate suctioning after the head is delivered—before delivery of the chest—may prevent significant meconium aspiration.

The air trapping, diffuse nodular densities, and areas of focal emphysema typical of meconium aspiration all reflect obstructions in the peripheral bronchial tree caused by the aspirated meconium particles. Aspirated meconium contributes to focal atelectasis by depleting pulmonary surfactant[4] and causes a chemical pneumonitis that predisposes to superimposed bacterial infection. Pleural effusions are present in approximately 10% of patients[2]; air block is a common complication, with pneumothorax reported in 25 to 40% of patients.[2,3] Figure 16D shows an intubated patient with meconium aspiration who developed a left tension pneumothorax despite the presence of a chest tube in the upper chest. Additional air in the mediastinum elevates the thymus and sharply outlines its inferior border. This is especially well seen on the right (arrows). Figures 16E and 16F depict a patient with severe air trapping related to meconium aspiration (notice rounded sternum, flattened diaphragms, and increased AP dimension of chest). A large left pneumomediastinum has lifted the left thymic lobe up to the apex of the left hemithorax (Fig. 16E, arrowheads). The tongue of opacity created by the elevated thymus is especially well seen on the lateral radiograph (Fig. 16F). Arrowheads point to the sharply outlined inferior thymic border.

Persistent fetal circulation (persistent pulmonary hypertension) is a known additional effect of meconium aspiration, caused in part by hypoxia-induced peripheral pulmonary arteriolar vasoconstriction.[4] Extracorporeal membrane oxygenation is employed as a method of oxygenation in severe cases where conventional management has failed. Differential diagnosis includes neonatal pneumonias and pulmonary hemorrhage.

PEARLS

- Rapid improvement after an initial film showing consolidation and air trapping in the clinical setting of meconium aspiration suggests that there was predominately aspiration of clear amniotic fluid.[4]

- If the initial film is normal and consolidation develops later, consider the possibility of neurogenic pulmonary edema related to an in utero hypoxemic episode.

- Clinical improvement precedes radiographic clearing, which may take weeks.

- Typical meconium aspiration infants have proximal humeral and/or coracoid epiphyses, hyperaerated lungs, asymmetrical infiltrates, and pneumothorax or pneumomediastinum.

PITFALLS

- Meconium aspiration, pneumonia, and wet lung may look identical on initial radiograph with hyperinflated lungs and bilateral asymmetrical infiltrates.

Further Reading

1. Kuhns LR, Sherman MP, Poznanski AK, Holt JF. Humeral-head and coracoid ossification in the newborn. *Radiology* 107:145–149, 1973.
2. Cleveland RH. A radiologic update on medical diseases of the newborn chest. *Pediatr Radiol* 25:631–637, 1995.
3. Hedlund GL, Kirks DR. Respiratory system. In: Kirks DR, ed. *Practical Pediatric Imaging. Diagnostic Radiology of Infants and Children,* 2nd ed. Boston: Little Brown & Co; 1991;6:599–601.
4. Swischuk LE. *Imaging of the Newborn, Infant and Young Child,* 3rd ed. Baltimore: Williams & Wilkins; 1989; 1:50–54.

CARDIAC
RADIOLOGY

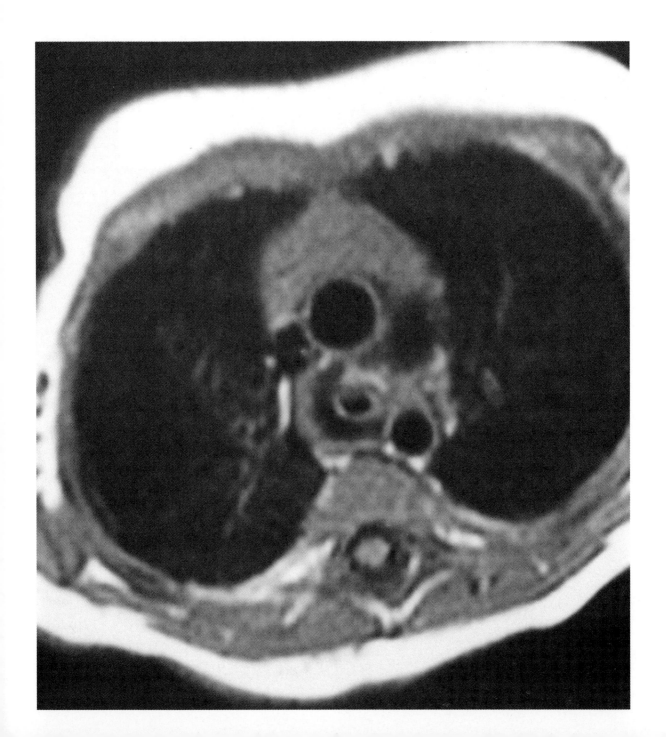

Case 1

Clinical Presentation

A 3-month-old infant with cyanotic heart disease.

Radiographic Studies

Chest radiograph (Fig. 1A) demonstrates prominent pulmonary arterial vascularity, cardiomegaly, and a prominent superior mediastinum. Venous phase of pulmonary arteriogram (Fig. 1B) shows anomalous pulmonary venous drainage into a left vertical vein (white arrow), which drains into the left innominate vein (black arrow) and finally into the superior vena cava.

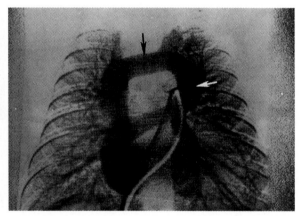

B

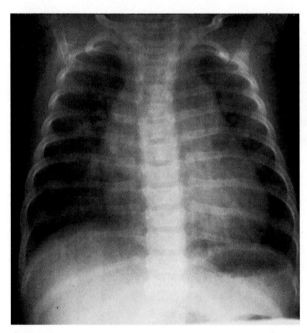

A

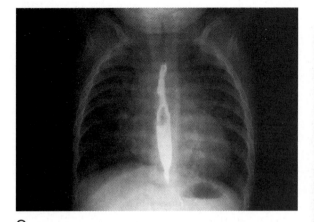

C

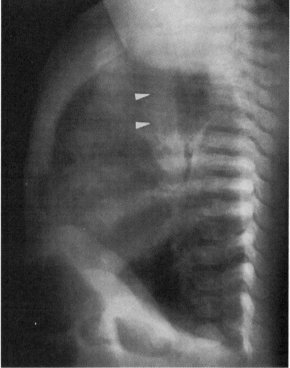

D

Diagnosis Supracardiac Total Anomalous Pulmonary Venous Return

Discussion and Differential Diagnosis

In total anomalous pulmonary venous return (TAPVR), the pulmonary veins do not return blood normally to the left atrium. TAPVR can be classified according to the site of pulmonary venous return. Categories include supracardiac (type I), cardiac (type II), infracardiac (type III), and mixed (type IV) types.[1]

In supracardiac TAPVR, the venous return is most commonly to an anomalous left vertical vein, also referred to as a left superior vena cava (SVC), which drains into the left innominate vein. Drainage can occasionally occur directly into the right superior vena cava or the azygos vein.[2] The cardiac type of TAPVR has an anomalous vein draining into the coronary sinus or directly into the right atrium. Infracardiac TAPVR has an anomalous vein that arises at the pulmonary venous confluence posterior to the heart and travels downward through the esophageal hiatus to drain into the ductus venosus or a portal vein or, much less commonly, a hepatic vein or the inferior vena cava (IVC). The anomalous draining vein can be obstructed or nonobstructed. In approximately three fourths of cases of types I, II, and IV, the connecting vein is widely patent.[3] Infracardiac TAPVR is almost invariably obstructed because blood flow must transit through the liver. Cardiac and supracardiac TAPVR are more commonly nonobstructed. Nonobstructed TAPVR is an admixture-type

- Thymic tissue can be mistaken for the head of the snowman. The lateral chest radiograph will show poststernal density if this is thymus. With TAPVR, the vertical vein appears as a pretracheal density superimposed on the superior vena cava.[7]

- Patients with cardiac TAPVR can have an enlarged coronary sinus.[8] The enlarged coronary sinus is inferior in location to the level of the left atrium on the lateral chest X ray but could be mistaken for an enlarged left atrium.

shunt lesion and therefore should show prominent pulmonary arterial vascularity. Increased blood volume to the right side of the heart causes cardiomegaly with enlargement of the right atrium, right ventricle, and main pulmonary artery. The left ventricle, left atrium, and aorta are inconspicuous.

"Snowman" or "figure-of-eight" is the classic description of the cardiac configuration of supracardiac TAPVR on the frontal chest radiograph. It is caused by enlargement of the left vertical vein, left innominate vein, and the SVC (Fig. 1C). On the lateral chest radiograph, there may be a density anterior to the trachea from superimposition of the SVC and left vertical vein that has been described as a finding in supracardiac TAPVR[4] (Fig. 1D). The left atrium is decreased in size in TAPVR.[5] Therefore, the presence of left atrial enlargement should help exclude TAPVR from the differential.

Axial and coronal cardiac gated T1-weighted angiography MR imaging is an effective method of evaluation for TAPVR.[6] MRA has also proved to be useful.[7] Echocardiography and angiography are often considered the gold standard for evaluation of congenital heart disease. However, evaluation of the pulmonary vein anomalies by echocardiography is often limited by restricted field of view.[7] Evaluation of pulmonary vein anomalies angiographically may also be difficult secondary to dilution of contrast.[7] Secondary to the above angiographic and echocardiographic limitations, some authors have suggested that MRI is a superior method for evaluation of pulmonary vein anomalies.[6,7]

Differential diagnosis for a cyanotic infant with cardiomegaly and increased pulmonary arterial vascularity would include other cyanotic bidirectional shunt lesions with cardiomegaly and increased pulmonary vascularity such as truncus arteriosus, transposition of the great arteries, single ventricle without pulmonary stenosis, double outlet right ventricle, and tricuspid atresia without pulmonary stenosis. The prominent left superior mediastinum, however, should make transposition an unlikely possibility. Without the history of cyanosis, additional considerations would be an atrial septal defect, which also typically shows right heart enlargement. Other noncyanotic shunt lesions with cardiomegaly and increased pulmonary vascularity such as ventricular septal defect, atrioventricular canal, and patent ductus arteriosus typically also have a component of left ventricular and left atrial enlargement.

Further Reading

1. Darling RC, Rothney WB, Craig JM. Total pulmonary venous drainage into the right side of the heart. Report of 17 autopsied cases not associated with other major cardiovascular anomalies. *Lab Invest* 6:44–64, 1957.
2. Delisle G, Ando M, Calder AL, et al. Total anomalous pulmonary venous connection: report of 93 autopsied cases with emphasis on diagnostic and surgical considerations. *Am Heart J* 91(1):99–122, 1976.
3. Amplatz K, Moller JH. Total anomalous pulmonary venous connection. In: *Radiology of Congenital Heart Disease*. St. Louis: Mosby Year Book; 1993: 805–826.
4. Weaver MD, Chen JT, Anderson PA, Lester RG. Total anomalous pulmonary venous connection to the left vertical vein. *Radiology* 118:670–683, 1976.

5. Coussement AM, Gooding CA, Carlsson E. Left atrial volume, shape, and movement in total anomalous pulmonary venous return. *Radiology* 107:139–143, 1973.
6. Choe YH, Lee HJ, Kim HS, Ko JK, Kim JE, Han JJ. MRI of total anomalous pulmonary venous connections. *J Comput Assist Tomogr* 18(2):243–249, 1994.
7. Cohen MC, Hartnell GG, Finn JP. Magnetic resonance angiography of congenital pulmonary vein anomalies. *Am Heart J* 127:954–955, 1994.
8. Fellows KE Jr, Sigmann J, Stern AM, Bookstein JJ. Coronary sinus enlargement in infants: a diagnostic note. *Radiology* 94:347–349, 1970.

Case 2

Clinical Presentation

A premature newborn infant with cyanosis.

Radiographic Studies

Chest radiograph (Fig. 2A) shows pulmonary edema without cardiomegaly. There is also a right pleural effusion. Pulmonary venous phase (Fig. 2B) of arteriogram shows abnormal pulmonary venous drainage.

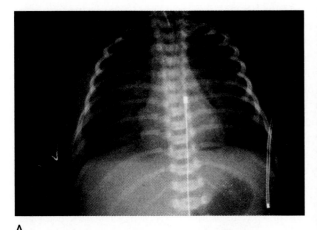

A

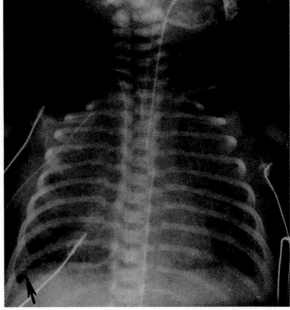

C

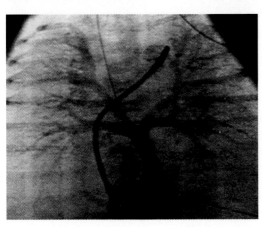

B

Diagnosis Infracardiac Total Anomalous Pulmonary Venous Return

Discussion and Differential Diagnosis

Anatomic classification of TAPVR has been discussed with the prior case. Obstruction can occur with infracardiac TAPVR or with the supradiaphragmatic types. Infracardiac TAPVR is almost invariably of the obstructed type.[1] The drainage is most commonly to the portal vein.[2] With closure of the ductus venosus, pulmonary venous drainage must travel through the capillary bed of the liver, causing severe obstruction. Additional causes of obstruction would include the esophageal hiatus or narrowing of the connecting vessel. Obstruction may occur in up to 50% of supracardiac TAPVR as well.[1]

In supracardiac TAPVR, obstruction can occur if the vertical vein travels between the left pulmonary artery and the left mainstem bronchus.[1] Stenosis can also occur at the junction of the vertical vein to the left innominate or at the junction of the innominate vein to the right superior vena cava.[1]

There is usually not significant cardiomegaly when TAPVR is of the obstructed type. With obstructed TAPVR, the right atrium and right ventricle are not dilated because the volume of pulmonary blood returned to the right ventricle is limited by high resistance to flow through the obstructing site.[3] Right ventricular hypertrophy does develop, but this does not usually cause significant cardiomegaly on a frontal radiograph.[3] However, with lesser degrees of obstruction, there may be some cardiomegaly. The pulmonary vascular pattern is venous congestion with diffuse pulmonary edema often with Kerley's B lines. Figure 2C is an additional example of obstructed TAPVR with mixed drainage above and below the diaphragm showing severe interstitial edema, pleural effusions, and Kerley's B lines (arrow).

The differential diagnosis of a cyanotic infant with a normal-sized heart and pulmonary edema should also include cor triatriatum and atresia of the common pulmonary vein, both of which are much more rare.

Further Reading

1. Delisle G, Ando M, Calder AL, et al. Total anomalous pulmonary venous connection: report of 93 autopsied cases with emphasis on diagnostic and surgical considerations. *Am Heart J* 91(1):99–122, 1976.
2. Duff DF, Nihill MR, McNamara DG. Infradiaphragmatic total anomalous pulmonary venous return. Review of clinical and pathological findings and results of operation in 28 cases. *Br Heart J* 39:619–626, 1977.
3. Amplatz K, Moller JH. Total anomalous pulmonary venous connection. In: *Radiology of Congenital Heart Disease*. St. Louis: Mosby Year Book; 1993: 805–826.
4. Choe YH, Lee HJ, Kim HS, Ko JK, Kim JE, Han JJ. MRI of total anomalous pulmonary venous connections. *J Comput Assist Tomogr* 18(2):243–249, 1994.

Case 3

Clinical Presentation

Three infants with stridor.

Radiographic Studies

Anteroposterior (AP) plain radiograph in the first patient shows the trachea is deviated to the left (Fig. 3A). Lateral radiograph from airway fluoroscopy in a second patient shows tracheal narrowing at the level of the aortic arch (Fig. 3B). Posteroanterior (PA) radiograph in a third patient shows a right-sided and slightly lower left-sided extrinsic impression on the esophagus at the level of the aortic arch (Fig. 3C). Lateral esophagram shows a focal posterior impression upon the esophagus (Fig. 3D). Axial and coronal T1-weighted MR images in this patient show a large right aortic arch and a smaller left aortic arch surrounding the trachea (Figs. 3E, 3F). Axial T1-weighted image above the level of the arch shows symmetric alignment of the carotid and subclavian vessels (arrowheads) surrounding the trachea (Fig. 3G).

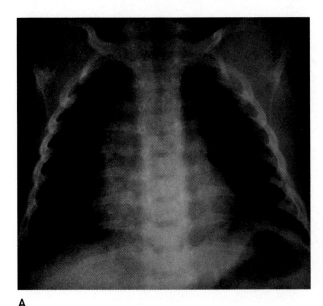

A

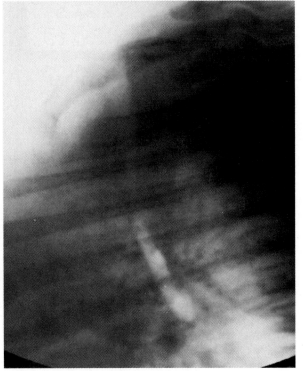

B

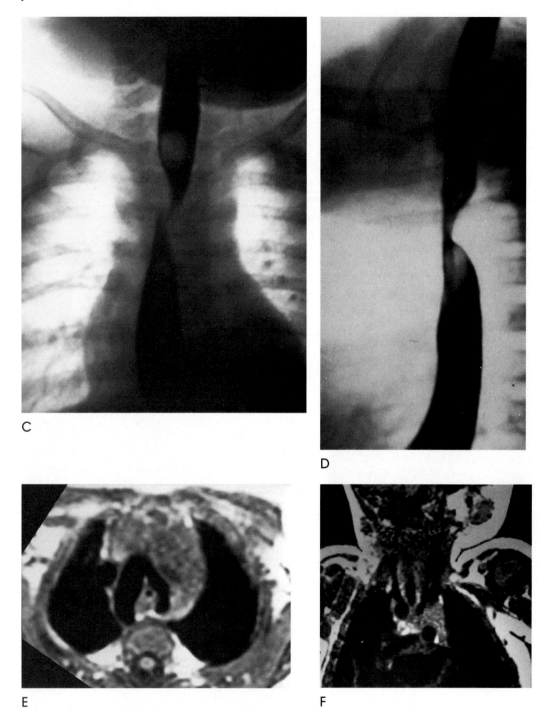

C

D

E

F

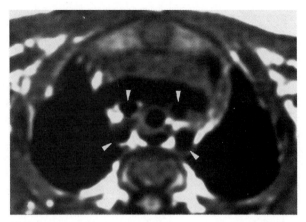

G

Diagnosis Double Aortic Arch

Discussion and Differential Diagnosis

Double aortic arch is the most common arch anomaly to require surgery for esophageal or tracheal compression.[1] The typical clinical presentation includes stridor in infants and feeding difficulties or dysphagia.[2] In the older child, respiratory symptoms are usually more prominent than esophageal symptoms.[3] Stridor occurs on both inspiration and expiration.[2] In infants, feedings may be long and difficult, with episodes of coughing and cyanosis.[2] Dysphagia may occur when solids are added to the diet.[4] Symptoms are usually present from the first few days of life.[2] The anomaly may also be seen as an incidental finding in older patients or adults.

Double aortic arch develops when neither of the fourth brachial arches regresses. Double aortic arch is typically not associated with other cardiac anomalies.[3,5] The right arch is usually higher, larger, and more posteriorly located than the left arch.[6] As a rule, the upper descending aorta is on the left.[3] Either arch may be atretic or both arches may be patent. However, it is rare to have an atretic right posterior arch.[7] The branches of the two arches are usually symmetrically arranged with a subclavian and common carotid artery branch from each arch.

On frontal chest radiograph, a prominent right mediastinum with a slight indentation on the right trachea suggests the possibility of a right arch or double aortic arch. If there is also a slightly lower, more subtle impression to the left of the trachea on frontal airway fluoroscopy or chest radiograph, this suggests the possibility of a double aortic arch.[3] Tracheal narrowing above the carina should be seen on the lateral radiograph.[8,9] The classic findings seen with double aortic arch on the lateral esophagram include a posterior esophageal impression with an anterior impression on the trachea.[10] Many authors consider MRI the preferred method for evaluation of vascular rings and aortic arch anomalies, particularly in older children with a less optimal echocardiograph window.[11–16] The number, size, and location of aortic lumens is well depicted on cardiac-gated T1-weighted MR sequences using multiple imaging planes. More recently, spiral CT angiography has also been shown to be useful for evaluation of vascular rings in children.[17,18] The "four-vessel sign" can be seen on axial CT or MR images just above the level of the aortic arch in patients with a double aortic arch.[19] There are four arteries seen on axial images just cephalad to the aorta as opposed to the normal three arteries (right brachiocephalic, left carotid, and left subclavian arteries). These vessels are right and left carotid arteries and right and left subclavian arteries. The two anterior carotid and two posterior subclavian arteries are arranged symmetrically around the trachea as opposed to the usual asymmetrical three-vessel configuration.

Further Reading

1. Shuford WH, Sybers RG, Weens HS. The angiographic features of double aortic arch. *Am J Roentgenol Radium Ther Nucl Med* 116(1):125–140, 1972.
2. Binet JP, Langlois J. Aortic arch anomalies in children and infants. *J Thorac Cardiovasc Surg* 73:248–252 1977.
3. Stewart JR, Kincaid OW, Edwards JE. *An Atlas of Vascular Rings and Related Malformations of the Aortic Arch System.* Springfield, IL: Charles C. Thomas; 1964: 14–43.
4. Stewart JR, Kincaid OW, Titus JL. Right aortic arch: plain film diagnosis and significance. *Am J Roentgenol Radium Ther Nucl Med* 97(2):377–389, 1966.
5. Machiels F, de Maeseneer M, Desprechins B, Osteaux M, Dewolf D. A functioning double aortic arch in an infant: a case report. *Pediatr Radiol* 24:76–77, 1994.
6. Predey TA, McDonald V, Demos TC, Moncada R. CT of congenital anomalies of the aortic arch. *Semin Roentgenol* 24(2):96–111, 1989.
7. McFaul R, Millard P, Nowicki E. Vascular rings necessitating right thoracotomy. *J Thorac Cardiovasc Surg* 82:306–309, 1981.
8. Jaffe RB. Radiographic manifestations of congenital anomalies of the aortic arch. *Radiol Clin North Am* 29(2):319–334, 1991.
9. Lowe GM, Donaldson JS, Backer CL. Vascular rings: 10-year review of imaging. *Radiographics* 11:637–646, 1991.
10. Berdon WE, Baker DH. Vascular anomalies and the infant lung: rings, slings, and other things. *Semin Roentgenol* 7(1):39–64, 1972.
11. Bisset GS III, Strife JL, Kirks DR, Bailey WW. Vascular rings: MR imaging. *Am J Roentgenol* 149:251–256, 1987.
12. Bisset GS III. Magnetic resonance imaging of congenital heart disease in the pediatric patient. *Radiol Clin N Am* 29(2):279–291, 1991.
13. Gomes AS, Lois JF, George B, Alpan G, Williams RG. Congenital abnormalities of the aortic arch: MR imaging. *Radiology* 165:691–695, 1987.
14. Fletcher BD, Jacobstein MD. MRI of congenital abnormalities of the great arteries. *Am J Roentgenol* 146:941–948, 1986.
15. Kersting-Sommerhoff BA, Sechtem UP, Fisher MR, Higgins CB. MR imaging of congenital anomalies of the aortic arch. *Am J Roentgenol* 149:9–13, 1987.
16. Burrows PE, MacDonald CE. Magnetic resonance imaging of the pediatric thoracic aorta. *Semin Ultrasound CT MR* 14(2):129–144, 1993.

17. Hopkins KL, Patrick LE, Simoneaux SF, Bank EF, Parks WJ, Smith SS. Pediatric great vessel anomalies: initial clinical experience with spiral CT angiography. *Radiology* 200:811–815, 1996.

18. Katz M, Konen E, Rozenman J, Szeinberg A, Itzchak Y. Spiral CT and 3D image reconstruction of vascular rings and associated tracheobronchial anomalies. *J Comput Assist Tomogr* 19(4):564–568, 1995.

19. McLoughlin MJ, Weisbrod G, Wise DJ, Yeung HP. Computed tomography in congenital anomalies of the aortic arch and great vessels. *Radiology* 138:399–403, 1981.

20. Simoneaux SF, Bank ER, Webber JB, Parks WJ. MR imaging of the pediatric airway. *Radiographics* 15:287–298, 1995.

Case 4

Clinical Presentation

Hypertension with weak femoral artery pulses.

Radiographic Studies

Posteroanterior chest radiograph (Fig. 4A) shows bilateral rib notching (arrowheads). The aortic knob is high and inconspicuous. The descending aorta appears prominent (arrow, Fig. 4A), suggesting some poststenotic dilatation. Lateral chest radiograph (Fig. 4B) shows prominent wavy retrosternal soft tissue density (arrowheads). Sagittal T1-weighted oblique MR images in the plane of the aortic arch (Figs. 4C, 4D) show focal narrowing of the aorta at the junction of the aortic arch and descending aorta (arrowhead, Fig. 4C) and prominent collateral vessels (arrows, Fig. 4D).

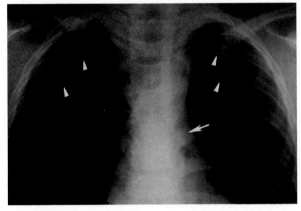

A

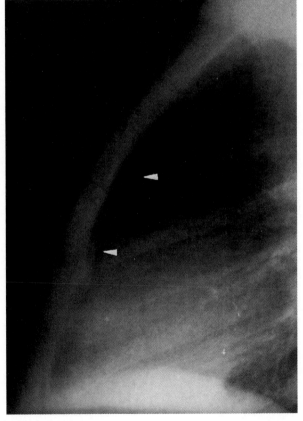

B

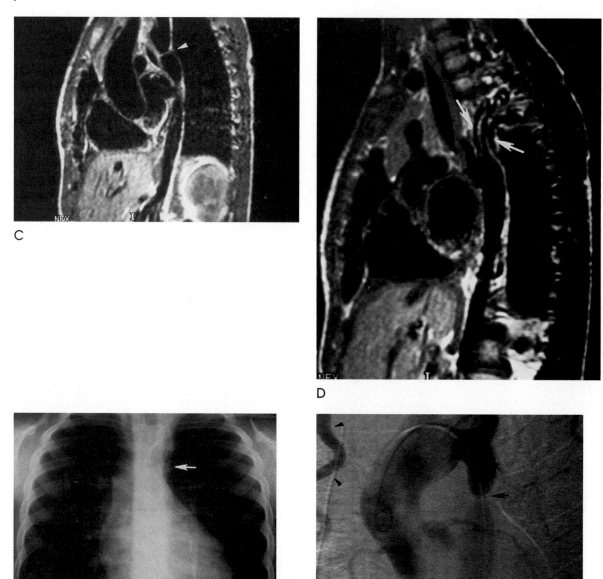

Diagnosis Coarctation of the Aorta

- Rib notching is rarely seen above the third or below the ninth ribs.[16]

- A low-appearing aortic knob on frontal chest radiograph is another described finding with coarctation. It is caused by nonvisualization of the superior aspect of the three sign with prominent poststenotic dilation in the lower half of the three sign.[17]

- Wavy retrosternal soft tissue on lateral chest radiograph (Fig. 4B) caused by enlarged mammary arteries can be seen in up to 30% of patients.[4] An enlarged internal mammary collateral (arrowheads, Fig. 4F) is shown on digital subtraction angiogram in a hypertensive patient with focal coarctation (arrow, Fig. 4F). Note associated dilated ascending aorta.

- A balloon angioplasty may be performed rather than surgical correction in some cardiovascular centers.[18,19]

Discussion and Differential Diagnosis

Coarctation of the thoracic aorta can be divided into two general types, tubular hypoplasia and localized coarctation. Tubular hypoplasia is also sometimes referred to as infantile, diffuse, or preductal coarctation. Localized coarctation is sometimes referred to as adult type or postductal coarctation. Localized coarctation may actually be in a preductal, juxtaductal, or postductal location. Some patients may have elements of both tubular hypoplasia and localized coarctation.[1]

Localized coarctation is caused by a shelf-like projection of media at the junction of the arch and the proximal descending aorta.[1] The abnormal shelf of media involves the anterior, posterior, and superolateral walls of the aorta while sparing the ductal side of the aortic wall. This causes the aortic lumen to be eccentrically narrowed. The aortic lumen often becomes significantly more narrow following closure of the ductus arteriosus[1] and patients become more symptomatic after ductal closure.

Patients may present early in life secondary to additional associated cardiac congenital anomalies. Infants diagnosed early without other anomalies classically present at the end of the first week of life or early in the second week of life when the ductus closes. They present with findings of heart failure,[1] cardiomegaly, and pulmonary edema. With closure of the ductus, the aortic lumen becomes significantly more narrow rather acutely, with abrupt increase in the left ventricular work load.[1] Lower extremity and upper extremity pulses remain relatively symmetric until after the ductus closes,[1] so coarctation may be missed in the newborn period. Older children and young adults typically present with upper extremity hypertension, murmur, or decreased femoral pulses discovered incidentally by physical exam. These patients are otherwise usually healthy.

There is a 50 to 85% association with bicuspid aortic valve.[2,3] The hemodynamic consequences of a bicuspid aortic valve can cause prominence of the ascending aorta. The ascending aorta is prominent on plain film in 30% of patients.[4] Coarctation has a marked male predominance with 80% of coarctations occurring in boys.[2] If coarctation is seen in a female, the diagnosis of Turner syndrome should be considered because coarctation occurs in 20% of patients with Turner syndrome.[5]

Coarctation can be associated with other forms of congenital heart disease, including patent ductus arteriosus, ventricular septal defect, transposition of the great arteries, Taussig-Bing form of double outlet right ventricle, and tricuspid atresia.[2] Associated acquired cardiovascular abnormalities include endocardial fibroelastosis, cardiomyopathy, mitral regurgitation, atherosclerosis, subacute bacterial endocarditis, aortic dissection, and thrombosis of the anterior spinal artery.[2,3] In addition, aneurysms of the circle of Willis occur in approximately 10% of patients.[2]

Radiographic abnormalities of the aortic knob contour that have been described with coarctation include an inconspicuous aortic knob, an enlarged aortic knob, or elevated aortic knob.[6] The figure three sign (arrow, Fig. 4E) can be seen by plain film in approximately 40% of patients.[6] This is caused by prestenotic and poststenotic dilatation of the aorta. The left ventricle may appear detectably enlarged by plain film in up to 40% of cases.[4] Rib notching is seen in up to 77% of patients older than two years of age with coarctation.[4] By esophogram, a bilobed impression on the esophagus called an "E" or reversed three sign can sometimes be seen caused again by the same pre- and poststenotic dilatation. MRI is an excellent noninvasive modality for the evaluation of coarctation. Some authors consider it the imaging modality of choice for evaluation of coarctation, particularly postoperatively[7] and in older children and adults.[7–12] For MRI evaluation of coarctation, T1-weighted axial and sagittal oblique images in the plane of the aortic arch are required.[7,10,11,13–15]

Further Reading

1. Talner NS, Berman MA. Postnatal development of obstruction in coarctation of the aorta: role of the ductus arteriosus. *Pediatrics* 56(4):562–569, 1975.
2. Elliott LP. *Cardiac Imaging in Infants, Children, and Adults.* Philadelphia: JB Lippincott Co; 1991:269–278.
3. Amplatz K, Moller JH. *Radiology of Congenital Heart Disease.* St. Louis: Mosby Year Book; 1993:469–498.
4. Figley MM. Accessory roentgen signs of coarctation of the aorta. *Radiology* 62:671–686, 1954.
5. Nora JJ, Torres FG, Sinha AK, McNamara DG. Characteristic cardiovascular anomalies of XO Turner syndrome, XX and XY phenotype and XO/XX Turner mosaic. *Am J Cardiol* 25:639–641, 1970.
6. Babbitt DP, Cassidy GE, Godard JE. Rib notching in aortic coarctation during infancy and early childhood. *Radiology* 110:169–171, 1974.
7. Rees S, Somerville J, Ward C, et al. Coarctation of the aorta: MR imaging in late postoperative assessment. *Radiology* 173:499–502, 1989.
8. Bank ER, Aisen AM, Rocchini AP, Hernandez RJ. Coarctation of the aorta in children undergoing angioplasty: pretreatment and posttreatment MR imaging. *Radiology* 162:235–240, 1987.
9. von Schulthess GK, Higashino SM, Higgins SS, Didier D, Fisher MR, Higgins CB. Coarctation of the aorta: MR imaging. *Radiology* 158:469–474, 1986.
10. Gomes AS, Lois JF, George B, Alpan G, Williams RG. Congenital abnormalities of the aortic arch: MR imaging. *Radiology* 165:691–695, 1987.
11. Amparo EG, Higgins CB, Shafton EP. Demonstration of coarctation of the aorta by magnetic resonance imaging. *Am J Roentgenol* 143:1192–1194, 1984.
12. Jaffe RB. Radiographic manifestations of congenital anomalies of the aortic arch. *Radiol Clin North Am* 29(2):319–334, 1991.
13. Bisset GS III. Magnetic resonance imaging of congenital heart disease in the pediatric patient. *Radiol Clin North Am* 29(2):279–291, 1991.
14. Burrows PE, MacDonald CE. Magnetic resonance imaging of the pediatric thoracic aorta. *Semin Ultrasound CT MR* 14(2):129–144, 1993.
15. Fletcher BD, Jacobstein MD. MRI of congenital abnormalities of the great arteries. *Am J Roentgenol* 146:941–948, 1986.
16. Woodring JH, Rhodes RA III. Posterosuperior mediastinal widening in aortic coarctation. *Am J Roentgenol* 144:23–25, 1985.
17. Poplausky MR, Haller JO. Radiological case of the month. Coarctation of the aorta. *Arch Pediatr Adolesc Med* 149:921–922, 1995.

18. Ho VB, Kinney JB, Sahn DJ. Contributions of newer MR imaging strategies for congenital heart disease. *Radiographics* 16(1):43–60, 1996.
19. Medellin GJ, DeSessa TG, Tonkin ILD. Interventional catheterization in congenital heart disease. *Radiol Clin North Am* 27(6):1223–1240, 1989.
20. Garman JE, Hinson RE, Eyler WR. Coarctation of the aorta in infancy: detection on chest radiographs. *Radiology* 85:418–422, 1965.

Case 5

Clinical Presentation

A cyanotic 15-month-old boy.

Radiographic Studies

Chest radiograph (Fig. 5A) shows a mildly enlarged heart with an upturned cardiac apex and concave main pulmonary artery segment. The pulmonary vascularity is normal to decreased. A right-sided aortic arch is present. Pulmonary arteriogram (Fig. 5B) from another patient shows a right-sided aortic arch with mirror-image branching. White arrowheads denote pulmonary infundibular stenosis, secondary to deviation of the infundibular septum. Left anterior oblique image with left ventricular injection (Fig. 5C) shows a ventricular septal defect with overriding of the aorta. Lateral view from angiogram in a third patient (Fig. 5D) shows pulmonary infundibular stenosis (arrow) to a better advantage.

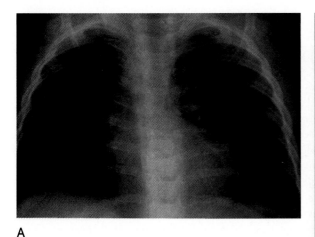

A

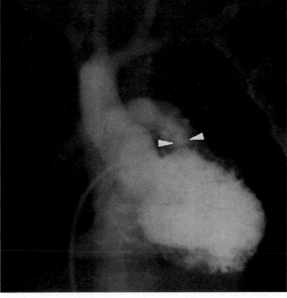

B

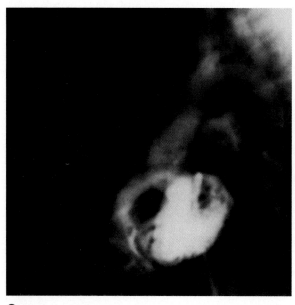

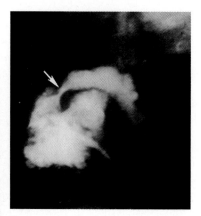

D

C

PEARLS

- Approximately 25% of patients with tetralogy of Fallot have a right arch. Right arch occurs most frequently in the patients with severe pulmonary stenosis or pulmonary atresia.[3]

- The right arch present with cyanotic heart disease is usually the mirror-image branching type that does not have a retroesophageal component by esophagram. In addition, the "mirror image" right arch of tetralogy does not have tracheal narrowing on the lateral radiograph as does the right arch associated with a vascular ring. However, tetralogy of Fallot may have a right arch with an aberrant left subclavian artery.

Diagnosis Tetralogy of Fallot

Discussion and Differential Diagnosis

The four components that make up tetralogy of Fallot consist of right ventricular outflow obstruction, subaortic ventricular septal defect, an overriding aorta, and right ventricular hypertrophy.[1]

Infundibular stenosis is the typical cause of right ventricular outflow obstruction in tetralogy of Fallot.[2] However, additional pulmonary valve abnormalities are seen in up to 90% of patients.[3] Most commonly, there is a bicuspid pulmonary valve that may also be stenotic.[1] Less commonly, the valve may be unicuspid or occasionally absent.[4] Stenosis or hypoplasia of the main pulmonary artery and/or pulmonary artery branches is also common.[1]

The classic cardiac configuration is described as boot-shaped or coeur en sabot.[1] With this configuration, the heart has an upturned cardiac apex and a concave main pulmonary artery segment. The boot-shaped configuration becomes more pronounced with greater degrees of pulmonary stenosis. The appearance is most marked in tetralogy with pulmonary atresia, also referred to as pseudotruncus or ventricular septal defect (VSD) with pulmonary atresia.

The aorta is typically enlarged with tetralogy. It is usually inversely proportional to the size of the infundibulum. Patients with a greater degree of pulmonary stenosis have more marked enlargement of the aorta. There is a right-to-left shunt across the VSD secondary to the pulmonary obstructive lesion. This causes cyanosis and decreased pulmonary arterial vascularity. The heart is usually normal in size to slightly enlarged. If it is markedly enlarged, other associated defects may be present.

• Up to 9% of patients with tetralogy will have coronary artery anomalies.[5] The most common variation in tetralogy patients is an anomalous anterior descending coronary artery that courses over the right ventricular outflow tract. It can be mistakenly ligated at surgery.[6]

PITFALLS

• Infundibular stenosis frequently progresses with advancing age.[1]

• In infants, the heart size and contour are most often normal. The classic boot-shaped heart may not be present until later childhood, adolescence, or even adulthood.[1,7,8]

• Tortuous bronchial collateral vessels, also called major aortopulmonary collateral arteries (MAPCA), may be confused for increased pulmonary vascularity.[7]

• Tetralogy with very mild pulmonary stenosis, sometimes referred to as pink tetralogy, may appear radiographically similar to a simple ventricular septal defect with increased pulmonary arterial vascularity and cardiomegaly.[7]

The differential diagnosis for a cyanotic newborn infant with normal to decreased flow without significant cardiomegaly would include transposition of the great arteries with intact ventricular septum and severe pulmonary valve obstruction, tricuspid atresia, pulmonary atresia with intact ventricular septum, and pseudotruncus. However, pulmonary atresia with intact ventricular septum usually shows cardiomegaly. Beyond infancy, as in this case, by far the most likely diagnosis would be tetralogy; other considerations—with decreased vascularity, normal-sized heart, and cyanosis—would include tricuspid atresia and pulmonary atresia with intact ventricular septum, as well as transposition with pulmonary stenosis, and single ventricle with pulmonary stenosis.

In the setting of right arch and cyanotic heart disease, two causes should come to mind—tetralogy and truncus arteriosus. Tetralogy of Fallot is much more common than truncus. In addition, tetralogy patients will have normal to decreased arterial pulmonary vascularity whereas patients with truncus more often have increased pulmonary vascularity.

Further Reading

1. Tonkin ILD, ed. *Pediatric Cardiovascular Imaging*. Philadelphia: WB Saunders Co; 1992:chap 2, 4.
2. Strife JL. Tetralogy of Fallot. *Semin Roentgenol* 20(2):160–168, 1985.
3. Amplatz K, Moller JH. *Radiology of Congenital Heart Disease*. St. Louis: Mosby Year Book; 1993: chap 30.
4. Greenberg SB, Faerber EN, Balsara RK. Tetralogy of Fallot: diagnostic imaging after palliative and corrective surgery. *J Thorac Imaging* 10(1):26–35, 1995.
5. O'Sullivan J, Bain H, Hunter S, Wren C. End-on aortogram: improved identification of important coronary artery anomalies in tetralogy of Fallot. *Br Heart J* 71:102–106, 1994.
6. White RI Jr, Frech RS, Castaneda A, Amplatz K. The nature and significance of anomalous coronary arteries in tetralogy of Fallot. *Am J Roentgenol Radium Ther Nucl Med* 114(2):350–354, 1972.
7. Walzem DE, Singleton EB. Tetralogy of Fallot: radiologic evaluation before and after surgical treatment. *Radiology* 81:760–768, 1963.
8. Elliot LP, ed. *Cardiac Imaging in Infants, Children, and Adults*. Philadelphia: JB Lippincott Co; 1991: 725–732.

Case 6

Clinical Presentation

A preterm infant with poor perfusion, respiratory distress, and muffled heart sounds.

Radiographic Studies

There is massive enlargement of the cardiac silhouette (Fig. 6A), which developed since chest radiograph of prior day (Fig. 6B).

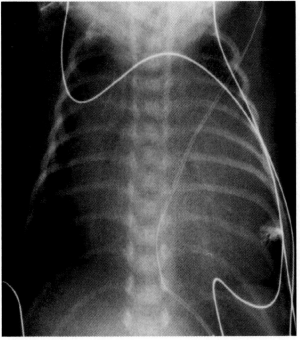

A

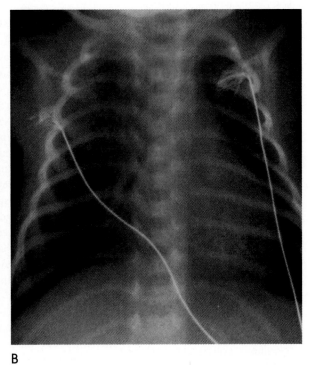

B

Diagnosis Pericardial Effusion

Discussion and Differential Diagnosis

The rapid development of massive cardiac enlargement over a short period of time without pulmonary edema makes pericardial effusion the obvious choice. On the lateral chest radiograph, if the normal pericardium is seen as a radiopaque line between the epicardial fat and pericardial fat, it should be less than 2 mm in thickness. If the pericardium appears thicker than 2 mm, a positive lateral epicardial fat pad sign is present, indicating that there is pericardial thickening or effusion.[1] Straightening of the left cardiac border on posteroanterior chest radiograph may be one of the earliest plain film findings to suggest the presence of pericardial effusion in children.[2] In some patients, widening of the subcarinal angle without other evidence of left atrial enlargement can be a clue to suggest the possibility of pericardial effusion on frontal chest radiograph.[3] Echocardiography is the standard imaging method to directly make the diagnosis of pericardial effusion. On MRI, the signal characteristic of pericardial effusion varies according to the type of fluid. Simple fluid (transudate) is low signal intensity on T1- and high signal intensity on T2-weighted images. Proteinaceous or hemorrhagic pericardial effusions often have areas of high or medium signal intensity on T1-weighted images.[4] CT can also show characteristic signs of pericardial effusion. Pericardial effusion is a frequent finding in patients who have undergone total correction of congenital heart disease.

Without a prior normal chest radiograph, and clinical history suggestive of pericardial effusion, a differential diagnosis of marked cardiomegaly should be considered. With a pericardial effusion, the heart appears enlarged, but the pulmonary vasculature is not increased or engorged. In the neonatal period, cardiomegaly and heart failure can be caused by left ventricular outflow lesions such as hypoplastic left heart, severe coarctation, or critical aortic stenosis, or by large shunt lesions such as vein of Galen aneurysm, hemangioendothelioma, large ventricular septal defect, or large patent ductus arteriosus. In those conditions, there will be pulmonary venous congestion or increased pulmonary arterial vascularity. In an older infant, some additional causes of generalized cardiomegaly and heart failure would include cardiomyopathy, infant of a diabetic mother, endocardial fibroelastosis, or an anomalous origin of coronary arteries from the pulmonary trunk. In addition, Ebstein's anomaly can cause massive cardiomegaly in the newborn. However, the patient should have a history of cyanosis with this degree of cardiomegaly. The pericardial effusion in this case was caused by central line placement. The most common causes of pericardial effusion are uremia, postviral pericarditis, and malignancy.[1] Other causes include trauma, congestive heart failure, myxedema, Dressler syndrome, collagen vascular disease, tuberculosis sarcoidosis, and bacterial pericarditis.[1]

PEARLS

- The epicardial fat pad can be seen on frontal chest radiograph in up to 20% of patients with pericardial effusion.[1]

- The heart appears enlarged, but the pulmonary vasculature is not engorged or increased in face of a pericardial effusion.

PITFALLS

- The classic water bottle configuration of the heart may not be seen unless the pericardial effusion is massive.

- The fat pad sign is often not seen in children with pericardial effusion.[2]

CONTROVERSY

- Some authors have discussed a differential density sign of pericardial effusion whereby the effusion can be seen as a band of less radiopaque density on PA and lateral chest radiographs,[5] whereas others attribute this appearance simply to the epicardial fat pad.[6]

Further Reading

1. Carsky EW, Mauceri RA, Azimi F. The epicardial fat pad sign. *Radiology* 137:303–308, 1980.
2. Stolz JL, Borns P, Schwade J. The pediatric pericardium. *Radiology* 112:159–165, 1974.
3. Chen JTT, Putman CE, Hedlund LW, Dahmash NS, Roberts L. Widening of the subcarinal angle by pericardial effusion. *Am J Roentgenol* 139:883–887, 1982.
4. White CS. MR evaluation of the pericardium and cardiac malignancies. *Magn Reson Imaging Clin N Am* 4(2):237–251, 1996.
5. Tehranzadeh J, Kelley MJ. The differential density sign of pericardial effusion. *Radiology* 133:23–30, 1979.
6. Torrance DJ. Demonstration of subepicardial fat as an aid in the diagnosis of pericardial effusion thickening. *Am J Roentgenol* 24(5):850–855, 1955.

Case 7

Clinical Presentation

A noncyanotic infant.

Radiographic Studies

The patient has cardiomegaly and prominent pulmonary arterial vascularity (Fig. 7A). Only 11 pairs of ribs are present. Two manubrial ossification centers (arrows) can be seen (Fig. 7B). The upper lumbar vertebral bodies appear tall (Fig. 7B). They have a narrow anteroposterior diameter and a straight anterior margin on the lateral image of the chest. Radiograph of the left acetabulum shows a decreased acetabular index (Fig. 7C).

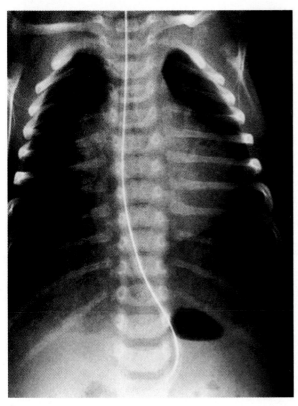

A

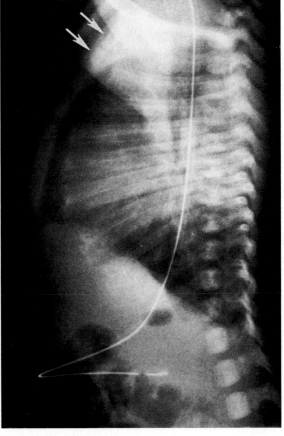

B

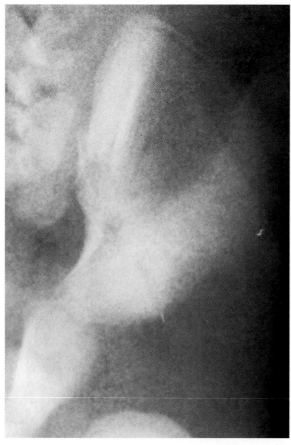

C

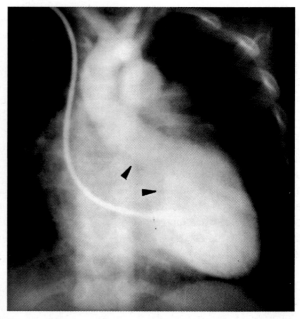

D

Diagnosis Down Syndrome with Atrioventricular (AV) Canal

Discussion and Differential Diagnosis

Approximately 40% of infants with Down syndrome will have associated congenital heart disease.[1] There is debate in the literature concerning the most common lesion associated with Down syndrome. Some authors claim ventricular septal defect (VSD) is more common than AV septal defect; others report AV canal is more common.[1–4] Other cardiac defects less frequently seen with Down syndrome include secundum type of atrial septal defect, tetralogy of Fallot, inlet type or posterior VSD, secundum atrial septal defect (ASD), and patent ductus.[3]

Persistent AV canal may be divided into complete, transitional or intermediate, and partial types.[3,5] With all three types, there is a defect in the inferior atrial septum (ostium primum type of atrial septal defect).[4] In addition, abnormalities of the tricuspid and mitral valves are usually present.[6] With complete AV canal, there is a contiguous defect involving the inferior atrial septum and the ventricular septum.

- Prominent conoid process of the clavicle has been recently described as roentgenologic finding seen in Down patients.[15]

PITFALLS

- Shunt vascularity in AV canal and ventriculoseptal defect may not be radiographically evident in the early neonatal period secondary to the high pulmonary artery pressures seen in the first few days of life.

- Decreased acetabular angles can also be seen in normal infants and in achondroplasia and Ellis-van Creveld syndrome.[10]

The mitral and tricuspid valves are at least partially fused with common anterior and common posterior leaflets. Complete AV canal can be further classified according to the degree of cleavage of the common leaflets and the manner in which they are or are not attached.[6] In the transitional type of AV canal, there is a bridge of tissue between the anterior and posterior atrioventricular valve leaflets.[3,5] The bridge of tissue is attached by short cordae tendonae to the ventricular septum creating a smaller interventricular communication than seen in complete AV canal.[5] In partial AV canal, also referred to as ostium primum atrioseptal defect, there are two distinct atrioventricular valves and valve rings.[5] There is an anomalous attachment of the anterior mitral leaflet to a deficient interventricular septum, which functionally prevents communication between the two ventricles.[5] There may be an associated cleft in the anterior mitral valve leaflet, which can result in mitral regurgitation.[7]

The most evident radiographic findings include cardiac enlargement and increased pulmonary arterial vascularity. Careful analysis of plain radiographs often will reveal additional findings suggesting the diagnosis of Down syndrome. Approximately 30% of trisomy 21 patients have 11 rib pairs compared to only 5% of non–trisomy 21 patients.[8] This finding is more common in girls.[9] Eighty percent of infants with trisomy 21 have multiple manubrial ossification centers; only 10% of non–trisomy 21 newborns have multiple manubrial ossification centers.[8] In infants, characteristic findings seen in the pelvis include flattening of the lower edges of the ilium with a reduced acetabular angle and widening and flaring of the iliac wings.[10] Abnormally tall lumbar vertebral bodies with reduced anteroposterior diameter in children under 2 years of age is an additional roentgenologic sign that suggests the diagnosis of Down syndrome.[11] In addition, the anterior margin of the lumbar vertebral bodies tends to be abnormally straight or may have increased concavity as opposed to the bullet-shaped or anteriorly convex anterior lumbar vertebral margin, which is often seen in small infants.[11] At angiography, the extent and degree of left to right shunting should be evaluated. In addition, a classic finding seen with AV canal in the frontal projection is the gooseneck deformity of the left ventricular outflow tract[6,12,13] (Fig. 7D, case courtesy of C. Joseph Chang, MD, Kansas City, Kansas).

The differential diagnosis for a noncyanotic infant with biventricular cardiomegaly and increased pulmonary arterial vascularity would include ventriculoseptal defect, atrioventricular canal, left ventricle right atrial communication, the noncyanotic type of double outlet right ventricle, and patent ductus. Patent ductus should cause primarily left heart enlargement. However, the prominent thymus in the newborn period makes evaluation for right heart enlargement on the lateral chest radiograph difficult. With right heart enlargement and increased pulmonary arterial vascularity in a noncyanotic patient, the primary considerations would include atrioseptal defect and partial AV canal without significant mitral regurgitation.

Further Reading

1. Rowe RD, Uchida IA. Cardiac malformation in mongolism: a prospective study of 184 mongoloid children. *Am J Med* 31:726–735, 1961.
2. Greenwood RD, Nadas AS. The clinical course of cardiac disease in Down's syndrome. *Pediatrics* 58(6):893–897, 1976.

3. Spicer RL. Cardiovascular disease in Down syndrome. *Pediatr Clin North Am* 31(6):1331–1343, 1984.

4. Tandon R, Edwards JE. Cardiac malformations associated with Down's syndrome. *Circulation* 47:1349–1355, 1973.

5. Elliott LP. Pathophysiology and roentgenologic findings in persistent common atrioventricular canal. In: Elliot LP, ed. *Cardiac Imaging in Infants, Children, and Adults.* Philadelphia: JB Lippincott Co; 1991:612–618.

6. Towbin R, Schwartz D. Endocardial cushion defects: embrology, anatomy, and angiography. *AJR Am J Roentgenol* 136:157–162, 1981.

7. Amplatz K, Moller JH, eds. *Radiology of Congenital Heart Disease.* St. Louis: Mosby Year Book; 1993:365–394.

8. Edwards DK III, Berry CC, Hilton SvW. Trisomy 21 in newborn infants: chest radio-graphic diagnosis. *Radiology* 167:317–318, 1988.

9. Beber BA, Litt RE, Altman DH. A new radiographic finding in mongolism. *Radiology* 86:332–333, 1966.

10. Caffey J, Ross S. Pelvic bones in infantile mongoloidism: roentgenographic features. *Am J Roentgenol* 80(3):458–467, 1958.

11. Rabinowitz JG, Moseley JE. The lateral lumbar spine in Down's syndrome: a new roentgen feature. *Radiology* 83:74–79, 1964.

12. Schwartz DC. Atrioventricular septal defects. *Semin Roentgenol* 20(3):226–235, 1985.

13. Tonkin ILD, ed. *Pediatric Cardiovascular Imaging.* Philadelphia: WB Saunders Co; 1992:83–176.

14. Kliewer MA, Hertzberg BS, Freed KS, et al. Dysmorphologic features of the fetal pelvis in Down syndrome: prenatal sonographic depiction and diagnostic implications of the iliac angle. *Radiology* 201:681–684, 1996.

15. Weinberg B, Maldjian C, Kass EG, Himelstein ES. The prominent conoid process of the clavicle: a new radiographic sign in Down's syndrome. *Am J Roentgenol* 160:591–592, 1993.

Case 8

Clinical Presentation

A noncyanotic 2-month-old infant with a murmur.

Radiographic Studies

Posteroanterior chest radiograph shows cardiomegaly and arterial shunt vascularity (Fig. 8A). On the lateral chest radiograph (Fig. 8B), there is filling in of the retrosternal air space suggesting right ventricular enlargement. The posterior inferior heart border is prominent, suggesting left ventricular enlargement. The left atrium also appears enlarged on the lateral view. Left ventricular angiogram from another patient shows perimembranous right ventricular contrast (Fig. 8C).

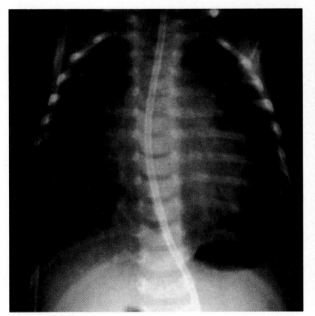

A

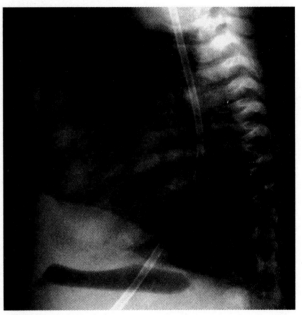

B

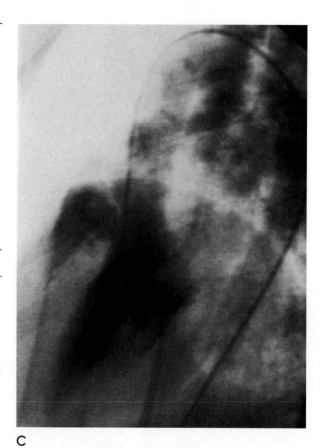

C

Diagnosis Ventricular Septal Defect (VSD)

Discussion and Differential Diagnosis

Isolated VSD is the most common form of congenital heart disease, excluding bicuspid aortic valve. It represents 20 to 30% of congenital heart disease.[1–3] In addition, VSD occurs as a component of many types of complex congenital heart diseases including transposition of the great vessels, tricuspid atresia, tetralogy of Fallot, persistent truncus arteriosus, double outlet right ventricle, single ventricle, and interruption of the aortic arch. VSD also coexists with a patent ductus or coarctation in a significant number of patients.[2]

The reported incidence of VSD has progressively increased with time.[4] The reported estimates ranged from approximately 2 per 1000 live births in 1941 up to 5.7 per 1000 live births in 1992.[4] One recent study with echocardiac screening of 1053 consecutively born neonates found muscular ventricular septal defects in 53 per 1000 live births.[5] However, approximately 90% of the lesions in this study closed spontaneously within 10 months.[5] The increasing rates are thought to be secondary to increased detection.[4–6] VSD has also been found to be more prevalent in premature infants.[7]

Ventricular septal defects can be divided into several types. The nomenclature varies somewhat among authors.[8] Classically, VSD has been divided into membranous or perimembranous, muscular, anterior conal or malalignment supracrystal, and atrioventricular canal types.[9] Membranous or perimembranous (Fig. 8C) and muscular VSDs are the most common types of isolated VSD.[7,10] A significant percentage of membranous and muscular VSDs will close spontaneously, most before the age of two.[11] Muscular VSDs spontaneously close more frequently than membranous VSDs.[11] Smaller lesions close more frequently than larger lesions.[11]

The plain film radiographic findings depend primarily on the size of the defect and the pulmonary vascular resistance. Patients with small VSDs have normal chest radiographs. With large VSDs and normal pulmonary vascular resistance, the heart appears enlarged. Usually there is biventricular and left atrial enlargement. There is prominent arterial shunt vascularity and prominence of the main pulmonary artery. The aortic knob should appear small to normal but not enlarged as in patent ductus arteriosus.

Echocardiography is the preferred method for evaluation of ventricular septal defect. However, cardiac gated spin echo MRI has been found to be 86 to 100% sensitive and 90% specific in the evaluation of VSDs, which is closely comparable to the sensitivity and specificity of echocardiography.[12] In addition, gated cine MRI can detect the turbulent flow of even very small VSDs and can provide quantification of the degree of shunting.[13,14]

The differential diagnosis for a noncyanotic patient with increased arterial pulmonary vascularity and biventricular and left atrial enlargement would include VSD, atrioventricular canal and left ventricular right atrial communication. Patent ductus typically causes only left ventricular and left atrial enlargement. However, the large amount of thymic tissue filling in the retrosternal tissue on the lateral chest radiograph in infants may give the appearance of right ventricular enlargement. Therefore, in infants, patent ductus arteriosus should be included in this differential. Atrial septal defect gives primarily right heart enlargement. In addition, the left atrium should not be enlarged with atrial septal defect as it can decompress through the defect.

Further Reading

1. Soto B, Bargeron LM Jr, Diethelm E. Ventricular septal defect. *Semin Roentgenol* 20(3):200–213, 1985.
2. Amplatz K, Moller JH. *Radiology of Congenital Heart Disease.* St. Louis: Mosby Year Book; 1993:243–272.
3. Spindola-Franco H, Fish BG. *Radiology of the Heart.* New York: Springer-Verlag; 1985:342–357.
4. Mehta AV, Chidambaram B. Ventricular septal defect in the first year of life. *Am J Cardiol* 70:364–366, 1992.
5. Roguin N, Du Z-D, Barak M, Nasser N, Hershkowitz S, Milgram E. High prevalence of muscular ventricular septal defect in neonates. *J Am Coll Cardiol* 26:1545–1548, 1995.

6. Martin GR, Perry LW, Ferencz C. Increased prevalence of ventricular septal defect: epidemic or improved diagnosis. *Pediatrics* 83(2):200–203, 1989.

7. Moe DG, Guntheroth WG. Spontaneous closure of uncomplicated ventricular septal defect. *Am J Cardiol* 60:674–678, 1987.

8. Van Praagh R, Kreutzer J. Ventricular septal defects: How shall we describe, name and classify them? *J Am Coll Cardiol* 14(5):1298–1299, 1989.

9. Tonkin ILD, ed. *Pediatric Cardiovascular Imaging.* Philadelphia: WB Saunders Co; 1992:83–176.

10. Ramaciotti C, Vetter JM, Bornemeier RA, Chin AJ. Prevalence, relation to spontaneous closure, and association of muscular ventricular septal defects with other cardiac defects. *Am J Cardiol* 75:61–65, 1995.

11. Shirali GS, O'Brian Smith E, Geva T. Quantitation of echocardiographic predictors of outcome in infants with isolated ventricular septal defect. *Am Heart J* 130:1228–1235, 1995.

12. Elliott LP. *Cardiac Imaging in Infants, Children, and Adults.* Philadelphia: JB Lippincott Co; 1991:565–584.

13. Sechtem U, Pflugfelder P, Cassidy MC, Holt W, Wolfe C, Higgins CB. Ventricular septal defect: visualization of shunt flow and determination of shunt size by cine MR imaging. *Am J Roentgenol* 149:689–692, 1987.

14. Ho VB, Kinney JB, Sahn DJ. Contributions of newer MR imaging strategies for congenital heart disease. *Radiographics* 16(1):43–60, 1996.

15. Coussement AM, Gooding CA. Objective radiographic assessment of pulmonary vascularity in children. *Radiology* 109:649–654, 1973.

Case 9

Clinical Presentation

A newborn with grunting and respiratory distress.

Radiographic Studies

Anteroposterior (AP) chest radiograph (Fig. 9A) reveals cardiomegaly with the heart apex on the left, increased pulmonary vascularity, and a right-sided stomach. Transverse ultrasound of the upper abdomen (Fig. 9B) shows a transverse liver. CT of the abdomen (Fig. 9C) from a different patient with a liver transplant for biliary atresia reveals absence of the hepatic portion of the inferior vena cava (IVC), a prominent azygos vein (white arrowhead), and multiple splenules (white arrows). Digital subtraction arteriogram (Fig. 9D) from a right heart catheterization in another patient shows an azygos vein the size of a normal IVC that crosses the midline in the chest to empty into the SVC. Technetium sulfur colloid imaging reveals absence of the spleen in a different patient (Fig. 9E).

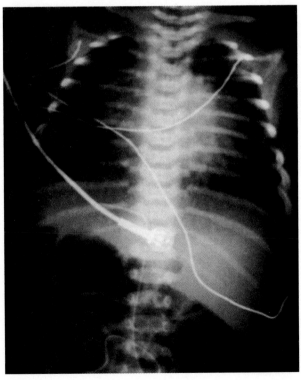

A

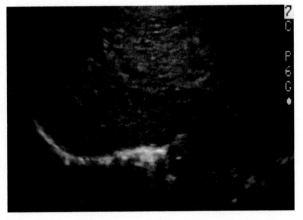

B

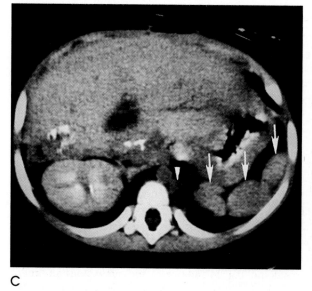

C

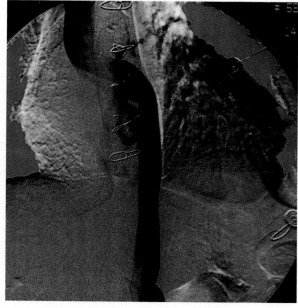

D

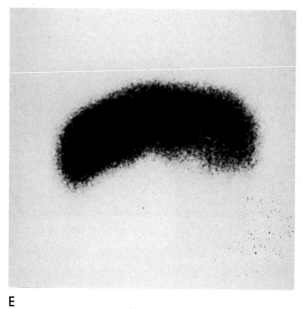

E

Diagnosis Asplenia/Polysplenia

Discussion and Differential Diagnosis

Situs ambiguous is a condition in which the atria and viscera have an inconsistent relationship and asymmetric structures become symmetric.[1] Polysplenia is one of the isomeric syndromes with bilateral left-sidedness. Its sister syndrome is asplenia or bilateral right-sidedness. In polysplenia, the anomalies involve the heart, the lungs, the systemic venous system, the liver and biliary system, and the GI tract. The cardiac disease in polysplenia is less common and less severe than with asplenia. The common cardiac anomalies include atrial septal defect, ventricular septal defect and partial anomalous pulmonary venous return with shunt vascularity usually present. The major extracardiac anomalies are interruption of the IVC with azygos or hemiazygos continuation, bilateral SVC, hepatic symmetry and multiple splenules. Two bilobed lungs are noted with bilateral hyparterial bronchi.

The diagnosis of polysplenia can be inferred on a posteroanterior (PA) and lateral chest radiograph. Radiographic findings in addition to situs ambiguous on the PA radiograph include equal length of the major bronchi, which appear to be two left main bronchi, no minor fissure, and widening of the paravertebral stripe due to a dilated azygos or hemiazygos vein. In addition, on the lateral view, absence of the IVC is noted along with an abnormal bronchus to pulmonary artery relationship with both major bronchi inferior and anterior to the right and left pulmonary arteries.[2] Ultrasound (US) of the abdomen is key in these patients and is an excellent noninvasive way to evaluate the abdominal vessels prior to heart catheterization.[1,3] With US, the liver and spleen are easily evaluated for symmetry (Fig. 9B), absence, and multiplicity as well as for associated biliary atresia[4] (Fig. 9C). The abdominal findings can also be seen with CT and MRI. Splenic scintigraphy and radionuclide venography with ^{99m}Tc sulfur colloid is used to evaluate IVC anomalies and to look for splenic abnormalities.[5] If further evaluation of the spleen is needed, dual radiopharmaceutical imaging can be performed with ^{99m}Tc-labeled IDA derivatives (DISIDA, mebrofenin) and sulfur colloid.[6] The image of the liver with DISIDA or mebrofenin can be subtracted from a sulfur colloid liver/spleen scan to optimally show the spleen. Technetium[99m] sulfur colloid SPECT imaging has also proven useful in finding splenic tissue not seen on planar sulfur colloid liver/spleen imaging.[7] Sulfur colloid scan with SPECT imaging can also demonstrate multiple spleens.[7]

The main item in the differential diagnosis of a patient with situs ambiguous and polysplenia is asplenia. Asplenia more often presents in the male newborn with severe cyanotic heart disease. The patient has no spleen in this bilateral right-sidedness disease (Fig. 7E). Howell-Jolly bodies may be present later because of the asplenia. The mortality is high because of the severe heart disease. All patients with asplenia have a common atrium, 50% have single ventricle, and 75% have transposition of the great vessels, usually with pulmonic stenosis and anomalous pulmonary venous return. The IVC and aorta are on the same side of the spine, whereas in polysplenia, the IVC/aorta relationship is usually normal. In asplenia, the lungs usually have decreased vascularity; in polysplenia, there is increased vascularity. The patient with asplenia has bilateral eparterial bronchi and bilateral minor fissures. In both, the liver is usually symmetrical and malrotation is almost always present.

Further Reading

1. Tonkin ILD, Tonkin AK. Visceroatrial situs abnormalities: sonographic and computed tomographic appearance. *Am J Roentgenol* 138:509–515, 1982.
2. Soto B, Pacifico AD, Souza AS Jr, Bargeron LM Jr, Ermocilla R, Tonkin IL. Identification of thoracic isomerism from the plain chest radiograph. *Am J Roentgenol* 131:995–1002.
3. Oleszczuk-Raschke K, Set PA, von Lengerke HJ, Tröger J. Abdominal sonography in the evaluation of heterotaxy in children. *Pediatr Radiol* 25:S150–S156, 1995.
4. Freedom RM, Treves S. Splenic scintigraphy and radionuclide venography in the heterotaxy syndrome. *Radiology* 107:381–386, 1973.
5. Abramson SJ, Berdon WE, Altman RP, Amodia JB, Levy J. Biliary atresia and noncardiac polysplenic syndrome: US and surgical considerations. *Radiology* 163:377–3791, 1987.
6. Rao BK, Shore RM, Lieberman LM, Polcyn RE. Dual radiopharmaceutical imaging in congenital asplenia syndrome. *Radiology* 145:805–810, 1982.
7. Oates E, Austin JM, Becker JL. Technetium-99m-sulfur colloid SPECT imaging in infants with suspected heterotaxy syndrome. *J Nucl Med* 36:1368–1371, 1995.
8. Amplatz K, Moller JH. *Radiology of Congenital Heart Disease.* St. Louis: Mosby Year Book; 1993:945–976.

Case 10

Clinical Presentation

Screening obstetrical ultrasound with cardiac abnormality.

Radiographic Studies

Axial images of the heart from prenatal ultrasound (Fig. 10A) and ultrasound images of the heart performed following delivery (Fig. 10B) show a single large echogenic mass involving the ventricular septum (arrow) as well as multiple smaller echogenic masses involving other portions of the myocardium (arrowheads). MR imaging with coronal T1-weighted (Fig. 10C) and coronal T2-weighted (Fig. 10D) images of the heart from another infant with the same diagnosis show a large cardiac mass. The mass is isointense to cardiac muscle on the T1-weighted image and hyperintense to cardiac muscle on the T2-weighted image. (Case reprinted with permission from *AJDC*, April 1991.)

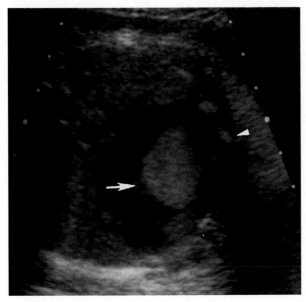

A

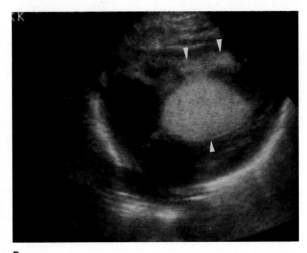

B

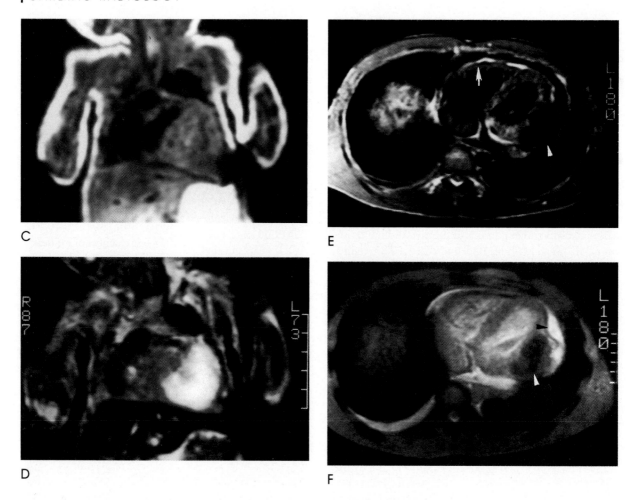

C

E

D

F

Diagnosis Cardiac Tumor (Rhabdomyoma)

Discussion and Differential Diagnosis

Three fourths of all primary cardiac tumors are benign.[1] When all age groups are considered, atrial myxoma is the most common intracardiac tumor and accounts for 50% of intracardiac tumors.[1,2] Rhabdomyoma represents only 8% of all cardiac neoplasms[3] and is only the fifth most common cardiac neoplasm.[3] However, rhabdomyoma is the most common cardiac tumor of fetal life,[4] infancy,[5] and childhood.[6] Fibromas are the second most common cardiac tumors in children.[7] Rhabdomyoma occurs three times more frequently in infants and children than does fibroma or teratoma.[8]

Fifty-one to 86% of cardiac rhabdomyomas are associated with TS.[9] The classic clinical triad of TS consists of seizures, mental retardation, and adenoma sebaceum.[10] Only 29% of patients display the classic triad.[10] Neurologic manifestations of TS include subependymal nodules,[11] cortical hamartomas, and giant cell astrocytoma.

<hr>

PEARLS

- Rhabdomyomas are usually echogenic on ultrasound.[12]

- Males predominate among patients with tuberous sclerosis (TS) and rhabdomyomas.[5]

Cutaneous lesions are present in 96% of TS patients.[11] Skin findings include adenoma sebaceum, hypopigmented ash leaf patches, shagreen rough skin patches, ungual fibromas, and fibrous plaques of the scalp.[11] Multiple cysts and angiomyolipomas occur in the kidneys.[11] The angiomyolipomas have a propensity to bleed.[11] Lung disease similar to lymphangiomyomatosis occurs in approximately 1% of patients with TS.[11] Retinal hamartomas called phakomas are seen in the eye in approximately 50% of patients. Sclerotic bone lesions may be seen in the pelvis, skull, and lumbar spine.[11] The typical signs of TS—including pale ash leaf skin spots, adenoma sebaceum, and periventricular hamartomatous gliomas of the brain—are usually absent in infancy.[12]

Rhabdomyomas of the heart are histologically benign lesions. They most commonly arise from the interventricular septum and adjacent ventricular walls.[4] Rhabdomyomas are usually multiple (90%).[4] Sixty-eight to 86% of patients with rhabdomyomas have multiple tumors involving more than one chamber of the heart.[9]

Fetal arrhythmia is the most frequent prenatal manifestation of cardiac rhabdomyoma.[9] It is also the most common reason for getting a prenatal ultrasound.[9] The masses typically appear echogenic as compared to the adjacent myocardium. Fetal hydrops may be an associated finding.[8]

The rhabdomyomas regress[5] and/or completely resolve[4] in 70 to 80% of patients seen before the age of four.[4,5] However, tumor regression occurs in only 17% of patients seen after the age of four.[5] Some authors suggest that the spontaneous regression of rhabdomyomas is related to the removal of maternal hormonal stimulation.[8]

Because a large percentage of rhabdomyomas spontaneously regress with time, surgery is usually indicated only for patients with life-threatening symptoms.[3,6] Surgery is indicated for tumors that significantly obstruct blood flow or cause significant valvular insufficiency.[3,13] When there are multiple tumors, only the symptomatic masses need be resected.[3] In addition, complete resection is not necessary. Only the obstructing portion of the tumor need be resected.[3] Surgery is also indicated for patients with arrhythmias that are refractory to medical management.[3,13] In patients with life-threatening symptoms, mortality is high.

When evaluating a mass in or around the heart by MR, it is important to perform both T1- and T2-weighted imaging sequences to characterize the mass. Fat suppression techniques or gradient echo sequences are also helpful in characterizing cardiac masses and distinguishing a solid mass from cardiac thrombus. The signal intensity of rhabdomyomas is reported to be high[14–17] or isointense on T2-weighted images as compared to that of normal myocardium.[17] Cardiac masses may enhance following gadolinium administration.[18,19] The signal intensity of fibroma is reported to be lower than that of normal myocardium, consistent with fibrous tissue.[15] A fat-suppressed axial T1-weighted MR image (Fig. 10E) shows a low signal fibroma (arrowhead) arising from the posterior wall of the left ventricle. An associated low signal intensity pericardial effusion causes posterior displacement of high signal intensity epicardial fat (arrow, Fig. 10E). A T2*-weighted axial MR image (Fig. 10F) shows the low signal fibroma (white arrowhead) and an associated high signal pericardial effusion (black arrowhead). The fibroma is lower in signal compared to myocardium on both the T1- and T2-weighted images.

The differential diagnosis for cardiac masses in a child would include rhabdomyoma, fibroma, myxoma, teratoma, or possible thrombus. Teratomas may be cystic and should be epicardial in location,[8,20] whereas rhabdomyomas usually extend into the cardiac chambers and have an extracavitory origin. Myxomas are ordinarily intracavitary. In addition, myxomas are rarely seen in children and are not seen in infants.[8] Multiple cardiac tumors in young children most likely represent rhabdomyomas because other cardiac tumors such as fibromas and myxomas are invariably solitary and are less common in childhood.[4]

Further Reading

1. Reynen K. Frequency of primary tumors of the heart. *Am J Cardiol* 77:107, 1996.
2. Go RT, O'Donnell JK, Underwood DA, et al. Comparison of gated cardiac MRI and 2D echocardiography of intracardiac neoplasms. *Am J Roentgenol* 145:221–225, 1985.
3. Jacobs JP, Konstantakos AK, Holland FW II, Herskowitz K, Ferrer PL, Perryman RA. Surgical treatment for cardiac rhabdomyomas in children. *Ann Thorac Surg* 58:1552–1555, 1994.
4. Seki I, Singh AD, Longo S. Pathological case of the month. Congenital cardiac rhabdomyoma. *Arch Pediatr Adolesc Med* 150:877–878, 1996.
5. Nir A, Tajik AJ, Freeman WK, et al. Tuberous sclerosis and cardiac rhabdomyoma. *Am J Cardiol* 76:419–421, 1995.
6. Smythe JF, Dyck JD, Smallhorn JF, Freedom RM. Natural history of cardiac rhabdomyoma in infancy and childhood. *Am J Cardiol* 66:1247–1249, 1990.
7. Abushaban L, Denham B, Duff D. 10 year review of cardiac tumours in childhood. *Br Heart J* 70:166–169, 1993.
8. Groves AMM, Fagg NLK, Cook AC, Allan LD. Cardiac tumours in intrauterine life. *Arch Dis Child* 67:1189–1192, 1992.
9. Harding CO, Pagon RA. Incidence of tuberous sclerosis in patients with cardiac rhabdomyoma. *Am J Med Genet* 37:443–446, 1990.
10. Menor F, Marti-Bomati L, Mulas F, Poyatos C, Cortina H. Neuroimaging in tuberous sclerosis: a clinicoradiological evaluation in pediatric patients. *Pediatr Radiol* 22:485–489, 1992.
11. Bell DG, King BF, Hattery RR, Charboneau JW, Hoffman AD, Houser OW. Imaging characteristics of tuberous sclerosis. *Am J Roentgenol* 156:1081–1086, 1991.
12. Deeg LH, Voigt HJ, Hofbeck M, Singer H, Kraus J. Prenatal ultrasound diagnosis of multiple cardiac rhabdomyomas. *Pediatr Radiol* 20:291–292, 1990.
13. Mühler EG, Turniski-Harder V, Engelhardt W, von Bernuth G. Cardiac involvement in tuberous sclerosis. *Br Heart J* 72:584–590, 1994.
14. Cohen MD, Edwards MK. *Magnetic Resonance Imaging of Children.* Philadelphia: BC Decker, 1990:575–584.
15. Winkler M, Higgins CB. Suspected intracardiac masses: evaluation with MR imaging. *Radiology* 165:117–122, 1987.

16. Allison JW, Stephenson CA, Angtuaco TL, Glasier CM, Wood BP. Radiological case of the month. Tuberous sclerosis with myocardial and central nervous system involvement at birth. *Am J Dis Child* 145:471–472, 1991.

17. Rienmüller R, Lloret JL, Tiling R, et al. MR imaging of pediatric cardiac tumors previously diagnosed by echocardiography. *J Comput Assist Tomogr* 13(4):621–626, 1989.

18. White CS. MR evaluation of the pericardium and cardiac malignancies. *Magn Reson Imaging Clin N Am* 4(2):237–251, 1996.

19. Smelka RC. Cardiac masses: signal intensity features on spin echo gradient echo gadolinium enhanced spin echo and turbo flash imaging. *J Magn Reson Imaging* 2:415–420, 1992.

20. Freedberg RS, Kronzon I, Rumancik WM, Liebeskind D. The contribution of magnetic resonance imaging to the evaluation of intracardiac tumors diagnosed by echocardiography. *Circulation* 77(1):96–103, 1988.

21. Smith HC, Watson GH, Patel RG, Super M. Cardiac rhabdomyomata in tuberous sclerosis: their course and diagnostic value. *Arch Dis Child* 64:196–200, 1989.

Case 11

Clinical Presentation

An 8-month-old boy with history of repeated attacks of respiratory distress. The patient had been refractory to treatment with bronchodilators at another hospital.

Radiographic Studies

Frontal chest radiograph (Fig. 11A) shows a right-sided impression on the trachea (arrowhead). The aortic arch descends on the left. Lateral esophagram (Fig. 11B) shows a focal anterior impression on the esophagus caused by a mass interposed between the trachea and the esophagus. Pulmonary arteriogram (Fig. 11C) shows the left pulmonary artery originates from the right pulmonary artery. Coronal and axial cardiac gated MR images in another patient display similar findings (case courtesy of Lane F. Donnelly, MD, Cincinnati, Ohio). On the coronal T1-weighted scan (Fig. 11D), the left pulmonary artery (arrow) abuts a narrowed right mainstem bronchus and narrowed distal trachea. Axial T1-weighted MR images (Figs. 11E, 11F) show the left pulmonary artery (arrow) passing to the right of and posterior to the trachea before coursing toward the left lung.

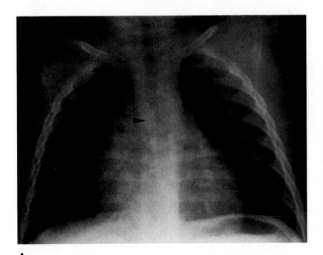

A

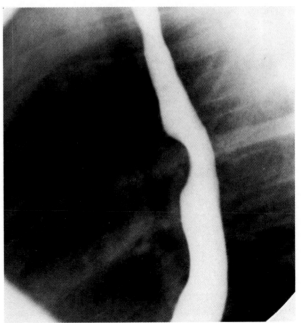

B

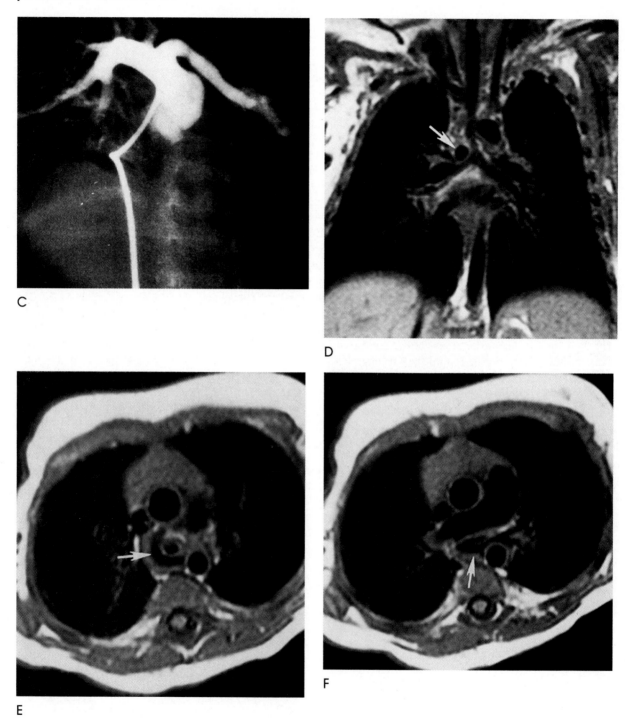

Diagnosis Pulmonary Sling

Discussion and Differential Diagnosis

Pulmonary artery sling is a rare vascular anomaly. With this anomaly, the left pulmonary artery arises from the posterior aspect of the right pulmonary artery. The vessel courses posteriorly over the right mainstem bronchus and then leftward between the trachea and esophagus. The left pulmonary artery then courses inferiorly and enters the hilum at a slightly lower position than normal.[1] The anomalous vessel often compresses the right side of the trachea and right mainstem bronchus. In addition, the ligamentum arteriosum or a patent ductus may nearly complete the vascular ring surrounding the trachea on its left side.[2]

Associated tracheobronchial abnormalities are extremely common with left pulmonary artery sling and occur in over 50% of patients.[3] Reported abnormalities of the tracheobronchial tree include compression of the lower trachea or main bronchi by the aberrant left pulmonary artery, tracheomalacia, tracheal stenosis, complete tracheal cartilaginous rings, and anomalous branching of the airway.[4] Complete cartilaginous tracheal rings with absence of the normal pars membranacea is sometimes referred to as a napkin ring trachea.[4] There is often a long segment of airway stenosis when complete tracheal rings are present. The stenosed segment is often much longer than the area compressed upon by the left pulmonary artery sling. Some authors have labeled the association of complete cartilaginous rings and pulmonary sling the "ring-sling" syndrome.[5]

One of the frequent branching anomalies associated with pulmonary sling is referred to as a bridging bronchus.[4] With this malformation, the right upper lobe of the lung is supplied by the right main bronchus, and the right middle and lower lobes are supplied by a bridging bronchus. The bridging bronchus originates from the left main bronchus and crosses to the right mediastinum forming a "pseudocarina."[4] Radiographically, the pseudocarina appears low, occurring at the T6–7 vertebral level. In children under 2 years of age, the carina is usually not lower than approximately T4–5.[4] In addition, the pseudocarina appears abnormally splayed, having an inverted T shape.[4] The left pulmonary artery sling crosses at the level of the pseudocarina and there is typically a long segment of tracheal hypoplasia between the bronchus supplying the right upper lobe and the pseudocarina.[4]

When an airway originates directly from the trachea to supply the right upper lobe, this bronchus has been previously referred to as bronchus suis, pig bronchus, tracheal accessory, or preeparterial bronchus.[4] It can occur with a normal bifurcation or in the presence of the bridging bronchus.[4]

Left pulmonary artery sling has recently been classified into two types with additional subtypes.[4,6] Type I left pulmonary artery sling has a normal carina with airway narrowing usually caused by compression from the anomalous left pulmonary artery.[4,6] Type II left pulmonary artery sling has an anomalous right bridging bronchus or pseudocarina, a long segment of tracheobronchial stenosis, and a low left pulmonary artery sling.[4,6] The two types are then further characterized according to the presence or absence of direct bronchial supply to the right upper lobe originating from the trachea. Types Ia and IIa both have a right upper lobe bronchus originating from the trachea. Types Ib and IIb do not have a tracheal origin of the right upper lobe bronchus.[4,6]

Approximately 50% of patients with pulmonary sling also have other cardiovascular anomalies.[3] Most commonly, the other anomalies include persistent left superior vena cava and ventricular septal defect.[7] However, most congenital heart defects have been reported.[8] Most patients present with severe respiratory distress in the first year of life, often in the first few months.[9] Very few patients will present after the age of two.[4] Among symptomatic infants, mortality approaches 90% without surgical intervention.[7]

Radiographically, patients with pulmonary sling often have altered pulmonary aeration involving primarily the right lung with findings including both obstructive emphysema or, less commonly, atelectasis.[10] Classically, there is hyperaeration of the right lung. If a tracheal bronchus is present, atelectasis may involve primarily the right middle and lower lobes.[10] In normal infants, the left pulmonary artery typically branches at the level of the main pulmonary artery. In infants with pulmonary sling, the left hilus appears low on frontal chest radiograph and is often seen to branch at a lower level than the main pulmonary artery.[10] Anterior bowing of the right mainstem bronchus on lateral chest radiograph is an additional sign that suggests the presence of pulmonary sling.[10] The left lung may appear hyperlucent as a result of decreased blood flow.[11] Tracheal narrowing is almost always seen on the lateral radiograph because of the associated tracheomalacia. Some authors consider MRI to be the preferred method for evaluation of pulmonary artery sling because of the ability of MRI to clearly evaluate both the tracheal and vascular anatomy and their relationship noninvasively.[6,8] Computed tomography may also be able to supply this information.[11-13]

The most common surgical repair consists of transection of the anomalous left pulmonary artery with reimplantation on the main pulmonary artery.[9] In the past, loss of patency of the left pulmonary artery was a problem.[9] However, improved surgical techniques appear to have decreased this complication.[9] In addition, there are reports of several cases of pulmonary sling that were repaired by transection of the trachea or a bronchus for removal of a stenosis with translocation of the left main pulmonary artery anterior to the trachea.[2,9]

Overall mortality and prognosis appear to be most closely related to the extent of tracheobronchial stenosis.[5,9] Patients with type I sling of the left pulmonary artery usually have good results following repair of the sling.[5] Patients with type II sling tend to have a high postoperative mortality rate, usually require extensive tracheoplasty, and often have residual tracheal stenosis.[4,5,9]

The differential diagnosis of chronic airway obstruction in infancy includes such entities as vascular rings, tracheomalacia, mediastinal tumors, foreign body aspiration, and laryngeal web.[7] The differential diagnosis for a mass density between the esophagus and trachea would include pulmonary sling, a bronchogenic cyst, or lymphadenopathy.

Further Reading

1. Campbell CD, Wernly JA, Koltip PC, Vitullo D, Replogle RL. Aberrant left pulmonary artery (pulmonary artery sling): successful repair and 24 year follow-up report. *Am J Cardiol* 45:316–320, 1980.
2. Jonas RA, Spevak PJ, McGill T, Castaneda AR. Pulmonary artery sling: primary repair by tracheal resection in infancy. *J Thorac Cardiovasc Surg* 97:548–550, 1989.
3. Sade RM, Rosenthal A, Fellows K, Castaneda AR. Pulmonary artery sling. *J Thorac Cardiovasc Surg* 69:333–346, 1975.
4. Wells TR, Gwinn JL, Landing BH, Stanley P. Reconsideration of the anatomy of sling left pulmonary artery: the association of one form with bridging bronchus and imperforate anus. Anatomic and diagnostic aspects. *J Pediatr Surg* 23(10):892–898, 1988.
5. Berdon WE, Baker DH, Wung J-T, et al. Complete cartilage-ring tracheal stenosis associated with anomalous left pulmonary artery: the ring-sling complex. *Radiology* 152:57–64, 1984.
6. Newman B, Meza MP, Towbin RB, Del Nido P. Left pulmonary artery sling: diagnosis and delineation of associated tracheobronchial anomalies with MR. *Pediatr Radiol* 26:661–668, 1996.
7. Rheuban KS, Ayres N, Still JG, Alford B. Pulmonary artery sling: a new diagnostic tool and clinical review. *Pediatrics* 69(4):472–475, 1982.
8. Phillips RR, Culham JAG. Pulmonary artery sling and hypoplastic right lung: diagnostic appearances using MRI. *Pediatr Radiol* 23:117–119, 1993.
9. Backer CL, Idriss FS, Holinger LD, Mavroudis C. Pulmonary artery sling. Results of surgical repair in infancy. *J Thorac Cardiovasc Surg* 103:683–691, 1992.
10. Capitanio MA, Ramos R, Kirkpatrick JA. Pulmonary sling. Roentgen observations. *Am J Roentgenol* 112(1):28–34, 1971.
11. Moncada R, Demos TC, Churchill R, Reynes C. Chronic stridor in a child: CT diagnosis of pulmonary vascular sling. *J Comput Assist Tomogr* 7(4):713–715, 1983.
12. McCray P, Grandgeorge S, Smith W, Wagener J, Frey E. Cine CT diagnosis of pulmonary artery sling. *Pediatr Radiol* 16:508–510, 1986.
13. Wells TR, Stanley P, Padua EM, Landing BH, Warburton D. Serial section-reconstruction of anomalous tracheobronchial branching patterns from CT scan images: bridging bronchus associated with sling left pulmonary artery. *Pediatr Radiol* 20:444–446, 1990.
14. Berdon WE, Baker DH. Vascular anomalies and the infant lung: rings, slings, and other things. *Semin Roentgenol* 7(1):39–64, 1972.
15. Siegel MJ, Shackelford GD, McAlister WH. Tracheobronchography in the evaluation of anomalous left pulmonary artery. *Pediatr Radiol* 12:235–238, 1982.

Acknowledgment

We are indebted to Ina Tonkin, MD, Department of Radiology at Le Bonheur Medical Center, for reviewing this cardiac section.

INTERVENTIONAL RADIOLOGY

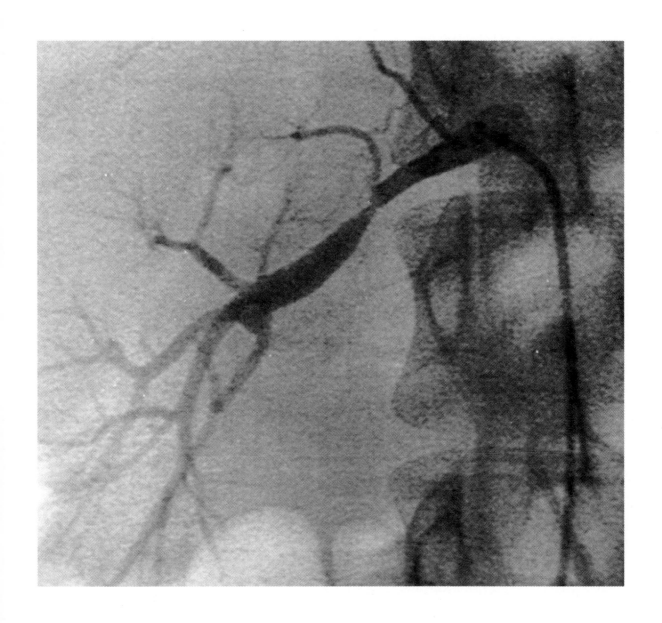

Case 1

Clinical Presentation

A 16-year-old boy presents with abdominal pain and nausea 1 week after epigastric blunt abdominal trauma.

Radiographic Studies

Ultrasound evaluation of the abdomen (Fig. 1A) shows a large, well-defined oval lesion located within the head of the pancreas. Moderate diffuse echoes are noted throughout the lesion. Enhanced CT exam of the abdomen reveals a well-defined low-attenuation oval lesion of the pancreatic head (arrowheads, Fig. 1B). Amylase value was elevated at 4300 U/L. Follow-up ultrasound 3 weeks after injury shows resolution of the internal echoes within the mass and increased through-transmission deep to the lesion (Fig. 1C). At this time, percutaneous drainage was indicated, due to increasing abdominal pain. CT shows the transgastric path of the sheathed needle into the mass (Fig. 1D). A 12 French van Sonnenberg sump drainage catheter was placed over a stiff 0.035-inch Amplatz guide wire after tract dilatation. CT performed after 10 days of low output drainage (Fig. 1E) shows collapse of the mass around the drainage catheter. The drain was removed after several days of uneventful oral feeding.

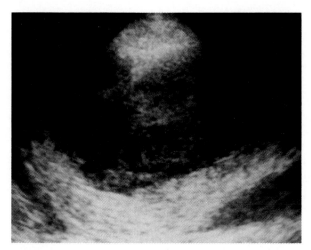

A

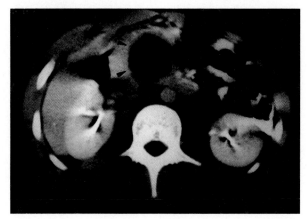

B

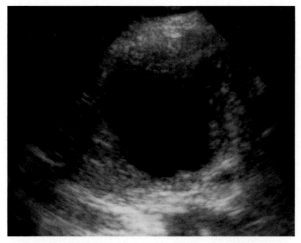

C

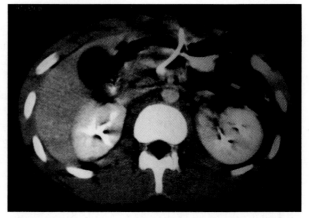

E

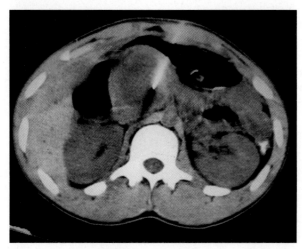

D

Diagnosis Pancreatic Pseudocyst

Discussion and Differential Diagnosis

Pediatric pancreatic pseudocysts are uncommon and are generally caused by accidental or nonaccidental blunt abdominal trauma. Pseudocysts are generally detected within 2 weeks of the traumatic event.[1] As pseudocysts can spontaneously resolve, percutaneous drainage is indicated when stable or increasing size is documented on follow-up imaging, superimposed infection is suspected, or clinical symptoms persist. Symptoms frequently encountered include abdominal pain, malaise, nausea, and vomiting. Drainage may be performed under CT, ultrasound, or fluoroscopic guidance. Both transperitoneal and transgastric percutaneous drainage routes have been advocated.[1–3] The transgastric route is advocated when this is the most direct

• Administration of the somatostatin analogue octreotide has been shown to decrease pseudocyst drainage duration.[4]

PITFALLS

• If communication of the cyst with the pancreatic duct is present, significantly longer percutaneous drainage may be required.

route and to attempt formation of a cyst-enterostomy.[2,3] Cessation of oral feeding is required and hyperalimentation is delivered.

For pseudocysts, unlike percutaneous abscesses, several weeks of drainage can be expected, particularly when communication with the pancreatic duct is demonstrated on fluoroscopic sinogram. Percutaneous drainage is complete when the symptoms and imaging findings resolve and the amylase value stabilizes. A trial of oral feeding without reaccumulation of the pseudocyst, amylase elevation, or symptom recurrence is encouraged before removal of the drainage catheter.[1,2]

Further Reading

1. Jaffe RB, Arata JA Jr, Matlak ME. Percutaneous drainage of traumatic pancreatic pseudocysts in children. *Am J Roentgenol* 152:591–595, 1989.
2. Amundson GM, Towbin RB, Mueller DL, Seagram CGF. Percutaneous transgastric drainage of the lesser sac in children. *Pediatr Radiol* 20(8):590–593, 1990.
3. van Sonnenberg E, D'Agostino HB, Casola G, Halasz NA, Sanchez RB, Goodacre BW. Percutaneous abscess drainage: current concepts. *Radiology* 181:617–626, 1991.
4. D'Agostino HB, van Sonnenberg E, Sanchez RB, Goodacre BW, Villaveiran RG, Lyche K. Treatment of pancreatic pseudocysts with percutaneous drainage and octreotide: work in progress. *Radiology* 187(3):685–688, 1993.

Case 2

Clinical Presentation

A 16-year-old with 6 days of massive hemoptysis unresponsive to medical therapy.

Radiographic Studies

Chest X ray (Fig. 2A) shows coarse interstitial disease, bronchiectasis, and segmental infiltrates. After identification of a common bronchial arterial trunk at the mid descending thoracic aorta, selective angiogram of markedly enlarged right (Fig. 2B) and left (Fig. 2C) bronchial artery branches was performed. Multiple tortuous and ectatic bronchial artery branches are visualized bilaterally. After selective bilateral bronchial artery embolization with polyvinyl alcohol particles (250 to 350 micrometer size), angiogram of the common bronchial artery trunk shows abrupt cutoff of the bronchial arteries (arrows, Fig. 2D) with occlusion of peripheral bronchial branches.

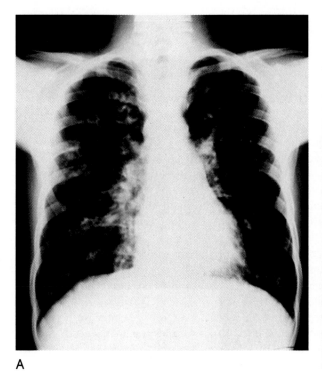

A

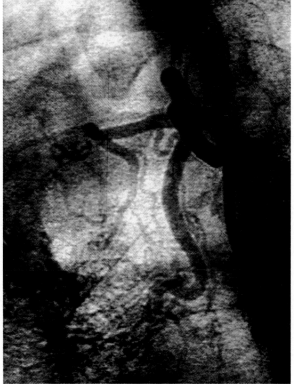

B

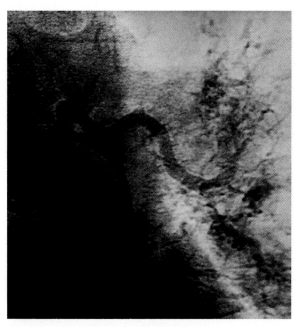

C

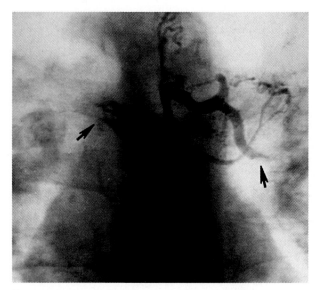

D

Diagnosis   Cystic Fibrosis/Embolization of Hemoptysis

Discussion and Differential Diagnosis

Initially, several days of high-dose intravenous antibiotics are administered to reduce bleeding relating to the pulmonary inflammatory disease in patients with cystic fibrosis. If massive hemoptysis (greater than 300 cm^3/day) continues, or if smaller volumes of hemoptysis limit postural drainage or affect the patient's lifestyle, angiography and bronchial artery embolization are indicated.[1–3] A majority of bronchial artery branches are found arising from the descending thoracic aorta from the T4 to T6 vertebral body levels.[2] However, search for multiple enlarged bronchial vessels is critical in any given patient. Known sites of origin of aberrant bronchial arteries include the thyrocervical trunk, the internal mammary arteries, and the intercostal arteries.[2,3] Angiograms prior to embolization should evaluate catheter stability, lack of aortic reflux of contrast, and origin of spinal artery branches from the bronchial vessels. Peripheral embolization with polyvinyl alcohol particles and absorbable gelatin pledgets are used most commonly, and control of hemoptysis is generally achieved.[1–3] Post-procedural chest pain, dysphagia, and fever are frequently encountered. Careful technique and fluoroscopic guidance of embolization is warranted to prevent inadvertent embolization of spinal artery branches. Late recurrence of hemoptysis may occur, and repeat embolization of previously embolized bronchial arteries may be needed.[1–3]

Further Reading

1. Fellows KE, Khaw KT, Schuster S, Shwachman H. Bronchial artery embolization in cystic fibrosis; technique and long-term results. *J Pediatr* 95(6):959–963, 1979.
2. Cohen AM, Doershuk CF, Stern RC. Bronchial artery embolization to control hemoptysis in cystic fibrosis. *Radiology* 175:401–405, 1990.
3. Tonkin ILD, Hanissian AS, Boulden TF, et al. Bronchial arteriography and embolotherapy for hemoptysis in patients with cystic fibrosis. *Cardiovasc Intervent Radiol* 14:241–246, 1991.

Case 3

Clinical Presentation

An 8-month-old infant presents with abdominal mass, fever, irritability, and decreased oral intake.

Radiographic Studies

Longitudinal renal ultrasound (Fig. 3A) shows a markedly dilated intrarenal collecting system without visualization of a dilated proximal ureter. Moderate echogenic debris implies infectious debris or hemorrhage in the collecting system. After ultrasound-guided entry into the collecting system, a 0.018-inch floppy-tip guide wire is passed through the 21-gauge needle under fluoroscopic guidance (Fig. 3B). Subsequent passage of a 4.5 French coaxial introducer allowed exchange for a 0.038-inch guide wire and placement of a 6 French pigtail nephrostomy catheter. Antegrade pyelogram (Fig. 3C) performed several days later, after the patient defervesced, showed delayed passage of contrast.

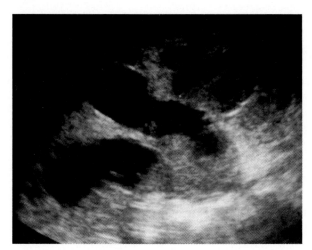

A

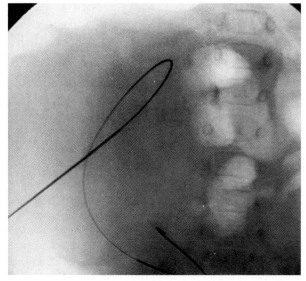

B

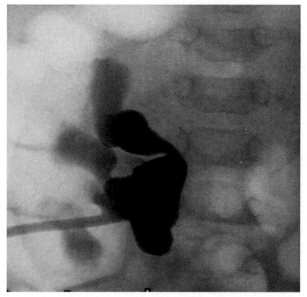

C

Diagnosis   Ureteropelvic Junction (UPJ) Obstruction

Discussion and Differential Diagnosis

Percutaneous urinary tract procedures can be performed safely in infants and children for a variety of congenital and acquired conditions. More commonly, pediatric urinary tract drainage is performed to temporarily control infection or to improve renal function prior to surgical treatment of an obstructing lesion.[1] In other instances, such as urinary diversion for urine leak or irrigation for urinary tract fungal infection, urinary drainage may provide definitive treatment.[1,2] Less commonly, percutaneous nephrostomy tract dilatation can be performed to accommodate percutaneous urinary tract procedures such as stone removal or pyeloplasty.

Preprocedural review of imaging studies is important because vesicoureteral reflux or neurogenic bladder may simulate urinary tract obstruction. In addition, anomalies such as horseshoe kidney or crossed fused ectopic kidney may require percutaneous access sites differing from the norm.[3] Preprocedural antibiotics are usually administered, and sedation appropriate for the patient's age and duration/pain of the procedure must be considered.[1,3] In instances of decreased renal function, marked ureteral dilatation, or high resting bladder pressure, a ureteral perfusion test (Whitaker test) may be useful to discriminate obstructive from nonobstructive dilatation.[4] In infants and small children, procedural heat loss, mobility of the kidney with gradual needle passage, smaller equipment size, and external fixation of the drainage catheters should be considered.[1,3] Though many procedures can be performed through an easily accessible lower pole calyx, some percutaneous procedures require specific mid or upper pole caliceal entry.[2,3,5] Complications from most percutaneous urinary drainage procedures are minor and self-limited (hematuria, asymptomatic urine leak, etc.).[6]

More significant complications (pneumothorax, hemothorax, etc.) may occur when an intercostal approach into the urinary tract is required.[7]

Further Reading

1. Ball WS Jr, Towbin R, Strife JL, Spencer R. Interventional genitourinary radiology in children: a review of 61 procedures. *Am J Roentgenol* 147:791–796, 1986.

2. Lee WJ, Leonidas JC, Rich M. Percutaneous management of ureteropelvic junction obstruction in children. *Semin Intervent Radiol* 8(3):179–187, 1991.

3. Papanicolaou N, Yoder IC, Pfister RC, Tung GA. Percutaneous nephrostomy in children. *Semin Intervent Radiol* 8(3):170–178, 1991.

4. Krebs TL, Papanicolaou N, Yoder IC, Tung GA, Pfister RC. Antegrade pyelography and ureteral perfusion in children with urinary tract dilatation. *Semin Intervent Radiol* 8(3):161–169, 1991.

5. Towbin RB, Wacksman J, Ball WS. Percutaneous pyeloplasty in children: experience in three patients. *Radiology* 163:381–384, 1987.

6. Pfister RC, Newhouse JH, Yoder IC, et al. Complications of pediatric percutaneous renal procedures: incidence and observations. *Urol Clin North Am* 10(3):563–571, 1983.

7. Hopper KD, Yakes WF. The posterior intercostal approach for percutaneous renal procedures: risk of puncturing the lung, spleen, and liver as determined by CT. *Am J Roentgenol* 154(1):115–117, 1990.

8. Towbin RB, Ball WS. New pediatric 5-F drainage system. *Radiology* 163(3):827, 1987.

Case 4

Clinical Presentation

Fever, elevated white blood cell count, and abdominal pain 5 days after surgery for appendicitis.

Radiographic Studies

Abdominal CT (Fig. 4A) shows a rim-enhancing right lower quadrant fluid collection with inflammatory changes of the overlying abdominal wall. Advancement of a 0.035-inch guide wire through a 19-gauge sheathed needle was performed using CT guidance (Fig. 4B). Follow-up CT (Fig. 4C) shows a collapsed cavity and resolving inflammatory changes of the abdominal wall.

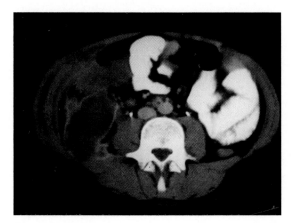

A

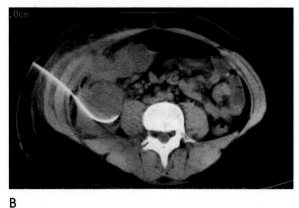

B

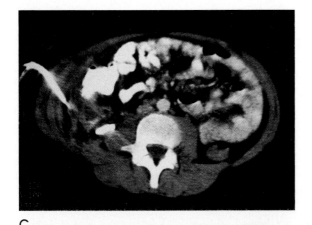

C

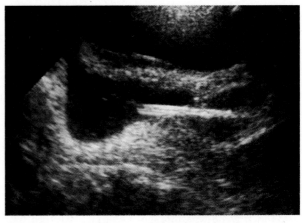

E

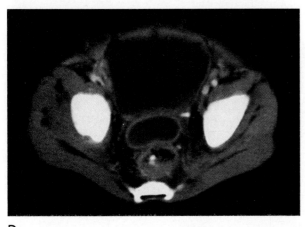

D

Diagnosis Abdominal Abscess

Discussion and Differential Diagnosis

A majority of pediatric abdominal abscesses arise in the postoperative child after appendiceal perforation. Other causes of abscess formation include Crohn's disease, prior bowel surgical procedures, and traumatic bowel injury. Indications for percutaneous abscess drainage continue to increase and include complicating features such as multilocular cavities, cavities with communications (fistulas), and cavities shielded by overlying structures.[1] Adequate fluid resuscitation, broad-spectrum antibiotics, and knowledge of coagulation status are imperative prior to the procedure.[2] Most pediatric abscess drainages can be performed with intravenous sedation, though general anesthesia may be needed in some instances.[2-4] Imaging and drainage can be performed under ultrasound guidance in many instances, with advantages of lower cost, lack of ionizing radiation, and real-time visualization of procedural maneuvers. However, CT has advantages for demonstration of multiplicity of fluid collections and when intervening bowel loops must be delineated.[1,2] Fluoroscopy is used as an adjunct to some drainage procedures and is particularly valuable in demonstrating fistulae and documenting cavity collapse.[1,4]

Though smaller single-lumen drain sizes (5 to 9 French) are adequate for less viscous serous collections, larger (12 to 14 French) double-lumen sump drainage catheters are required for more viscous abscess cavities.[1] Dependent position of the drainage catheter, placement of multiple drainage catheters when necessary, and daily saline irrigation of the drainage catheter will decrease drainage duration. A vast majority of pediatric abscess drainages are successful though occasional incomplete drainage is encountered in cavities associated with fistulae, phlegmons, or underlying tumors.[1,2]

Abscess cavities in the deep pelvic recesses (Fig. 4D) are often more challenging because an anterior approach of percutaneous drainage may be precluded by overlying bladder, ureters, and bowel loops. Imaging-directed means of deep pelvic abscess treatment include ultrasound-guided transrectal drainage (Fig. 4E) (transrectal sheathed needle shown within deep pelvic abscess), CT-guided transgluteal needle aspiration, and CT-guided transgluteal drainage.[5]

Further Reading

1. van Sonnenberg E, D'Agostino HB, Casola G, Halasz NA, Sanchez RB, Goodacre BW. Percutaneous abscess drainage: current concepts. *Radiology* 181(3):617–626, 1991.
2. Chair P, Towbin R. Percutaneous abscess drainage. *Semin Intervent Radiol* 8(3):195–197, 1991.
3. van Sonnenberg E, Wittich GR, Edwards DK, et al. Percutaneous diagnostic and therapeutic interventional radiologic procedures in children: experience in 100 patients. *Radiology* 162(3):601–605, 1987.
4. Alexander AA, Eschelman DJ, Nazarian LN, Bonn J. Transrectal sonographically guided drainage of deep pelvic abscesses. *Am J Roentgenol* 162:1227–1230, 1994.
5. van Sonnenberg E, Wittich G, Walser E. Re: Transrectal sonographically guided drainage of deep pelvic abscesses. Commentary. *Am J Roentgenol* 162:1231–1232, 1994.

Case 5

Clinical Presentation

A 16-year-old girl presents with sudden onset of hypertension and seizures.

Radiographic Studies

Selective digital angiogram of the right main renal artery shows focal high-grade stenosis (arrow, Fig. 5A) of the mid right main renal artery. Angiogram of the left renal artery was normal. After intravenous administration of 2500 units of heparin, the stenosis was crossed with a guide wire and angioplasty was performed. The 6-mm balloon was inflated once with relief of the balloon waist (Fig. 5B). Postangioplasty angiogram of the right main renal artery shows resolution of the renal artery stenosis (Fig. 5C). The patient is asymptomatic and has normal blood pressure without medication 2 years after the angioplasty procedure.

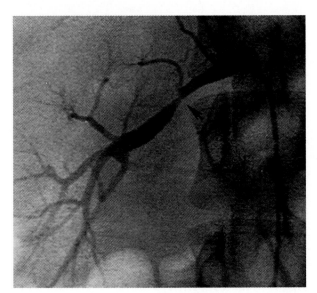

A

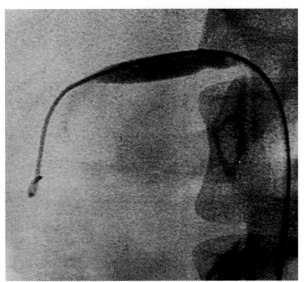

B

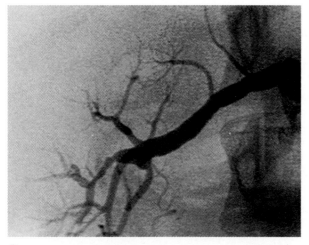

C

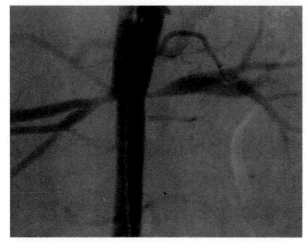

D

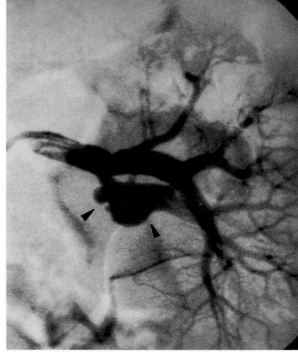

E

Diagnosis Renovascular Hypertension

Discussion and Differential Diagnosis

When nonvascular causes of hypertension are not established or when pediatric hypertension is progressive or difficult to control, angiography is indicated to evaluate for renal arterial causes of hypertension. The range of causes of renal artery stenosis is greater in children than in adult patients and includes developmental abnormalities of the abdominal aorta/renal artery origins, inflammatory aortoarteritis with renal artery involvement, and fibromuscular dysplasia of the mid and distal renal arteries.[1-3] Angiographic considerations include transcatheter aortic pressure recordings for detection of a pressure gradient, lateral views of the abdominal aorta for detection of coexisting visceral artery stenoses, selective renal artery injections for detection

PEARLS

• Globular irregular aneurysms (arrowheads, Figure 5E) may accompany pediatric segmental renal artery stenoses.[2]

of peripheral branch artery stenoses, and renal vein renin sampling. Bilateral smooth stenoses of the renal artery origins (Fig. 5D) may accompany congenital segmental narrowing or hypoplasia of the abdominal aorta (note infrarenal aortic caliber change, Fig. 5D).[2] A similar appearance may be seen in patients with clinical stigmata of neurofibromatosis or Williams syndrome.[1] These ostial lesions respond poorly to angioplasty balloon inflation, and surgical revision may be required. Systemic symptoms such as fever, rash, and myalgia and laboratory findings such as an elevated erythrocyte sedimentation rate (ESR) may suggest an inflammatory arteritis of the aorta and renal arteries.[1,3] Balloon angioplasty may relieve the hypertension in some of these patients.[3] Mid main renal artery or segmental branch renal artery stenoses are common in pediatric patients with renovascular hypertension and may relate to fibromuscular disease.[1,2,4] Technical success of balloon angioplasty in segmental renal artery stenoses in middle-aged patients and of microballoon angioplasty with or without segmental embolization in pediatric segmental renal artery stenoses has been reported.[5,6]

Further Reading

1. Robinson L, Gedroyc W, Reidy J, Saxton HM. Renal artery stenosis in children. *Clin Radiol* 44:376–382, 1991.
2. Stanley JC. Renal vascular disease and renovascular hypertension in children. *Urol Clin North Am* 11:451–463, 1984.
3. Kumar S, Mandalam KR, Rao VR, et al. Percutaneous transluminal angioplasty in nonspecific aortoarteritis (Takayasu's disease): experience of 16 cases. *Cardiovasc Intervent Radiol* 12(6):321–325, 1990.
4. Mali WP, Puijlaert CB, Kouwenberg HJ, et al. Percutaneous transluminal renal angioplasty in children and adolescents. *Radiology* 165(2):391–394, 1987.
5. Cluzel P, Raynaud A, Beyssen B, Pagny JY, Gaux JC. Stenoses of renal branch arteries in fibromuscular dysplasia: results of percutaneous transluminal angioplasty. *Radiology* 193:227–232, 1994.
6. Towbin RB, Kaye RD. Treatment of segmental renal artery stenosis in children. Presented at the 38th Annual Meeting, The Society for Pediatric Radiology, Washington, DC, April 27–30, 1995.

Case 6

Clinical Presentation

Abdominal distention and vomiting following gastrostomy tube feeds.

Radiographic Studies

Upper GI study performed through the surgically placed gastrostomy tube (Fig. 6A) shows high-grade obstruction of the third duodenum at the expected course of the superior mesenteric artery (SMA). Conversion to a percutaneous gastrojejunal feeding tube was accomplished under fluoroscopic guidance to allow feeding of the jejunum beyond the SMA-obstructing lesion (arrow, Fig. 6B).

Another patient with intermittent gastroesophageal reflux and aspiration pneumonia on gastrostomy tube feeds is shown in Figure 6C. Curved catheter and floppy 0.035-inch guide wire combination is used to access the small bowel through the gastrostomy site. Subsequent placement of a percutaneous gastrojejunal feeding tube over the guide wire and formation of the gastic retention pigtail loop (arrowheads, Fig. 6D) was performed.

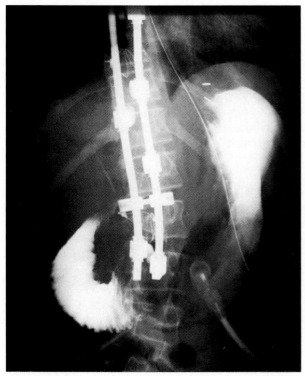

A

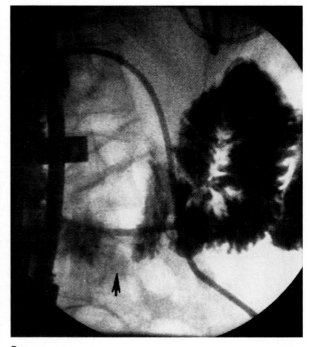

B

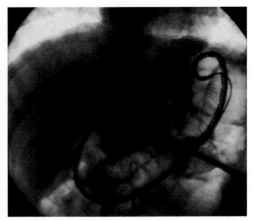

D

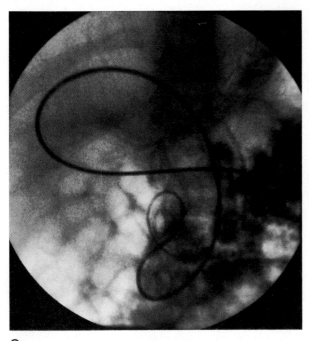

C

PEARLS

• Most gastrostomy tubes can be placed under local anesthesia and intravenous sedation.

• Image left lobe of liver with ultrasound and transverse colon with barium before procedure.

PITFALLS

• Antegrade approach may not be used if there is nasopharyngeal or esophageal obstruction.

Diagnosis Percutaneous Feeding

Discussion and Differential Diagnosis

Percutaneous feeding in the pediatric population consists of primary gastrostomy tube placement when long-term nutrition is inadequate and conversion of a previously placed gastrostomy tube to a gastrojejunal feeding tube when gastroesophageal reflux persists despite antireflux procedures. Conversion of a prior mature gastrostomy tract to gastrojejunal feeding is achieved by advancing a floppy guide wire across the pylorus with a curved directional angiographic catheter. The guide wire–catheter combination is subsequently advanced beyond the duodenal jejunal junction. Subsequently, a gastrojejunal feeding tube is advanced over the guide wire and positioned near the duodenal jejunal junction. Exchange for a stiff guide wire prior to tube placement may be necessary to avoid undesirable guide wire loops in the stomach.

Primary pediatric radiologic gastrostomy placement has progressed as a quick and safe procedure in infants and children of all sizes.[1–4] Pediatric indications for long-term nutrition include severe central nervous system impairment, failure to thrive, malignancy, chronic chest or gastrointestinal diseases, and craniofacial abnormalities.[1,4] Most gastrostomy tubes can be placed under local anesthesia and intravenous sedation. Both retrograde placement of a gastrostomy tube through the anterior abdominal wall and antegrade placement of gastrostomy tubes through the mouth have been described in pediatric patients.[1–4] Regardless of approach, a majority of pediatric interventionalists image the left lobe of the liver with ultrasound and the transverse colon with barium before gastric puncture.[1,2,4] The stomach is distended with air via nasogastric tube, and gastric motility is decreased with intravenous glucagon. In the retrograde insertion technique, retention suture placement prevents retraction of the stomach from the anterior abdominal wall during tract dilation and tube placement.[4] Proponents of the antegrade technique cite lack of tube dislodgments and decreased need for later tube exchanges.[1] Rarely, the antegrade technique is not feasible because of nasopharyngeal or esophageal obstruction.[1] Major complications after percutaneous gastrostomy placement such as hemorrhage or peritonitis are decreased compared to surgical rates.[1] Localized skin infection and tube migration may occur but are easily treated.[2-4] Feeding begins after return of bowel sounds and lack of complications are documented. In the absence of gastroesophageal reflux, the gastrostomy tube may be exchanged for a lower-profile button after tract maturation.[4]

Further Reading

1. Towbin RB, Ball WS Jr, Bissett GS III. Percutaneous gastrostomy and percutaneous gastrojejunostomy in children: antegrade approach. *Radiology* 168:473–476, 1988.
2. Cory DA, Fitzgerald JF, Cohen MD. Percutaneous nonendoscopic gastrostomy in children. *Am J Roentgenol* 151:995–997, 1988.
3. Malden ES, Hicks ME, Picus D, Darcy MD, Vesely TM, Kleinhoffer MA. Fluoroscopically guided percutaneous gastrostomy in children. *J Vasc Intervent Radiol* 3:673–677, 1992.
4. King SJ, Chait PG, Daneman A, Pereira J. Retrograde percutaneous gastrostomy: a prospective study in 57 children. *Pediatr Radiol* 23:23–25, 1993.

Case 7

Clinical Presentation

An infant with cutaneous hemangiomas and mild symptoms of congestive heart failure.

Radiographic Studies

CT scan of the abdomen following intravenous contrast (Fig. 7A) shows multiple oval lesions throughout the liver with intense peripheral enhancement. On repeat imaging through the liver several minutes later (Fig. 7B) the lesions are equal in attenuation to the surrounding liver parenchyma. Another infant with mild tachycardia (Fig. 7C) presents with a dominant lesion in the right lobe of the liver that shows decreased attenuation compared with the surrounding liver parenchyma. After administration of intravenous contrast, a majority of the lesion enhances, although portions of this complex mass are nonenhancing (arrow, Fig. 7D). Digital hepatic arteriogram (Fig. 7E) shows hepatic artery enlargement and dense nodular enhancement along the periphery of this right hepatic lobe mass. No arteriovenous shunting was identified.

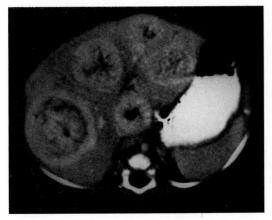

A

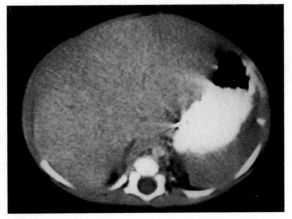

B

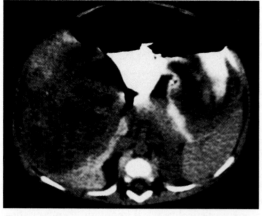

C

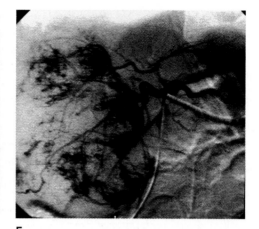

E

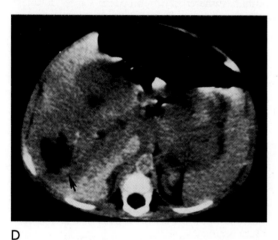

D

Diagnosis Hemangioendothelioma

Discussion and Differential Diagnosis

Hemangioendothelioma is a rare vascular tumor of the liver generally diagnosed in the first 6 months of life.[1] The lesion can present as a single mass, multifocal masses, or diffuse nodular lesions throughout both lobes of the liver.[1–3] Clinical presentation is generally that of a right upper quadrant mass or generalized hepatomegaly in an infant who may have cutaneous hemangiomas.[1,4] Given the vascularity of the lesions, high-output congestive heart failure occurs in a significant proportion of patients.[2,4] The lesions generally proliferate in the first 18 months of life before spontaneous involution. Aggressive treatment of the lesions is required when congestive heart failure does not respond to medical treatment with digoxin, diuretics, or a trial of corticosteroids. Treatment options include radiation therapy, surgical resection of localized lesions, hepatic artery ligation, or percutaneous transcatheter embolization.[5,6] More recently, daily subcutaneous administration of interferon has had success in treating life-threatening hemangiomatous lesions throughout the body.[7]

Imaging shows single or multiple well-defined lesions or diffuse ill-defined heterogeneity of the liver. Calcification of lesions may be detected.[1] On ultrasound, lesions may be hypoechoic or hyperechoic relative to normal liver parenchyma, and enlargement of associated arteries and veins may be seen. Variable Doppler findings of altered flow within the lesions can be demonstrated and decreased flow after treatment can be documented.[2] On CT, lesions are low attenuation relative to adjacent liver before contrast administration. After administration of intravenous contrast, early peripheral enhancement of the lesion that is isotense to surrounding liver on delayed scans is suggestive of hemangioendothelioma.[1,4] Angiographic findings include decrease in aortic caliber beyond the celiac artery origin, enlarged tortuous feeding vessels, and intense capillary staining, with subtle or absent arteriovenous shunting.[1,6] Identification of the frequently present collateral vessels is important if embolization is undertaken.[6] Long procedure times, catheter sizes appropriate for the newborn or infant access artery, and potential complications of embolization procedures should be thoroughly considered.[3,6]

Further Reading

1. Dachman AH, Lichtenstein JE, Friedman AC, Hartman DS. Infantile hemangioendothelioma of the liver: a radiologic-pathologic clinical correlation. *Am J Roentgenol* 140:1091–1096, 1983.
2. Paltiel HJ, Patriquin HB, Keller MS, Babcock DS, Leithiser, RE Jr. Infantile hepatic hemangioma: Doppler US. *Radiology* 182:735–742, 1992.
3. Burrows PE, Rosenberg HC, Chuang HS. Diffuse hepatic hemangiomas: percutaneous transcatheter embolization with detachable silicone balloons. *Radiology* 156:85–88, 1985.
4. Holcomb GW III, O'Neill JA Jr, Mahboubi S, Bishop HC. Experience with hepatic hemangioendothelioma in infancy and childhood. *J Pediatr Surg* 23(7):661–666, 1988.
5. Moazam F, Rodgers BM, Talbert JL. Hepatic artery ligation for hepatic hemangiomatosis of infancy. *J Pediatr Surg* 18(2):120–123, 1983.
6. Fellows KE, Hoffer FA, Markowitz RI, O'Neill, JA Jr. Multiple collaterals to hepatic infantile hemangioendotheliomas and arteriovenous malformations: effect on embolization. *Radiology* 181:813–818, 1991.
7. Ezekowitz RA, Mulliken JB, Folkman J. Interferon alpha-2a therapy for life-threatening hemangiomas of infancy. *N Engl J Med* 326(22):1456–1463, 1992.

Case 8

Clinical Presentation

A 3-year-old girl with upper GI bleeding.

Radiographic Studies

Ultrasound imaging of the porta hepatis (Fig. 8A) shows multiple small serpiginous vessels. Color flow ultrasound (Fig. 8B, Color Plate 9) confirms flow within collateral vessels. Venous phase of superior mesenteric artery angiogram displays the periportal collateral vessels (arrowheads, Fig. 8C) and filling of varices at the gastroesophageal junction (arrow, Fig. 8C).

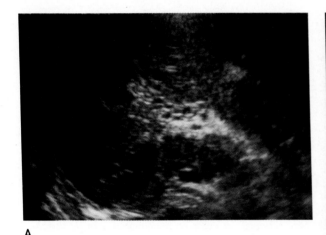

A

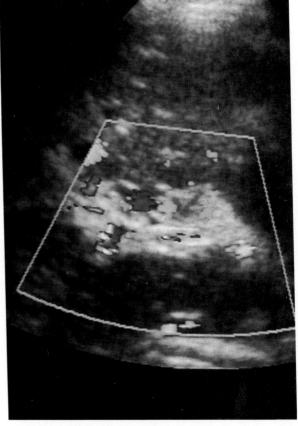

B

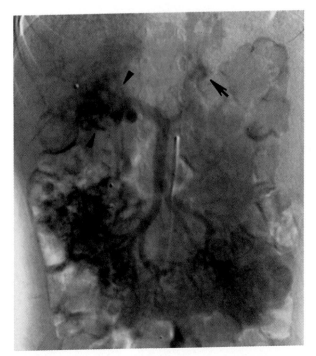

C

Diagnosis Portal Vein Thrombosis

Discussion and Differential Diagnosis

In the pediatric patient, portal hypertension is frequently caused by extrahepatic occlusion of the portal vein.[1] Though an exact cause of portal vein occlusion is often unknown, causes such as prior umbilical venous catheterization, dehydration, coagulopathy, or extrinsic portal vein compression by mass lesions or adjacent inflammatory processes have been noted.[1,2] Clinical presentation includes bleeding esophageal varices, anemia, or splenomegaly generally without jaundice or ascites.[1,3] Following portal vein occlusion, development of periportal collateral venous channels (cavernous transformation of the portal vein) provides flow toward the liver.[1,2] Given increased resistance to flow at the portal hepatis, hepatofugal portosystemic collateral venous flow away from the liver develops.[1]

Noninvasive imaging with ultrasound should document lack of intrahepatic alterations of cirrhosis, an occluded extrahepatic portal vein, and hepatopetal periportal collateral venous flow. Subsequent documentation of the caliber and flow direction in expected portosystemic collateral routes throughout the abdomen and pelvis is performed.[3] Major pathways include left gastric, short gastric veins to lower esophageal veins, splenorenal collaterals, splenic-retroperitoneal venous collaterals, and inferior mesenteric pelvic hemorrhoidal venous collaterals.[2,3] As extent of portal vein occlusion and collateral pathways may be incomplete on ultrasound, more invasive imaging with arterial portography or splenoportography provides complementary

SYNDROMES

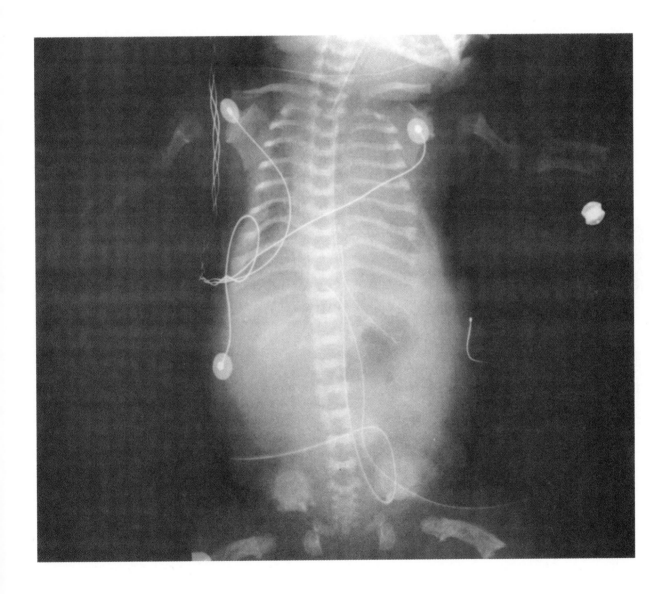

information needed during surgical planning. The goal of these procedures is to delineate complete extent of portal vein occlusion, to identify additional sites of portosystemic collaterals, and to define patent vessels appropriate for surgical shunt procedures.[1]

Further Reading

1. Rosch J, Dotter CT. Extrahepatic portal obstruction in childhood and its angiographic diagnosis. *Am J Roentgenol Radium Ther Nucl Med* 112:143–149, 1971.
2. Patriquin H, Lafortune M. Syllabus: Doppler sonography of the liver. In: Seibert JJ, ed. *Current Concepts: A Categorical Course in Pediatric Radiology.* Chicago: RSNA; 1994:207–220.
3. Patriquin H, Lafortune M, Burns PN, Dauzat M. Duplex Doppler examination in portal hypertension: technique and anatomy. *Am J Roentgenol* 149:71–76, 1987.

Case 1

Clinical Presentation

A 15-year-old girl with history of increasing bone pain in the limbs, especially the lower legs; waddling gait; and decrease in muscle mass.

Radiographic Studies

The radiographs show a marked cortical diaphyseal sclerosis of short and long tubular bones (Fig. 1A, 1B, 1C). The increased bone formation is endosteal rather than periosteal. This sclerosis is associated with an increase in isotope uptake (Fig. 1D). The vertebral bodies show marked increase in density, especially in the pedicles and posterior arch (Fig. 1E).

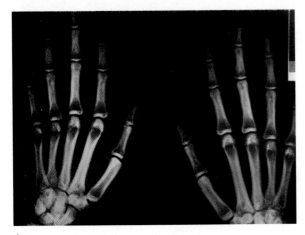

A

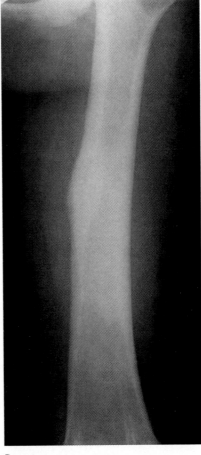

B

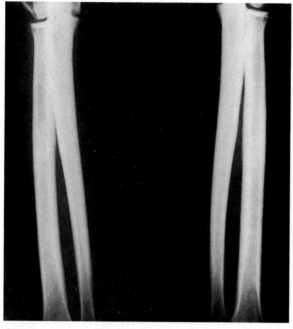

C

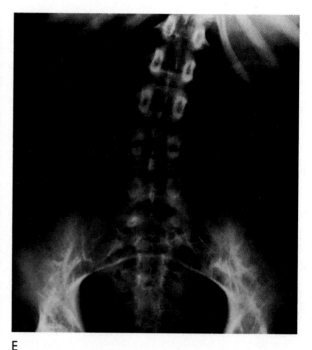

E

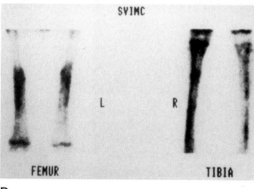

D

Diagnosis Engelmann Disease, Camurati-Engelmann Disease, Progressive Diaphyseal Dysplasia (PDD)

Discussion and Differential Diagnosis

Engelmann disease is a hereditary disorder with an autosomal dominant transmission. The symptoms usually become manifest early in life, commonly before the age of 10, with neuromuscular dystrophy. The diagnosis is made primarily on the basis of radiologic examination. Symmetric sclerosis is observed often with a fusiform enlargement of the diaphysis of the long bones, especially the femur and tibia. In children, the enlargement of the cortex produces a narrowed medullary cavity, which,

PEARLS

- CT may show vertebral sclerosis confined to the posterior elements and arches of vertebral bodies.[5]

- Ribbing disease is a milder form of diaphyseal dysplasia with irregular cortical sclerosis of the diaphysis. Ribbing disease presents in middle age, is either unilateral or asymmetrically bilateral, has no gait or neurological abnormality or anemia, and involves only long bones. It may be confused with a stress fracture.[6]

PITFALLS

- Increased bone activity on scintigraphy may be discordant with radiographic findings in Engelmann disease.[7]

if severe, may lead to extramedullary hematopoiesis and eventual hepatosplenomegaly. The osteosclerosis is irregular and inhomogeneous. The metaphyses and epiphyses are spared. Sclerotic changes at the skull base may produce cranial nerve abnormality.[1,2] Serum chemistries are usually normal. The etiology of the disorder is obscure, but the pain may be relieved by steroids.[3,4] Other diseases in the differential diagnosis include van Buchem syndrome, Paget's disease, craniodiaphyseal dysplasia, and familial hyperphosphatemia.

Further Reading

1. Naveh Y, Kaftori JK, Alon U, et al. Progressive diaphyseal dysplasia: genetics and clinical and radiologic manifestations. *Pediatrics* 74:399–405, 1984.
2. Applegate LJ, Applegate GR, Kemp SS. MR of multiple cranial neuropathies in a patient with Camurati-Engelmann disease: case report. *Am J Neuroradiol* 12:557–559, 1991.
3. Naveh Y, Alon U, Kaftori JK, Berant M. Progressive diaphyseal dysplasia: evaluation of corticosteroid therapy. *Pediatrics* 75:321–323, 1985.
4. Verbruggen LA, Bossuyt A, Schreuer R, Somers G. Clinical and scintigraphic evaluation of corticosteroid treatment in a case of progressive diaphyseal dysplasia. *J Rheumatol* 12(4):809–813, 1985.
5. Kaftori JK, Kleinhaus U, Naveh Y. Progressive diaphyseal dysplasia (Camurati-Engelmann): radiographic follow-up and CT findings. *Radiology* 164:777–782, 1987.
6. Seeger LL, et al. Ribbing Disease (Multiple Diaphyseal Sclerosis): Imaging and Differential Diagnosis. *Am J Radiol* 167:689–694, 1996.
7. Kumar B, Murphy WA, Whyte MP. Progressive diaphyseal dysplasia (Engelmann disease): Scintigraphic-radiographic-clinical correlations. *Radiology* 140:87–92, 1981.

Case 2

Clinical Presentation

An 8-year-old with recent fracture.

Radiographic Studies

Radiographs of tibia and femurs (Fig. 2A, 2B, 2C) show a fracture (arrow, Fig. 2C) of the tibia in uniformly dense long bones. The ribs are dense (Fig. 2D) with splaying at their ends. There is a bone-within-a-bone appearance in the dense spine (Fig. 2E). All bones show osteosclerosis with obliteration of corticomedullary junctions.

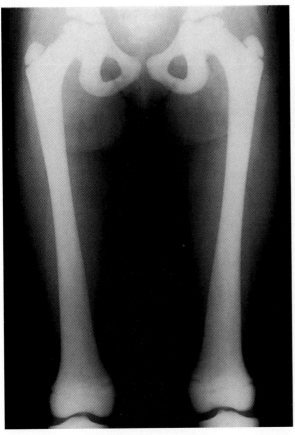

A

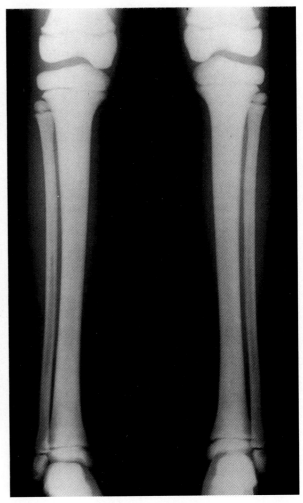

B

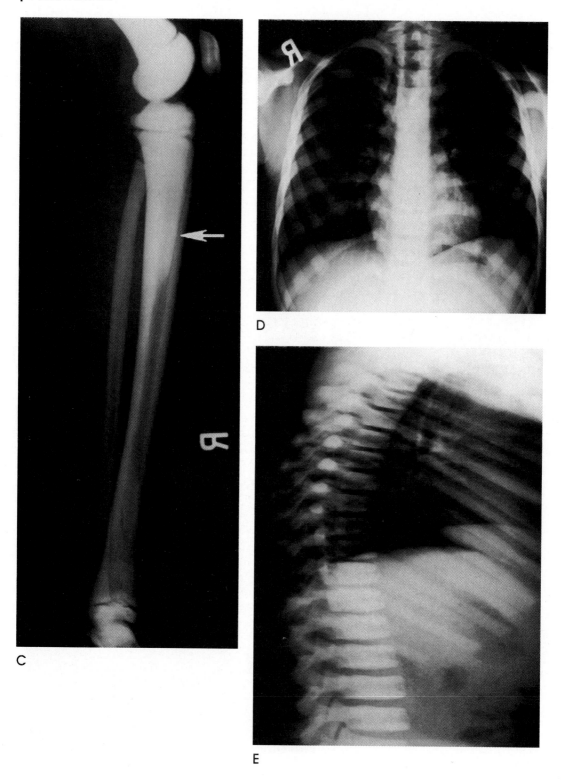

C

D

E

Diagnosis Osteopetrosis, Marble Bone Disease, Albers-Schönberg Disease

Discussion and Differential Diagnosis

Osteopetrosis is a genetic disorder characterized by generalized increased density in the bones. Three types are recessive, and the delayed type is dominant.[1] The infantile form may present as anemia and hepatosplenomegaly because of marrow encroachment. Patients have frequent fractures and osteomyelitis. The adult form may be asymptomatic except for bone pain. Impingement on neural and vascular foramina at the skull base may produce debilitating clinical symptoms.[2] Bone marrow transplant is proving a successful therapy.[3,4]

Further Reading

1. Taybi H, Lachman RS. *Radiology of Syndromes, Metabolic Disorders, and Skeletal Dysplasias,* 4th ed. St. Louis: Mosby; 1996:886–891.
2. Al-Mefty O, Fox JL, Al-Rodhan N, Dew JH. Optic nerve decompression in osteopetrosis. *J Neurosurg* 68(1):80–84, 1988.
3. Nisbet NW. Bone marrow transplantation in precocious osteopetrosis. *Br Med J (Clin Res Ed)* 294:463–464, 1987.
4. Orchard PJ, Dickerman JD, Mathews CH, et al. Haploidentical bone marrow transplantation for osteopetrosis. *Am J Pediatr Hematol Oncol* 9:335–340, 1987.
5. McAlister WH. Syllabus: an approach to skeletal dysplasias. In: Seibert JJ, ed. *Current Concepts: A Categorical Course in Pediatric Radiology.* Chicago: RSNA; 1994:115.
6. Oliveira G, Boechat MI, Amaral SM, Young LW. Osteopetrosis and rickets: an intriguing association. *Am J Dis Child* 140:377–378, 1986.
7. Donnelly LF, Johnson JF III, Benzing G. Infantile osteopetrosis complicated by rickets. *Am J Roentgenol* 154:968–970, 1995.

PEARLS
- Characteristic features are irregular and inhomogeneous cortical thickening and sclerosis of the diaphyses of tubular bones.
- Endosteal involvement is greater than periosteal.
- The medullary cavity is narrowed.[5]

PITFALLS
- Rickets may occur in patients with osteopetrosis, producing an intriguing radiograph of very dense bones in the diaphyses with flared irregular demineralized metaphyses.[6,7]

Case 3

Clinical Presentation

A 7-month-old infant with large head, large anterior fontanelle, wide sutures, and droopy shoulders.

Radiographic Studies

Lateral radiograph of skull (Fig. 3A) shows characteristic large anterior fontanelle, wide sutures, and multiple wormian bones (arrow). Anteroposterior (AP) radiograph of the chest (Fig. 3B) shows absence of the clavicles. AP radiograph of pelvis (Fig. 3C) of older child with the same condition shows delayed ossification of the pubic bones, wide pubic symphysis, hypoplastic vertical iliac wings, and coxa vara. AP radiograph of hands (Fig. 3D) shows tapered terminal phalanges.

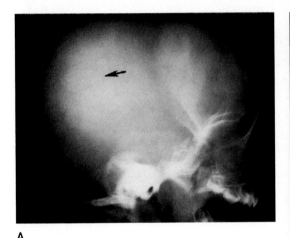

A

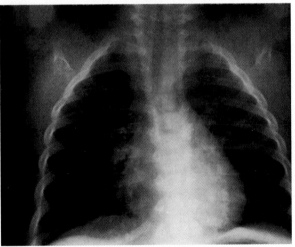

B

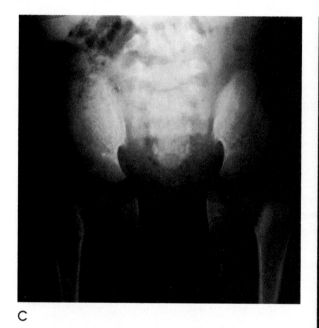

C

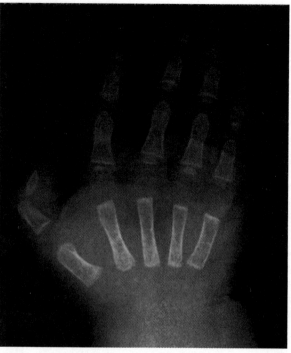

D

Diagnosis Cleidocranial Dysplasia

Discussion and Differential Diagnosis

Cleidocranial dysplasia is an autosomal dominant disorder characterized by ossification defects, especially in the midline. The anterior fontanelle may remain open in adults; the mandible is broad, with resulting prognathism. There is slow appearance of permanent teeth, with frequent dental caries. Various anomalies of the bones of the hands are also present, including long second and fifth metacarpals, pseudoepiphyses of the metacarpals, short middle phalanges, and the tapering terminal phalanges[1] demonstrated in this patient. Middle ear conductive hearing loss secondary to structural abnormalities of the ossicles has been reported in cleidocranial dysplasia.[2] Other conditions with ossification defects in the skull include pyknodysostosis, osteogenesis imperfecta, and hypophosphatasia.

Further Reading

1. Jarvis JL, Keats TE. Cleidocranial dysostosis: a review of 40 new cases. *Am J Roentgenol Radium Ther Nucl Med* 121(1):5–16, 1974.
2. Hawkins HB, Shapiro R, Petrillo CJ. The association of cleidocranial dysostosis with hearing loss. *Am J Roentgenol Radium Ther Nucl Med* 125(4):944–947, 1975.
3. Taybi H, Lachman RS. *Radiology of Syndromes, Metabolic Disorders, and Skeletal Dysplasias.* 4th ed. St. Louis: Mosby; 1996:788–789.

PEARLS

• First described in Homer's *Iliad*.[3]

• All or any portion of the clavicle may be missing, usually the middle third.

• The ossification of pubic bones is commonly delayed but usually becomes normal.

PITFALLS

• There is considerable intrafamilial variability.[3]

Case 4

Clinical Presentation

A newborn short-limbed dwarf who died shortly after birth.

Radiographic Studies

Radiographs (Fig. 4A) show rhizomelic (upper arms, upper legs) shortening of all long bones with metaphyseal irregularity, flaring, bowing, and widening.[1] The femurs look like "French telephone receivers," with a prominent medial spur on inner proximal margin of bowed upper femur (Fig. 4B). The sacrosciatic notches are small with small iliac wings and horizontal acetabular roofs (Fig. 4B). There is severe flattening of vertebral bodies (Fig. 4C) with apparent disc space widening and generalized narrowing of the interpediculate spaces. This produces a "u-" or "h-shaped" appearance of the vertebral bodies on the frontal projection (Fig. 4A).[2] The tubular bones of the hands and feet are extremely short and broad (Fig. 4D). The chest is small with very short ribs (Fig. 4A, 4C).

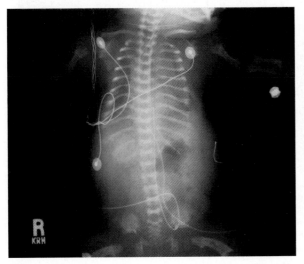

A

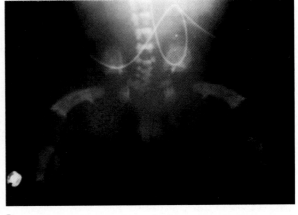

B

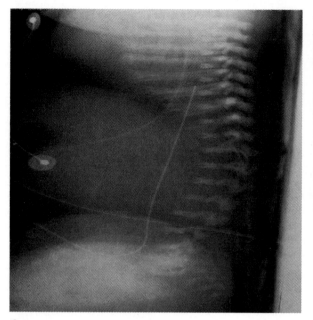

C

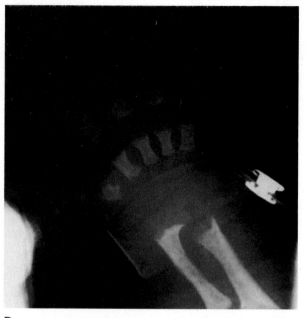

D

Diagnosis Thanatophoric Dysplasia

Discussion and Differential Diagnosis

Thanatophoric dysplasia is the most common neonatal lethal skeletal dysplasia, affecting one in 20,000 live births. It is characterized by severe dwarfism. Thanatophoric dwarfism may closely resemble homozygous achondroplasia. The history of two parents with achondroplasia should differentiate the two.[3] Thanatropic dysplasia may be diagnosed in the second trimester. A term intrauterine radiograph may be helpful for obstetrical management.[2]

Further Reading

1. McAlister WH. Current concepts: An approach to skeletal dysplasias. In: Seibert JJ, ed. *A Categorical Course in Pediatric Radiology.* Chicago: RSNA; 1994:101.
2. Taybi H, Lachman RS. *Radiology of Syndromes, Metabolic Disorders, and Skeletal Dysplasias,* 4th ed. St. Louis: Mosby; 1996:939–941.
3. Greenfield GB. *Radiology of Bone Diseases,* Philadelphia: JB Lippincott Co; 1990:276–277.

PEARLS

• Type 2 is associated with clover leaf deformity of skull or kleeblattschädel, and type 1 is not.

• This disorder is a new autosomal dominant mutation; gene location, chromosome 4p16.[2] Thanatophoric dysplasia, achondroplasia, and hypochondroplasia all share the same gene defect.

PITFALLS

• Thanatophoric dwarf with kleeblattshädel usually has straight femurs.[2]

Case 5

Clinical Presentation

1. A neonate with bent legs and soft head.
2. A 14-week abortus with short limbs.

Radiographic Studies

1. Lateral skull radiograph (Fig. 5A) of the newborn shows multiple wormian bones and decreased mineralization. Frontal radiograph of the chest (Fig. 5B) shows multiple lateral rib fractures on the right. Radiographs of the lower extremities (Fig. 5C) demonstrate fractures of the mid shaft of the femurs with abundant callus formation. There are fractures of the distal metaphyses of the femurs, bowing of the left tibia and fibula, and metaphyseal fractures of both proximal tibias.

2. Full-body radiograph of a 14-week abortus (Fig. 5D). The bones are short and broad, with multiple fractures. The femora are accordion-shaped. The long bones are crumpled. The ribs are broad, crumpled, and beaded.

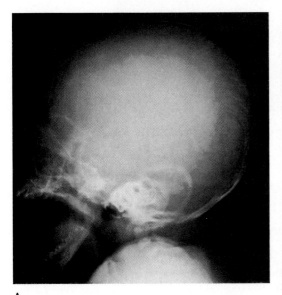

A

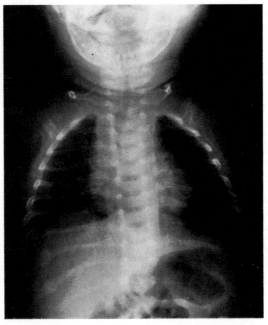

B

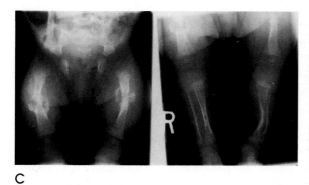

C

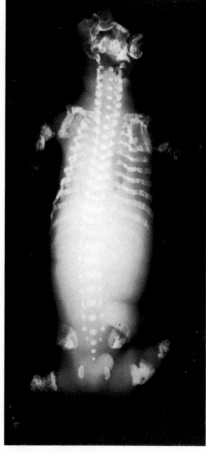

D

Diagnosis

1. Osteogenesis Imperfecta, Type III
2. Osteogenesis Imperfecta, Type IIA

PEARLS

• Osteogenesis imperfecta is the most common second-trimester ultrasound diagnosis for fetus with short bent limbs.[3,6]

Discussion and Differential Diagnosis

Osteogenesis imperfecta (OI) is a genetic disorder characterized by fragile bones, frequent fractures, blue sclera, deafness, poor dentition, ligamentous laxity, abnormal temperature regulation, and easy bruising. There are four major types. Type I is the most common type with no to moderately severe bone fragility, hearing loss (50% by age 40), blue sclerae throughout life, and autosomal dominant inheritance. There are two groups, one with normal dentition (group A) and one with abnormal teeth (group B). Fractures as severe as those seen in this first case usually do not present at birth in type I. Type II is characterized by broad, crumpled, accordion-like long bones and almost no ossification of the skull; is usually lethal in the perinatal period; and primarily represents a new dominant mutation (Fig. 5D is a 14-week abortus with OI type IIA). The first case is an example of the rarer autosomal recessive type III, which is progressive and nonlethal. Older children with this type may have metaphyseal and diaphyseal widening, "popcorn" calcifications, and hyperplastic callus.[1,2] Patients affected with autosomal dominant type IV have normal sclera and are also divided into two groups depending on the presence of normal or abnormal dentition. Type IV is similar to type I except for the absence of bleeding disorder, less deafness, and usually greater bone deformity. Twenty-five percent of patients with OI, especially types I and IV, have basilar invagination.[3,4]

The most frequent differential is child abuse or battered child syndrome. Other considerations would be steroid-induced osteoporosis, juvenile osteoporosis, camptomelic dysplasia, copper deficiency, and hyperimmunoglobulinemia E syndrome.[5]

Further Reading

1. Campbell JB. Case report 217. Hyperostosis of the calvaria in osteogenesis imperfecta. *Skeletal Radiol* 9:141–143, 1982.
2. Goldman AB, Davidson D, Pavlov H, Bullough PG. "Popcorn" calcifications: a prognostic sign in osteogenesis imperfecta. *Radiology* 136:351–358, 1980.
3. Taybi H, Lachman RS. *Radiology of Syndromes, Metabolic Disorders, and Skeletal Dysplasias,* 4th ed. St. Louis: Mosby; 1996:876–882.
4. Ablin DS, Greenspan A, Reinhart M, Grix A. Differentiation of child abuse from osteogenesis imperfecta. *Am J Roentgenol* 154:1035–1046, 1990.
5. Taybi H, Lachman RS. *Radiology of Syndromes, Metabolic Disorders, and Skeletal Dysplasias,* 4th ed. St. Louis: Mosby; 1996:880.
6. Romero R, et al. *Prenatal Diagnosis of Congenital Anomalies,* Norwalk, CT: Appleton & Lange; 1987:354–357.

Case 6

Clinical Presentation

A 1-year-old with coarse features, dwarfism, hepatosplenomegaly, corneal clouding, and mental retardation.

Radiographic Studies

The pelvis (Fig. 6A) shows that the iliac wings flare excessively, but the body of the iliac bone is small (ping pong paddle–shaped). The acetabular roof is oblique. The spine (Fig. 6B) shows a thoracolumbar gibbus with inferior beaking of the lower lumbar vertebrae with the characteristic broad hook deformity. The hand of a more severely affected child (Fig. 6C) shows marked osteoporosis, widened metacarpals, and phalanges with no diaphyseal constriction. The metacarpals are pointed proximally. The phalanges, especially the distal ones, are short. The carpal bones are small and irregular.

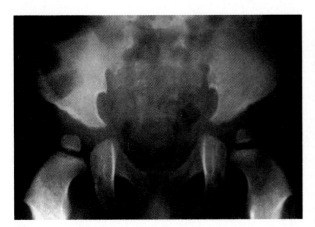

A

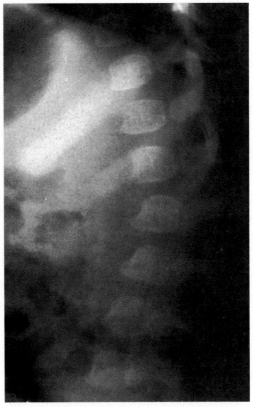

B

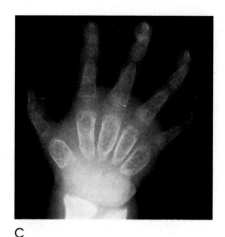

C

Diagnosis Mucopolysaccharidosis Type I, Hurler Syndrome, Dysostosis Multiplex

Discussion and Differential Diagnosis

The mucopolysaccharidoses (MPS) are a group of hereditary metabolic disorders caused by a deficiency of specific lysosomal enzymes that take part in the degradation of mucopolysaccharides. These lysosomal storage disorders result in subsequent intracellular accumulation of acid mucopolysaccharides in connective tissue, bone, skin, central nervous system tissue, and sometimes heart and blood vessels, and excess excretion of acid mucopolysaccharides in the urine.[1,2] The specific diagnosis is confirmed by fibroblast culture that discloses the specific enzyme deficiency. MPS I, the Hurler syndrome, is the best known and most common of the mucopolysaccharidoses. This progressive autosomal recessive disease is detected clinically in patients by 1 to 2 years of age with hepatosplenomegaly, hernias, a gibbus spine deformity, recurrent respiratory infections, rhinorrhea, and coarsening facial features.[3] The earliest radiographic finding may be osteoporosis. The skull is large and thickened with a J-shaped sella turcica. Bones are expanded, shortened, and pointed at one end, resulting in short pointed metacarpals, "oar-shaped" ribs (narrow posterior ribs near spine, which flare laterally), steep acetabular roofs, and "ping pong paddle" pelvis. Hunter (MPS II) has less severe findings than Hurler and is X-linked recessive. Sanfilippo (MPS III) has four types with mild skeletal abnormalities, no or mildly coarse features, and severe neurological degeneration. Morquio (MPS IV) is detected between the first and third year of age with short-trunk dwarfism secondary to universal platyspondyly with a central beak protruding from the vertebral bodies. Frequently, the odontoid process is small or disappearing with resulting atlantoaxial subluxation. Maroteaux-Lamy (MPS VI) is characterized by kyphosis at thoracic lumbar regions with wedged-shaped vertebra and irregular fragmentation of the femoral head (aseptic necrosis).

Further Reading

1. Eggli KD, Dorst JP. The mucopolysaccharidoses and related conditions. *Semin Roentgenol* 21(4):275–294, 1986.
2. Grossman H, Dorst JP. The mucopolysaccharidoses and mucolipidoses. In: *Progress in Pediatric Radiology, IV.* Basel: Karger; 1973:495–544.
3. Taybi H, Lachman RS. *Radiology of Syndromes, Metabolic Disorders, and Skeletal Dysplasias,* 4th ed. St. Louis: Mosby; 1996:669–682.
4. Taccone A, Tortori Donati P, Marzoli A, Dell'Acqua A, et al. Mucopolysaccharidosis: thickening of the dura mater at the craniocervical junction and other CT/MRI findings. *Pediatr Radiol* 23(5):349–352, 1993.
5. Fang-Kircher S. Mucopolysaccharidoses—current aspects of diagnosis and therapy. *Wien Klin Wochenschr* 107(22):698–701, 1995.

Case 7

Clinical Presentation

A newborn with short limbs.

Radiographic Studies

Anteroposterior chest radiograph (Fig. 7A) shows symmetrical short humeri bilaterally with punctate calcific deposits in the epiphyses of proximal and distal humeri and along the spine. The shortening of the extremities is much greater in the humeri than in the radius and ulna (Fig. 7B). Diffuse coronal clefts are noted in the spine as well as the calcific deposits in the upper cervical spine (Fig. 7C, 7D). The larynx and sternum are also calcified (Fig. 7D).

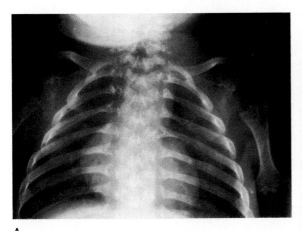

A

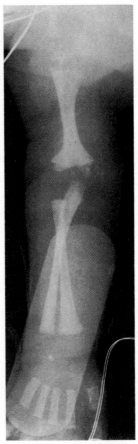

B

599

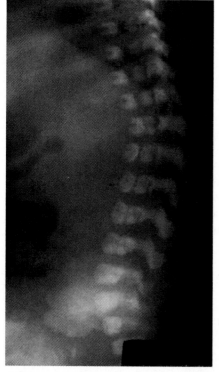

C

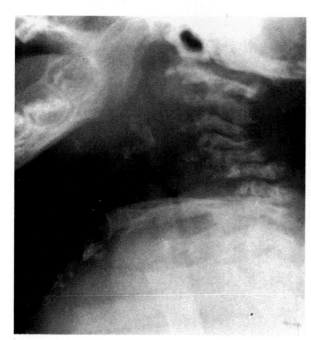

D

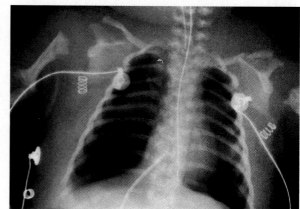

E

F

Diagnosis Stippled Epiphyses, Chondrodysplasia Punctata, Rhizomelic, Recessive Type

Discussion and Differential Diagnosis

Stippled epiphyses were first thought to be the result of two forms of a bone dysplasia, one recessive and one dominant. It is now known that many forms of this bone dysplasia exist and there are many other causes of punctate calcification in bones other than bone dysplasias.[1] The two most common forms of the bone dysplasia of chondrodysplasia punctata are the X-linked dominant form called Conradi-Hunermann and the often lethal recessive rhizomelic-type form sometimes called chondrodysplasia punctata congenita. The Conradi-Hunermann type usually is associated with normal intelligence, a characteristic flat nose, asymmetrical shortening of the limbs, and less incidence of cataracts (17%). The usually lethal rhizomelic form is characterized by severe psychomotor retardation and a higher incidence of cataracts (72%). The rhizomelic form less commonly is associated with laryngeal and tracheal calcifications and more often with coronal clefts in the vertebral bodies. C1–2 instability, spinal stenosis, and tracheal stenosis may be later sequelae, particularly of the Conradi type of dysplasia. A milder form called the Sheffield type typically presents in infancy as failure to thrive, typical facies, mild mental retardation with the calcaneus replaced by diffuse stippling.[2] Syndromes other than bone dysplasias presenting as stippling include warfarin embryopathy, alcohol embryopathy, Zellweger syndrome, and chromosome 15 and 21 syndromes.[3]

Further Reading

1. Poznanski AK. Punctate epiphyses: a radiological sign not a disease. *Pediatr Radiol* 24:418–424, 1994.
2. Sheffield LJ, Danks DM, Mayne V, Hutchinson LA. Chondrodysplasia punctata—23 cases of a mild and relatively common variety. *J Pediatr* 89(6):916–923, 1976.
3. Taybi H, Lachman RS. *Radiology of Syndromes, Metabolic Disorders, and Skeletal Dysplasias*, 4th ed. St. Louis: Mosby; 1996:776–786.
4. Leicher-Duber A, Schumacher R, Spranger J. Stippled epiphyses in fetal alcohol syndrome. *Pediatr Radiol* 20(5):369–370, 1990.

Case 8

Clinical Presentation

A robust, short-limbed neonatal dwarf with rhizomelic shortening and a large head with a prominent forehead.

Radiographic Studies

Anteroposterior radiograph of the spine demonstrates short, flat vertebral bodies with a decrease in the interpediculate distance from upper to lower lumbar spine (Fig. 8A, arrows). The iliac wings are squared (elephant ear), the sciatic notch is short and narrow, and the acetabular roof is flat. The lower extremities (Fig. 8B) are short, thick with V-shaped growth plates with a long fibula. There is rhizomelic shortening, more evident in the humerus (Fig. 8C).

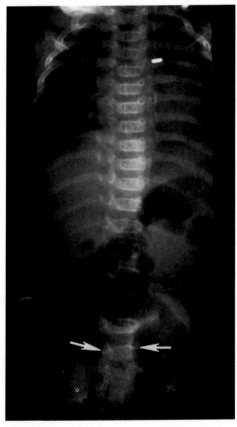
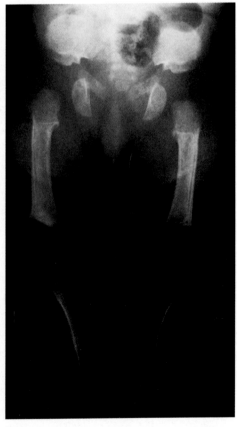

A   B

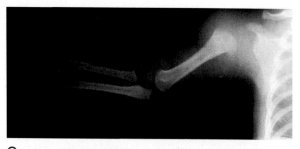

C

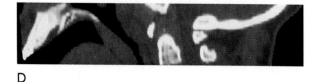

D

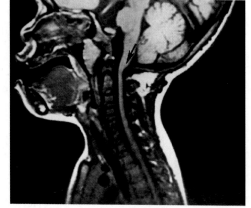

E

Diagnosis Achondroplasia

Discussion and Differential Diagnosis

Achondroplasia is the most common nonlethal skeletal dysplasia (1 in 26,000 live births).[1,2] It is the most common rhizomelic dwarfism (greatest shortening in the "roots" of the long bones, the humeri and femurs). The underlying abnormality in this most common genetic form of dwarfism is a defect in the maturation of the cartilage growth plate of long bones. This autosomal dominant disorder is accompanied by a high incidence of neurologic complications such as hydrocephalus, brainstem compression by a small foramen magnum (Fig. 8D; 8E, arrow) with sleep apnea and sudden infant death, and spinal cord compression due to spinal stenosis.[3–7] The major differential diagnosis is with hypochondroplasia, in which the face and hands are normal and the other stigmata of achondroplasia are milder.[8,9] Hypochondroplastic patients are largely normal in appearance except for their disproportionately short limbs.

Further Reading

1. Taybi H, Lachman RS. *Radiology of Syndromes, Metabolic Disorders, and Skeletal Dysplasias,* 4th ed. St. Louis: Mosby; 1996:749–755.
2. Langer LO Jr, Baumann PA, Gorlin RJ. Achondroplasia. *Am J Roentgenol Radium Ther Nucl Med* 100(1):12–26, 1967.
3. Waters KA, Everett F, Sillence DO, et al. Treatment of obstructive sleep apnea in achondroplasia: evaluation of sleep, breathing, and somatosensory-evoked potentials. *Am J Med Genet* 59(4):460–466, 1995.
4. Pauli RM, Horton VK, Glinski LP, Reiser CA. Prospective assessment of risks for cervico-medullary-junction compression in infants with achondroplasia. *Am J Hum Genet* 56(3):732–744, 1995.

5. Rimoin DL. Cervicomedullary junction compression in infants with achondroplasia: when to perform neurosurgical decompression. *Am J Hum Genet* 56(4):824–827, 1995.

6. Kao SC, Waziri MH, Smith WL, et al. MR imaging of the craniovertebral junction, cranium and brain in children with achondroplasia. *Am J Roentgenol* 153:565–569, 1989.

7. Ryken TC, Menezes AH. Cervicomedullary compression in achondroplasia. *J Neurosurg* 81:43–48, 1994.

8. Hall BD, Spranger J. Hypochondroplasia: clinical and radiological aspects in 39 cases. *Radiology* 133:95–100, 1979.

9. Heselson NG, Cremin BJ, Beighton P. The radiographic manifestations of hypochondroplasia. *Clin Radiol* 30:79–85, 1979.

10. Patel MD, Filly RA. Homozygous achondroplasia: US distinction between homozygous, heterozygous, and unaffected fetuses in the second trimester. *Radiology* 196(2):541–545, 1995.

11. Saleh M, Burton M. Leg lengthening: patient selection and management in achondroplasia. *Orthop Clin North Am* 22(4):589–599, 1991.

Case 9

Clinical Presentation

A short-limbed dwarf with postaxial polydactyly, hypoplastic nails and teeth, sparse hair, fusion of the upper lip and gum, small chest, and heart disease.

Radiographic Studies

A radiograph of the shortened lower extremities (Fig. 9A) shows premature ossification of the proximal femoral epiphysis (arrow), shortening of tibia more than the femur, and marked shortening of the fibula. The iliac wings are hypoplastic with a small sciatic notch and "trident" or three-pointed, "saw-toothed" acetabular roof. The acetabular angle is reversed so that the inferior margin of the acetabulum is convex. A radiograph of the shortened upper extremities (Fig. 9B) shows an enlarged proximal ulna and distal radius in a patient with polydactyly and short tubular bones of the hand. There is a short medial and long lateral slope to the metaphysis of the proximal humerus and a bony spike on the medial side of the distal humeral metaphysis. Frontal radiograph of the chest and abdomen (Fig. 9C) shows a small chest, an enlarged heart, small sacrosciatic notch, saw-toothed acetabulum, and ossification of the proximal femur. Lateral radiograph of the chest (Fig. 9D) shows the short ribs.

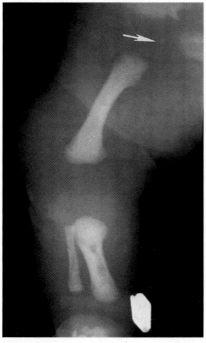
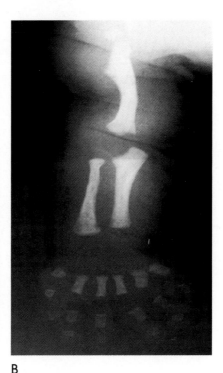

A

B

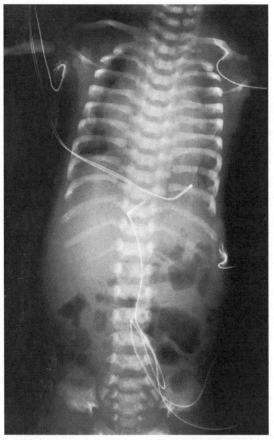

C

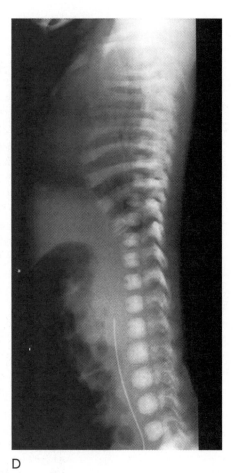

D

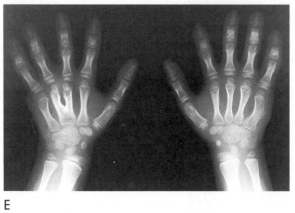

E

Diagnosis Chondroectodermal Dysplasia, Ellis–van Creveld (EVC) Syndrome

Discussion and Differential Diagnosis

Ellis–van Creveld syndrome is an autosomal recessive ectodermal dysplasia character-ized by mesomelic dwarfism (shortening in the "middle" long bones) with shortening in the radius/ulna, tibia/fibula as well as acromelic shortening (hands and feet). It is one of the short rib polydactyly syndromes. The major differential diagnosis of this disorder is with asphyxiating thoracic dystrophy (ATD) or Jeune syndrome, which will have similar radiographic findings with no or only mild ectodermal dysplasia. The incidence of heart disease and polydactyly is less than with thoracic dystrophy. The respiratory distress, small chest, hypoplastic lungs, and shortened ribs are usually more severe in ATD. Survivors with ATD develop a progressive nephropathy and hepatic dysfunction that are not seen in EVC. The carpal abnormal-ities seen in later life in EVC are absent in ATD.[1,2] Polycarpaly or a ninth carpal bone is present in all patients older than 5 years. It is located in the distal row, medial to the hamate and proximal to the fifth and sixth metacarpal.[5]

Further Reading

1. Hanissian AS, Riggs WW Jr, Thomas DA. Infantile thoracic dystrophy—a variant of Ellis–van Creveld syndrome. *J Pediatr* 71(6):855–864, 1967.
2. Cortina H, Beltran J, Olague R, et al. The wide spectrum of the asphyxiating thoracic dysplasia. *Pediatr Radiol* 8:93–99, 1979.
3. Qureshi F, Jacques SM, Evans MI, et al. Skeletal histopathology in fetuses with chondroectodermal dysplasia (Ellis–van Creveld syndrome). *Am J Med Genet* 45(4):471–476, 1993.
4. Taybi H, Lachman RS. *Radiology of Syndromes, Metabolic Disorders, and Skeletal Dysplasias,* 4th ed. St. Louis: Mosby; 1996:786–788.
5. Taylor GA, Jordan CE, Dorst SK, Dorst JP. Polycarpaly and other abnormalities of the wrist in chondroectodermal dysplasia: the Ellis–van Creveld syndrome. *Radiology* 151:393–396, 1984.
6. Silverman FN. A differential diagnosis of achondroplasia. *Radiol Clin North Am* 6(2):223–237, 1968.

PEARLS

- Ellis–van Creveld syndrome should be suspected on prenatal ultrasound when growth retardation, short limbs, small chest, heart disease, and polydactyly are observed.[3]

- In EVC, unlike achondroplasia, the skull and spine are normal.[4]

- The terminal phalanges in adults are so short that affected persons cannot make a closed fist.

- Carpal fusion is a frequent observation in older children as well as cone-shaped epiphyses of the middle phalanges 2-5 (Fig. 9E).

PITFALLS

- The characteristic pelvis seen in infancy becomes normal in childhood.[6]

Case 10

Clinical Presentation

A 5-year-old child who first presented with swelling, reddening, and hardening after minor trauma, which then progressed to stiffness in the shoulder with severe limitation of joint movement.

Radiographic Studies

Radiograph (Fig. 10A) shows ectopic ossification adjacent to and extending around muscles of the proximal humerus. Radiograph (Fig. 10B) of the feet shows short great toe caused by a monophalangic great toe resulting from synostosis between the hypoplastic proximal phalanx and the first metatarsal. Hallux valgus is also present. Anteroposterior radiograph of both hands (Fig. 10C) shows clinodactyly of the fifth finger and a hypoplastic first metacarpal.

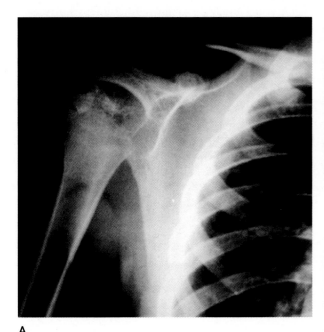

A

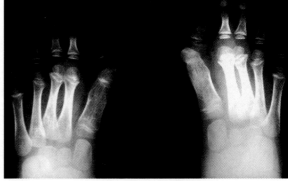

B

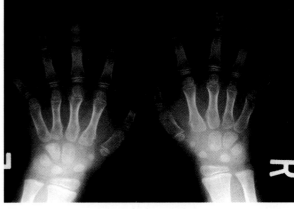

C

Diagnosis Myositis Ossificans Progressiva, Fibrodysplasia Ossificans Progressiva

Discussion and Differential Diagnosis

Fibrodysplasia ossificans progressiva is an autosomal dominant mesodermal disorder characterized by swelling and progressive ossification of the fasciae, aponeuroses, ligaments, tendons, and connective tissue of skeletal muscle.[1] The patient's average age at onset is 5 years, with the heterotopic ossification proceeding from the axial to appendicular skeleton as well as in a cranial to caudal and proximal to distal direction. Radionuclide imaging and computed tomography are sensitive for new bone formation.[2–4] The diagnosis may be confused with traumatic myositis ossificans, multiple exostoses, tuberculous cervical spondylitis, torticollis, or osteomyelitis.[5]

Further Reading

1. Taybi H, Lachman RS. *Radiology of Syndromes, Metabolic Disorders, and Skeletal Dysplasias,* 4th ed. St. Louis: Mosby; 1996:180–182.
2. Bridges AJ, Hsu KC, Singh A, et al. Fibrodysplasia (myositis) ossificans progressiva. *Semin Arthritis Rheum* 24(3):155–164, 1994.
3. Guze BH, Schelbert H. The nuclear medicine bone image and myositis ossificans progressiva. *Clin Nucl Med* 14(3):161–162, 1989.
4. Reinig JW, Hill SC, Fang M, et al. Fibrodysplasia ossificans progressiva: CT appearance. *Radiology* 159:153–157, 1986.
5. Seibert JJ, Morrissy RT, Fuller J, Young LW. Radiological case of the month: fibrodysplasia ossificans progressiva. *Am J Dis Child* 137:77–78, 1983.
6. Singleton EB, Holt JF. Myositis ossificans progressiva. *Am J Roentgenol* 62:47–54, 1954.
7. Thickman D, Bonakdar-pour A, Clancy M, et al. Fibrodysplasia ossificans progressiva. *Am J Roentgenol* 139:935–941, 1982.
8. Rogers JG, Geho WB. Fibrodysplasia ossificans progressiva. *J Bone Joint Surg Am* 61(6A):909–914, 1979.

Case 11

Clinical Presentation

Thrombocytopenia, bilaterally deformed forearm and hand, with hand at right angles to the forearm.

Radiographic Studies

Anteroposterior radiographs of forearms and hands (Fig. 11A, 11B) demonstrate bilateral absent radii with thumbs present. Noncontrast CT scan of the head demonstrates multiple small intracranial hemorrhages (Fig. 11C).

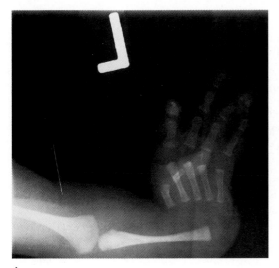

A

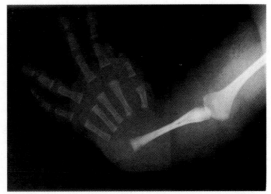

B

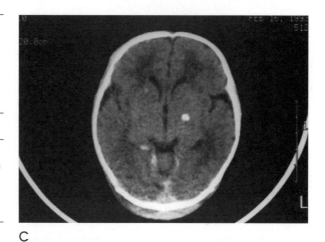

C

Diagnosis Thrombocytopenia–Absent Radius (TAR) Syndrome

Discussion and Differential Diagnosis

TAR is a syndrome characterized by bilateral absent radii with associated thrombocytopenia secondary to myeloid leukemoid reaction and hypercellular bone marrow with absent or markedly reduced megakaryocytes.[1] Three other diseases should be included in the differential diagnosis: Fanconi anemia, Holt-Oram, and Roberts syndrome.[2] Fanconi anemia patients have thrombocytopenia, absent, hypoplastic, or supernumerary thumbs, and renal anomalies. Patients with Holt-Oram have thumb, upper extremity, and cardiac defects with no hematological disorder. Patients with Roberts syndrome have no thrombocytopenia, cleft lip and palate, and reduction anomalies of the hands and feet.[1,2]

Further Reading

1. Taybi H, Lachman RS. *Radiology of Syndromes, Metabolic Disorders, and Skeletal Dysplasias,* 4th ed. St. Louis: Mosby; 1996:484.
2. Hedberg VA, Lipton JM. Thrombocytopenia with absent radii: a review of 100 cases. *Am J Pediatr Hematol Oncol* 10:51–64, 1988.

Case 12

Clinical Presentation

A newborn with epicanthal folds, downward-slanting palpebral fissures, low-set ears, low posterior hairline, short neck, funnel-shaped chest with pectus excavatum, cubitus valgus, and murmur of pulmonary stenosis.

Radiographic Studies

Anteroposterior radiograph of chest and abdomen (Fig. 12A) shows enlarged heart, barium from upper gastrointestinal series in colon on left side of abdomen with small bowel on the right in this malrotated neonate. Lateral view of the chest (Fig. 12B) shows pectus excavatum deformity of chest with the classic deformity of the sternum. There is elongation of the manubrium, and the body of the sternum is short with premature fusion of the ossification centers of the body of the sternum.

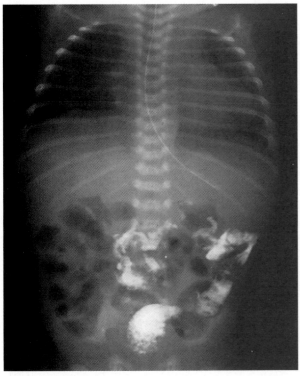
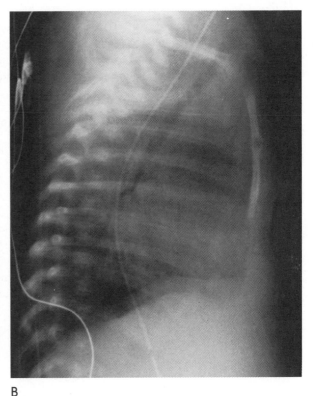

A

B

Diagnosis Noonan Syndrome, Male Turner Syndrome

Discussion and Differential Diagnosis

In 1963, Noonan and Emke first described an autosomal dominant syndrome characterized by short stature, mild mental retardation, webbed neck, cryptorchidism, cubitus valgus, pectus excavatum, pulmonic stenosis, vertebral anomalies, low posterior hairline, characteristic facies, and low-set ears. It was initially called male Turner syndrome because the physical appearance of the children was similar to that of patients with Turner syndrome, but the karyotype was normal.[1] Patients with Turner syndrome more often have left heart obstructive lesions such as aortic stenosis and coarctation whereas Noonan patients more commonly have right heart lesions such as pulmonic stenosis. Mental retardation and dental malocclusion is rare in Turner syndrome but common in Noonan syndrome. The short stature constantly seen in Turner syndrome is more variable in Noonan syndrome.[2,3] Fifty percent of patients with Noonan syndrome have a cardiac lesion. Noonan syndrome is the most common nonchromosomal syndrome among children with congenital heart disease.[3] Over 90% of patients with Noonan syndrome have a chest deformity, such as pectus carinatum or pectus excavatum.[3]

Two other syndromes should be considered in the differential diagnosis: Williams syndrome and cardiofacial-cutaneous syndrome. Williams syndrome patients have short stature, mild mental retardation, typical facies, normocalcemia or hypercalcemia, and, typically, supravalvular aortic stenosis.[1]

Further Reading

1. Taybi H, Lachman RS. *Radiology of Syndromes, Metabolic Disorders, and Skeletal Dysplasias,* 4th ed. St. Louis: Mosby; 1996:352–355, 528–530.
2. Riggs W Jr. Roentgen findings in Noonan's syndrome. *Radiology* 96:393–395, 1970.
3. Noonan JA. Noonan syndrome: an update and review for the primary pediatrician. *Clin Pediatr* 33:548–555, 1994.
4. Hoeffel JC, Juncker P, Remy J. Lymphatic vessels dysplasia in Noonan's syndrome. *Am J Roentgenol* 134:399–401, 1980.
5. Hernandez RJ, Stern AM, Rosenthal A. Pulmonary lymphangiectasis in Noonan syndrome. *Am J Roentgenol* 134:75–80, 1980.

Case 13

Clinical Presentation

A neonate with heart failure and previous arterial thrombosis in lower extremity.

Radiographic Studies

Chest radiograph in this neonate demonstrates mild cardiomegaly and rounded calcification of the aorta and pulmonary arteries (arrows, Fig. 13A). Ultrasound of the abdomen in sagittal (Fig. 13B) and transverse (Fig. 13C) planes demonstrates hyperechoic walls of the aorta representing diffuse, linear, and circular calcification in the abdominal aorta. The patient also demonstrated nephrocalcinosis in the papillary areas of the kidney.

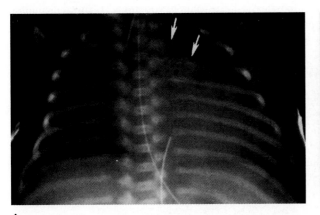

A

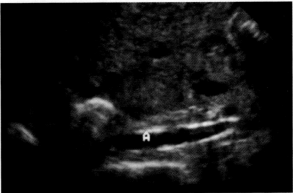

B

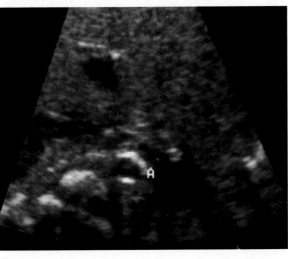

C

Diagnosis Arterial Calcification of Infancy

PEARLS

• Vessels of the brain are often spared.

• Renal infarcts are often seen.[3]

• Hypertension may be the first presentation.

PITFALLS

• Calcification may spontaneously resolve and only be seen in infancy.

Discussion and Differential Diagnosis

Arterial calcification of infancy is a rare disorder characterized by dystrophic calcification in major arteries in infants. Death usually occurs before the first year as the result of coronary artery involvement.[1] Calcifications may be seen in the periarticular area of extremities and ear lobes as well as the kidneys. Spontaneous remission has been reported. The infants can be treated with steroids, estrogen, and diphosphonate, an inhibitor of calcium salt precipitation.[2–4] Generalized arterial calcification in infants can be caused by hypervitaminosis D and primary or secondary hyperparathyroidism—laboratory examination will demonstrate abnormalities of calcium metabolism. Calcium is normal in idiopathic arterial calcification. Older children with aortic calcification may have Singleton-Merten syndrome, characterized by generalized muscular weakness with hip and feet deformities, progressive calcification of the thoracic aorta in childhood, dysplasia of the teeth, osteoporosis, expanded medullary cavities of the metacarpals, and psoriasiform skin lesions.[5,6]

Further Reading

1. Rosenbaum DM, Blumhagen JD. Sonographic recognition of idiopathic arterial calcification of infancy. *Am J Roentgenol* 146:249–250, 1986.
2. Vera J, Lucaya J, Garcia-Conesa JA, et al. Idiopathic infantile arterial calcification: unusual features. *Pediatr Radiol* 20:585–587, 1990.
3. Green DW, Laughlin WR. Pathological case of the month: idiopathic arterial calcification of infancy. *Arch Pediatr Adolesc Med* 150:101–102, 1996.
4. Taybi H, Lachman RS. *Radiology of Syndromes, Metabolic Disorders, and Skeletal Dysplasias,* 4th ed. St Louis: Mosby; 1996:30–31.
5. Gay BB Jr, Kuhn JP. A syndrome of widened medullary cavities of bone, aortic calcification, abnormal dentition, and muscular weakness (the Singleton-Merten syndrome). *Radiology* 118:389–395,1976.
6. Singleton EB, Merten DF. An unusual syndrome of widened medullary cavities of the metacarpals and phalanges, aortic calcification and abnormal dentition. *Pediatr Radiol* 1:2–7,1973.

Case 14

Clinical Presentation

Two 12-year-old girls with enlargement of face on left.

Radiographic Studies

Coronal CT (Fig. 14A) through the paranasal sinuses of one girl shows marked thickening of the left maxilla with a ground-glass density of the expanded bone. Anteroposterior radiograph (Fig. 14B) and CT (Fig. 14C, 14D) of the second patient show expansion of the bones of the face, orbit, sinuses, and temporal bones with a ground-glass density.

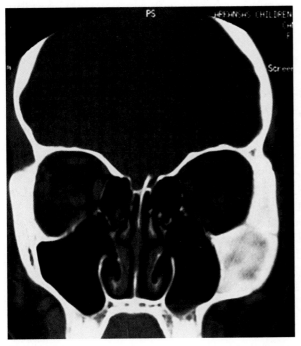

A

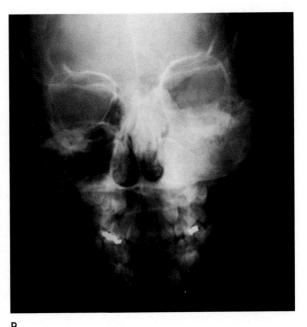

B

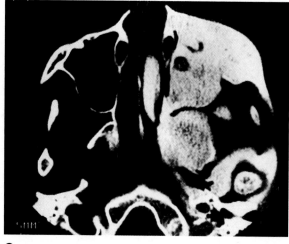

C

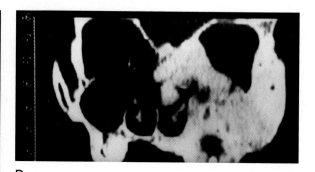

D

Diagnosis   Fibrous Dysplasia

Discussion and Differential Diagnosis

Fibrous dysplasia is a developmental abnormality of the bone-forming mesenchyme resulting in replacement of spongiosa and filling of the medullary cavity by fibrous tissue. There is an excessive proliferation of spindle cell fibrous tissue in bone, incorporating distorted trabeculae of primitive bone.[1] This fibrous tissue may undergo osseous metaplasia, producing poorly calcified "smoky" new bone. If fibrous tissue predominates, the bone lesion will be predominately lytic. The lesions vary in appearance from completely radiolucent to homogeneously ground glass or "smoky." The medullary canal is replaced; the bone is expanded, with well-defined sclerotic margins between normal bone and the lesion. The cortex is often thickened. The femur is the most often involved long bone. The child may present with a leg length discrepancy. There are several types of fibrous dysplasia, but the two major ones are the monostotic, with single bone involvement, and the polyostotic, with multiple lesions. There is a triad in females of multiple lesions, patchy cutaneous pigmentation (café au lait spots), and endocrine dysfunction associated with sexual precocity described by McCune and Albright.[2] In the skull, the outer table is often expanded with minimal involvement of the inner table. The lesions begin in young individuals and are often asymptomatic. There is no familial tendency. Differential diagnosis in children includes histiocytosis X, simple bone cyst, enchondroma, and aneurysmal bone cyst.

Involvement of the skull with fibrous dysplasia is primarily in the facial bones and base of skull, frontal, ethmoid, and sphenoid bones, with encroachment on the orbit, whereas histiocytosis X more often involves the calvarium. CT of the skull may be helpful for demonstrating the amorphous "ground glass" texture of the lesion as well as for defining the extent of the disease.[3] Most lesions show increased uptake on bone scintigraphy.[4] On MRI, the lesions are characterized by an expanded bony contour with a decreased signal on T1-weighted images. The T2-weighted scan is variable.[5]

PITFALLS

- Epiphyseal involvement has been described in the polyostotic type before closure of the growth plate.[6]

- Fibrous dysplasia of the tibia often simulates ossifying fibroma and adamantinoma histologically and radiographically.[7]

- True chondrosarcomatous transformation of fibrous dysplasia is rare (0.5%).[8] An unusual complication of fibrous dysplasia, especially in the femoral neck, is fibrocartilaginous dysplasia, which may be misdiagnosed as malignant. There is rapid growth of the lesion, increase in density within the lesion, and extensive calcifications.[9]

Further Reading

1. Taybi H, Lachman RS. *Radiology of Syndromes, Metabolic Disorders, and Skeletal Dysplasias,* 4th ed. St. Louis: Mosby; 1996:183–184.
2. Rieth KG, Comite F, Shawker TH, Cutler GB Jr. Pituitary and ovarian abnormalities demonstrated by CT and ultrasound in children with features of the McCune-Albright syndrome. *Radiology* 153:389–393, 1984.
3. Daffner RH, Kirks DR, Gehweiler JA Jr. Heaston DK. Computed tomography of fibrous dysplasia. *Am J Roentgenol* 139:943–948, 1982.
4. Machida K, Makita K, Nishikawa J, Ohtake T, Masahiro I. Scintigraphic manifestation of fibrous Med 11(6):426–429, 1986.
5. Utz JA, Kransdorf MJ, Jelinek JS, Moser RP Jr, Berrey BH. MR appearance of fibrous dysplasia. *J Comput Assist Tomogr* 13(5):845–851, 1989.
6. Nixon GW, Condon VR. Epiphyseal involvement in polyostotic fibrous dysplasia: a report of two cases. *Radiology* 106:167–170, 1973.
7. Resnick D, Sartoris D. *Bone Disease, IV.* Reston, VA: American College of Radiology; 1989:637–638.
8. Drolshagen LF, Reynolds WA, Marcus NW. Fibrocartilaginous dysplasia of bone. *Radiology* 156:32, 1985.
9. Pelzmann KS, Nagel DZ, Salyer WR. Case report 114. *Skeletal Radiol* 5:116–118, 1980.

Acknowledgment

I would like to thank Dr. William McAlister for reviewing this section on syndromes.

INDEX